EVIDENCE-BASED PRACTICE FOR NURSES

Appraisal and Application of Research

THE PEDAGOGY

Evidence-Based Practice for Nurses: Appraisal and Application of Research, Fourth Edition, drives comprehension through various strategies that meet the learning needs of students while also generating enthusiasm about the topic. This interactive approach addresses different learning styles, making this the ideal text to ensure mastery of key concepts. The pedagogical aids that appear in most chapters include the following:

CHAPTER OBJECTIVES

At the end of this chapter, you will be able to:

- Define evidence-based practice (EBP)
- List sources of evidence for nursing practice
- Identify barriers to the adoption of EBP and pinpoint strategies to overcome them
- Explain how the process of diffusion facilitates moving evidence into nursing practice
- Define research
- Discuss the contribution of research to EBP
- Categorize types of research
- Distinguish between quantitative and qualitative research approaches

- Describe the sections found in research articles
- Describe the cycle of scientific development
- Identify historical occurrences that shaped the development of nursing as a science
- Identify factors that will continue to move nursing forward as a science
- Discuss what future trends may influence how nurses use evidence to improve the quality of patient care
- Identify five unethical studies involving the violation of the rights of human subjects

KEY TERMS

abstract	inductive reasoning	qualitative research
applied research	innovation	quantitative research
barriers	introduction	replication study
basic research	Jewish Chronic Disease	research
cycle of scientific	Hospital study	research utilization
development	laggards	results section
deductive reasoning	list of references	review of literature
descriptive research	methods section	theoretical framework
discussion section	model of diffusion of	theory
early adopters	innovations	Tuskegee study
empirical evidence	Nazi experiments	Willowbrook studies
evidence-based practice	Nuremberg Code	
(EBP)	predictive research	
explanatory research	pyramid of evidence	

Chapter Objectives
These objectives provide instructors and students with a snapshot of the key information they will encounter in each chapter. They serve as a checklist to help guide and focus study.

Key Terms
Found in a list at the beginning of each chapter and in bold within the chapter, these terms will create an expanded vocabulary in evidence-based practice.

Critical Thinking Exercises

As an integral part of the learning process, the authors present scenarios and questions to spark insight into situations faced in practice.

CRITICAL THINKING EXERCISE 5-2

A nurse on a surgical floor observes that several new approaches are being used to dress wounds. She observes that some methods appear to promote healing faster than others do. While reviewing the research literature, she is unable to locate any research about the dressings she is using. How might she go about testing her theory that some methods are better than others? Can this be done deductively, inductively, or using mixed methods? Are any theories presently available related to wound healing, and if so, where might she locate these? What concepts might be important in forming the question?

treatment of human response, and advocacy in the care of individuals, families, communities, and populations" (ANA, 2003, p. 6). From the early days of the profession, students have been taught that a scientific attitude and method of work combined with "experience, trained senses, a mind trained to think, and the necessary characteristics of patience, accuracy, open-mindedness, truthfulness, persistence, and industry" (Harmer, 1933, p. 47) are essential components of good practice. Harmer goes on to say, "Each time this habit of looking, listening, feeling, or thinking is repeated it is strengthened until the habit of observation is firmly established" (p. 47). This still holds true today. Benner (1984) studied nurses in practice and concluded that to become an expert nurse one has to practice nursing a minimum of 5 years. There are no shortcuts to becoming an expert in one's field. The development of knowledge and skill takes time and work. As nurses encounter new situations, learning takes place. Nursing knowledge develops and is refined as nurses practice (Waterman, Webb, & Williams, 1995). In this way, nurses adapt theories to fit their practices. Unfortunately, much that is learned about theory during practice remains with the nurse because nurses rarely share their practice expertise through conference presentations and publications. The discipline will be enriched when nurses engage more formally in disseminating their knowledge about theory in practice.

The Relationships Among Theory, Research, and Practice

Practice relies on research and theory and also provides the questions that require more work by theorists and researchers. Each informs and supports the other in the application and development of nursing knowledge. When the relationships among theory, research, and practice are in harmony, the discipline is best served, ultimately resulting in better patient outcomes (Maas, 2006). The relationships are dynamic and flow in all directions.

FYI

After an outcome has been selected and measured, data are compiled and evaluated to draw conclusions. Evaluation is facilitated when appropriate outcomes and associated indicators are chosen—conversely, if the outcome is not clearly defined, then the measurements and subsequent evaluation will be flawed.

After an outcome has been selected and measured, data are compiled and evaluated to draw conclusions. Demonstrating the effectiveness of an innovation is a challenge, and conclusions must not extend beyond the scope of the data. Evaluation is facilitated when appropriate outcomes and associated indicators are chosen. If the outcome is not clearly defined, then the measurements and subsequent evaluation will be flawed. For example, suppose that you are a member of an interdisciplinary team that has developed a nursing protocol that reduces the amount of time the patient remains on bed rest after a cardiac catheterization procedure from 6 hours to 4 hours. The outcome selected is absence of bleeding from the femoral arterial puncture site. No other indicators are measured. The results obtained after implementing the protocol revealed that there was an increase in bleeding at the femoral arterial site in the 4-hour bed rest patients compared to the 6-hour bed rest patients. Before concluding that a shorter bed rest time leads to an increase in femoral bleeding, a few additional questions need to be considered. First, was absence of bleeding defined in a measurable way? Because bleeding might be interpreted in several different ways, a precise definition of bleeding should have been provided to ensure consistency in reporting. Second, when should patients be assessed for absence of bleeding? Is the absence of bleeding to be assessed when the patient first ambulates or at a later time? Input from the staff prior to changing the nursing protocol could have clarified these questions, resulting in more reliable results.

Another consideration in outcome evaluation is to obtain data relative to current practice for comparison purposes. To document the need for a practice change and to support a new protocol, baseline data might need to be collected

TEST YOUR KNOWLEDGE 18-3

True/False

1. Baseline data are unimportant in outcome measurement.
2. Precise description of indicators is essential.
3. For complex analyses, the assistance of a statistician may be needed.
4. Input from staff can help clarify outcome measurement.

How did you do? 1. F; 2. T; 3. T; 4. T

FYI

Quick tidbits and facts are pulled out in chapter margins to highlight important aspects of the chapter topic.

Test Your Knowledge

These questions serve as benchmarks for the knowledge acquired throughout the chapter.

apparent. Organizing the review with a grid is a positive strategy to overcome the barrier of lack of time because it reduces the need to repeatedly sort through articles during future discussions. Also, within this text's digital resources, you will find a grid to use for this exercise. Two articles (Cohen & Shastay, 2008; Tomietto, Sartor, Mazzocoli, & Palese, 2012) are summarized as an example.

Read Kliger, Blegen, Gootee, and O'Neil (2009). Enter information about this article into the first two columns. In column 1, use APA format, like in the example, because this is the most commonly used style for nursing publications.

RAPID REVIEW

» Today's work environment requires that nurses be adept at gathering and appraising evidence for clinical practice and assisting patients with healthcare information needs.

» Literature reviews provide syntheses of current research and scholarly literature. A well-done literature review can provide support for EBP.

» An understanding of the scientific literature publication cycle provides a basis for making decisions about the most current information on a topic.

» Primary sources are original sources of information presented by the people who created them. Secondary sources are resulting commentaries, summaries, reviews, or interpretations of primary sources.

» Many research journals involve peer review.

» There are many ways to categorize sources. Scholarly, trade, and popular literature is one way. Another categorizing system involves periodicals, journals, and magazines.

» There are four types of review: narrative, integrative, meta-analysis, and systematic.

» Understanding how sources are structured can simplify a search of the literature.

» Sources can be identified through both print indexes and electronic databases. Topics, subject matter, and format may vary but all include citation information.

» Helpful strategies to use when conducting a search include citation chasing, measurements of recall and precision, keyword and controlled vocabulary searches, Boolean operators, truncation,

Rapid Review
This succinct list at the end of the chapter compiles the most pertinent and key information for quick review and later reference.

Apply What You Have Learned
This outstanding feature applies newly acquired knowledge to specific evidence-based practice scenarios and research studies.

APPLY WHAT YOU HAVE LEARNED

Sign into a database for nursing literature (i.e., CINAHL, ProQuest, PubMed). For this chapter, you will need to obtain the following two articles:

Pipe, T. B., Kelly, A., LeBrun, G., Schmidt, D., Atherton, P., & Robinson, C. (2008). A prospective descriptive study exploring hope, spiritual well-being, and quality of life in hospitalized patients. *MEDSURG Nursing*, *17*, 247–257.

Flanagan, J. M., Carroll, D. L., & Hamilton, G. A. (2010). The long-term lived experience of patients with implantable cardioverter defibrillators. *MEDSURG Nursing*, *19*, 113–119.

One of these articles used qualitative methods, and the other used quantitative methods. Identify which is which. After you have done that, for each article identify the various sections that make up a research article. You may want to share these articles with nurses during your next clinical experience and consider ways the recommendations can be incorporated into practice.

REFERENCES

Aitken, L. M., Hackwood, B., Crouch, S., Clayton, S., West, N., Carney, D., & Jack, L. (2011). Creating an environment to implement and sustain evidence based practice: A developmental process. *Australian Critical Care*, *24*, 244–254.

American Medical Association. (1998). *Information from unethical experiments* (CEJA Report 5–A-98). Retrieved from http://www.ama-assn .org/resources/doc/code-medical-ethics/230a.pdf

American Nurses Association. (2010). National Database of Nursing Quality Indicators: Guidelines for data collection on the American Nurses Association's National Quality forum endorsed measures: Nursing Care Hours per Patient Day, Skill Mix, Falls, Falls with Injury. Retrieved from http://www.odh.ohio.gov/~/media/ODH/ASSETS/Files/dspc/health%20 care%20service/nursestaffing7-13-10materials.ashx

Barnsteiner, J., & Prevost, S. (2002). How to implement evidence-based practice. Some tried and true pointers. *Reflections on Nursing Leadership*, *28*(2), 18–21.

Barta, K. M. (1995). Information-seeking, research utilization, and barriers to research utilization of pediatric nurse educators. *Journal of Professional Nursing*, *11*, 49–57.

Benner, P. (1984). *From novice to expert: Excellence and power in clinical nursing practice*. Menlo Park, CA: Addison-Wesley.

Case Examples
Found in select chapters, these vignettes illustrate research questions and studies in actual clinical settings and provide critical thinking challenges.

Some researchers claim their work is nursing research because the researcher is a nurse or because the researcher studied nurses. But it is the focus on nursing practice that defines nursing research. The mere fact that the research was conducted by a nurse or that nurses were studied does not necessarily qualify the research as nursing research. Historically, and even today, approaches to practice are often based on "professional opinion" when research is absent. Case Example 5-1 provides such a historical illustration. It also demonstrates the value of systematically studying the effects of interventions.

CASE EXAMPLE 5-1

Early Methods of Resuscitation: An Example of Practice Based on Untested Theory

Throughout the past century, nursing students have been taught how to resuscitate patients who stop breathing. As early as 1912, students were taught a variety of methods for providing artificial respiration. It was theorized that moving air in and out of the lungs would be effective. One of these techniques was designed for resuscitating infants. Byrd's Method of Infant Resuscitation (Goodnow, 1919) directed the nurse to hold the infant's legs in one hand, and the head and back in the other. The nurse would then double the child over by pressing the head and the knees against the chest. Then the nurse would extend the knees to undouble the child. This would be repeated, but "not too rapidly" (Goodnow, 1919, p. 305). At intervals, the nurse would dip the child into a mustard bath in the hope that this would also stimulate respiration. The nurse would continue this until help arrived.

Other methods of artificial respiration taught included Sylvester's method for adults (Goodnow, 1919). The patient was placed flat on his back. The nurse would grasp the patient's elbows and press them close to his sides, pushing in the ribs to expel air from the chest. The arms would then be slowly pulled over the head, allowing the chest to expand. The arms would be lowered to put pressure on the chest, and the cycle was then repeated. This was to be done at the rate of 18 to 20 cycles per minute.

By 1939, postmortem examinations after unsuccessful resuscitations showed veins to be engorged while the arteries were empty (Harmer & Henderson, 1942). Although this evidence indicated other factors needed to be considered, resuscitation techniques continued to focus only on the respiratory system. The same methods of resuscitation that were in use in 1919 were still being taught in 1942. Although students were still being taught the Sylvester method, they were also learning the new "Schäfer method" (Harmer & Henderson, 1942, p. 9401). This method involved placing the patient in a prone position. The nurse would straddle the thighs, facing the patient's head, and alternately apply and remove pressure to the thorax.

Eventually, it was noted that what was believed to be best practice was not effective. Results of postmortem examinations indicated that something was missing in the techniques, and therefore research was begun to determine best practice. Today, nursing students are taught cardiopulmonary resuscitation techniques based on updated research and theories.

fully operational in 1996. It aims to improve the effectiveness of nursing practice and healthcare outcomes. Some initiatives include conducting systematic reviews, collaborating with expert researchers to facilitate development of practice information sheets, and designing, promoting, and delivering short courses about EBP.

2.2 Keeping It Ethical

At the end of this section, you will be able to:
‹ Discuss international and national initiatives designed to promote ethical conduct
‹ Describe the rights that must be protected and the three ethical principles that must be upheld when conducting research
‹ Explain the composition and functions of IRBs at the organizational level
‹ Discuss the nurse's role as patient advocate in research situations

Ethical research exists because international, national, organizational, and individual factors are in place to protect the rights of individuals. Without these factors, scientific studies that violate human rights, such as the Nazi experiments, could proceed unchecked. Many factors of ethical research, which evolved in response to unethical scientific conduct, are aimed at protecting human rights. *Human rights* are "freedoms, to which all humans are entitled, often held to include the right to life and liberty, freedom of thought and expression, and equality before the law" (Houghton Mifflin, 2007). Rights cannot be claimed unless they are justified in the eyes of another individual or group of individuals (Haber, 2006). When individuals have rights, others have *obligations*, that is, they are required to act in particular ways. This means that when nursing research is being conducted, subjects participating in studies have rights, and all nurses are obligated to protect those rights.

KEY TERMS
human rights:
Freedoms to which all humans are entitled

obligations:
Requirements to act in particular ways
·····················

International and National Factors: Guidelines for Conducting Ethical Research

One of the earliest international responses to unethical scientific conduct was the Nuremberg Code. This code was contained in the written verdict at the trial of the German Nazi physicians accused of torturing prisoners during medical experiments. Writers of the Nuremberg Code (Table 2-3) identified that voluntary consent was absolutely necessary for participation in research. Research that avoided harm, produced results that benefited society, and allowed participants to withdraw at will was deemed ethical. The Nuremberg Code became the standard for other codes of conduct.

Keeping It Ethical
Relevant ethical content concludes each chapter to ensure that ethics are a consideration during every step of the nursing process.

FOURTH EDITION

EVIDENCE-BASED PRACTICE FOR NURSES

Appraisal and Application of Research

Edited by

Nola A. Schmidt, PhD, RN, CNE
Professor
College of Nursing and Health Professions
Valparaiso University
Valparaiso, Indiana

Janet M. Brown, PhD, RN
Professor Emeritus
College of Nursing and Health Professions
Valparaiso University
Valparaiso, Indiana

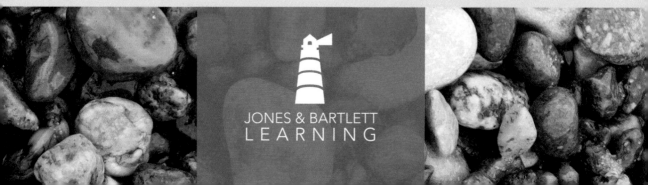

JONES & BARTLETT
LEARNING

World Headquarters
Jones & Bartlett Learning
5 Wall Street
Burlington, MA 01803
978-443-5000
info@jblearning.com
www.jblearning.com

Jones & Bartlett Learning books and products are available through most bookstores and online booksellers. To contact Jones & Bartlett Learning directly, call 800-832-0034, fax 978-443-8000, or visit our website, www.jblearning.com.

Substantial discounts on bulk quantities of Jones & Bartlett Learning publications are available to corporations, professional associations, and other qualified organizations. For details and specific discount information, contact the special sales department at Jones & Bartlett Learning via the above contact information or send an email to specialsales@jblearning.com.

12352-4

Production Credits
VP, Executive Publisher: David D. Cella
Director of Product Management: Amanda Martin
Product Assistant: Christina Freitas
Associate Production Editor: Alex Schab
Senior Marketing Manager: Jennifer Scherzay
Production Services Manager: Colleen Lamy
Product Fulfillment Manager: Wendy Kilborn
Composition: S4Carlisle Publishing Services
Cover Design: Kristin Parker
Rights & Media Specialist: Wes DeShano
Media Development Editor: Troy Liston
Cover Image (Title Page, Part Opener, Chapter Opener): © Madredus/Shutterstock
Printing and Binding: LSC Communications
Cover Printing: LSC Communications

Library of Congress Cataloging-in-Publication Data
Names: Schmidt, Nola A., editor. | Brown, Janet M. (Janet Marie), 1947– editor.
Title: Evidence-based practice for nurses : appraisal and application of research / [edited by] Nola A. Schmidt and Janet M. Brown.
Description: Fourth edition. | Burlington, Massachusetts : Jones & Bartlett Learning, [2019] | Includes bibliographical references and index.
Identifiers: LCCN 2017036581 | ISBN 9781284122909
Subjects: | MESH: Nursing Research--methods | Evidence-Based Nursing
Classification: LCC RT81.5 | NLM WY 20.5 | DDC 610.73072--dc23
LC record available at https://lccn.loc.gov/2017036581

6048

Printed in the United States of America
21 20 19 18   10 9 8 7 6 5 4 3 2 1

DEDICATION

For Mom, whose love and support are endless.

—*N. A. S.*

To my husband, my children, and my granddaughters and grandson, who enrich my life in every way.

—*J. M. B.*

CONTENTS

CONTRIBUTORS

Susie Adams, PhD, RN, PMHNP, FAANP
Professor and Director PMHNP Program
School of Nursing
Vanderbilt University
Nashville, Tennessee

Janet M. Brown, PhD, RN
Professor Emeritus
Valparaiso University
Valparaiso, Indiana

Amy C. Cory, PhD, MPH, RN, CPNP, PC
Associate Professor
College of Nursing and Health Professions
Valparaiso University
Valparaiso, Indiana

Jan Dougherty, MS, RN, FAAN
Director
Family and Community Services
Banner Alzheimer's Institute
Phoenix, Arizona

Moira Fearncombe, MEd, BS
Lake Barrington, Illinois

Diane McNally Forsyth, PhD, RN
Professor
Graduate Programs in Nursing
Winona State University
Rochester, Minnesota

Emily Griffin, MSN, ARNP, FNP-BC
Lecturer
College of Nursing
University of Iowa
Iowa City, Iowa

Elsabeth Jensen, PhD, RN
Associate Professor and Graduate
    Program Director
School of Nursing
Faculty of Health
York University
Toronto, Ontario

Carol O. Long, PhD, RN, FPCN, FAAN
Geriatric and Palliative Care Educator
   and Researcher
Capstone Healthcare Group
Adjunct Faculty
College of Nursing and Health Innovation
Arizona State University
Phoenix, Arizona

**Kristen L. Mauk, PhD, DNP, RN, CRRN,
   GCNS-BC, GNP-BC, FAAN**
Director RN-BSN and MSN Programs
Colorado Christian University
Lakewood, Colorado

Patricia Mileham, MA
Associate Professor of Library Services, Director
   of Public Service
Christopher Center for Library & Information
   Resources
Valparaiso University
Valparaiso, Indiana

Rosalind M. Peters, PhD, RN, FAAN
Associate Professor
College of Nursing
Wayne State University
Detroit, Michigan

Kathleen A. Rich, PhD, RN, CCNS-CSC, CNN
Cardiovascular Clinical Specialist
Patient Care Services
La Porte Hospital
La Porte, Indiana

Cynthia L. Russell, PhD, RN, ACNS-BC, FAAN
Professor
School of Nursing and Health Studies
University of Missouri—Kansas City
Kansas City, Missouri

Nola A. Schmidt, PhD, RN, CNE
Professor
College of Nursing and Health Professions
Valparaiso University
Valparaiso, Indiana

Marita G. Titler, PhD, RN, FAAN
Associate Dean for Practice and Clinical
   Scholarship
Rhetaugh G. Dumas Endowed Chair
Department Chair Systems, Populations
   and Leadership
University of Michigan School of Nursing
Ann Arbor, Michigan

Ann H. White, PhD, MBA, RN, NE-BC
Dean
College of Nursing and Health Professions
University of Southern Indiana
Evansville, Indiana

Maria Young, PhD, RN, ACNS-BC
Assistant Professor
Indiana University Northwest
College of Health and Human Services
Gary, Indiana

REVIEWERS

Billie Blake, EdD, MSN, BSN, RN, CNE
Associate Dean of Nursing
BSN Director
Professor
St. John's River State College
Orange Park, Florida

Tish Conejo, PhD, RN
Professor
MidAmerica Nazarene University
Olathe, Kansas

Patricia Grust, PhD, RN, CLNC
Clinical Associate Professor
Hartwick College
Oneonta, New York

Susan Montenery, DNP, RN, CCRN
Assistant Professor of Nursing
Coastal Carolina University
Conway, South Carolina

Chantel H. Murray, MSN, MBA, RN
Professor/Clinical Expert
Eastern University
St. Davids, Pennsylvania

Catherine A. Schmitt, PhD, RN, CNOR
Assistant Professor
University of Wisconsin, Oshkosh
Menasha, Wisconsin

Cynthia Softhauser, PhD, MSN, RN, AHN-BC, CNE
Associate Professor
Indiana University South Bend
Mishawaka, Indiana

Susan Steele-Moses, DNS, APRN-CNS, AOCN
Academic Research Director
Our Lady of the Lake College
Baton Rouge, Louisiana

Cathy J. Thompson, PhD, RN, CCNS, CNE
Visiting Professor
University of Colorado, Colorado Springs
South Fork, Colorado

PREFACE

We are most pleased to offer the *Fourth Edition* of this text. For this revision, we have extensively altered the "Apply What You Have Learned" feature. The new topic is adherence with hand hygiene, changed from medication errors in the last edition. We selected this clinical problem because it involves all healthcare providers in all settings and significantly impacts patient outcomes. Additionally, nurse educators are well-positioned to help students gain an appreciation for hand hygiene guidelines and build good hand hygiene habits. This feature continues to unfold in a manner that integrates chapter content with each step of the EBP process. Concrete strategies, in the form of exemplars and checklists, allow readers to master competencies needed to perform these activities in the clinical setting.

A new feature of the textbook includes two diagrams that summarize statistical analyses (Chapter 13) and designs (back cover). In response to user feedback, we updated the "Hierarchy of Evidence" to include types of evidence for each level. In Chapter 12, we made edits to the 5 Ss to better distinguish this hierarchy from the Hierarchy of Evidence.

We are even more committed to the premise that baccalaureate-prepared nurses, given the emphasis on leadership, critical thinking, and communication in their curricula, are ideally positioned to advance best practices. Therefore, nursing faculty must teach students educational strategies that develop a lifelong commitment to examining nursing practice critically in light of scientific advances. Although many texts and references deal with the principles, methods, and appraisal of nursing research, few sources address the equally important aspect of integrating evidence into practice. Because there is a growing expectation by accrediting bodies that patient outcomes are addressed through best practice, it is imperative that books be available to prepare nurses for implementing best practices. This edition of this textbook continues to provide substantive strategies to assist students with applying evidence at the point of care.

The American Association of Colleges of Nursing (AACN) charges nursing programs with preparing baccalaureate nurses with the basic understanding of the processes of nursing research. This book includes content related to methods, appraisal, and utilization, which is standard in many other texts. Furthermore, the AACN expects BSN-prepared nurses to apply research findings from nursing and other disciplines in their clinical practice. The framework for this text is the model of diffusion of innovations (Rogers, 2003), which gives readers a logical and useful means for creating an EBP. Readers are led step-by-step through the process of examining the nursing practice problem of hand hygiene using the innovation–decision process (IDP). It is recommended that faculty use this text with students to guide them through assignments that might effect actual change in patient care at a healthcare facility. Schmidt and Brown (2007) described this teaching strategy more fully. Because students typically express that research content is uninteresting and lacks application to real life, we have tried to create a textbook that is less foreboding and more enjoyable through the use of friendly language and assignments to make content more pertinent for students.

The primary audience for this textbook is baccalaureate undergraduate nursing students and their faculty in an introductory nursing research course. All baccalaureate nursing programs offer an introductory research course, for which this text would be useful. Because the readership has grown, we recognize that nursing graduate programs are also using this textbook.

This edition continues to follow the five steps of the IDP: knowledge, persuasion, decision, implementation, and confirmation. This organizational approach allows the research process to be linked with strategies that promote progression through the IDP. The chapters follow a consistent format: chapter objectives, key terms, major content, test your knowledge, case study, rapid review, and reference list. Critical thinking exercises and user-friendly tables and charts are interspersed throughout each chapter to allow readers to see essential information at a glance. Textbook users will be pleased to find more consistency between chapters in this edition. The Hierarchy of Evidence and questions to consider when appraising nursing studies are printed inside the back cover for easy reference.

The unique feature of integrating ethical content throughout the chapters remains. Organizing content in this manner helps students to integrate ethical principles into each step of the research process.

As a learning strategy, chapters are subdivided so that content is presented in manageable "bites." Students commented that they liked this feature. As in the *Third Edition*, chapters begin with a complete list of all objectives addressed in the chapter. Objectives are repeated for each subsection and are followed by content, and each subsection ends with a section called "Test Your Knowledge." Multiple-choice and true-or-false questions, with an answer key, reinforce the objectives and content. Chapters also include critical thinking exercises that challenge readers to make decisions based on the content. Users will find significant alterations to the digital resources available to readers.

New challenges arose while we wrote this *Fourth Edition*. Publishers are becoming less inclined to allow their materials to be reproduced. Therefore, we are disappointed that we can no longer offer the full-text reference articles within this text's digital resources. In response to this challenge, we have significantly transformed the Apply What You Have Learned exercise for Chapter 4. Students are provided with directions so that they can search for the articles themselves, thereby reinforcing behaviors that will be required of baccalaureate-prepared nurses, who need to keep up with the ever-changing healthcare environment. We are pleased with the result because this alteration has actually strengthened the exercise. For readers' convenience, we have included a table below containing the evidence used throughout the Apply What You Have Learned exercises.

We hope that the variety of strategies incorporated in this textbook meet your learning needs and generate enthusiasm about EBP. We wish you the best as you begin your professional career as an innovator who provides care based on best practices.

Citation	Chapter(s)	Search Terms (Limiters)
Articles to Search in CINAHL		
Al-Hussami, M., Darawad, M., & Almhairat, I. I. (2011). Predictors of compliance handwashing practice among healthcare professionals. *Healthcare Infection, 16,* 79–84.	4, 7	Al-Hussami (author) "handwashing practice" (all fields)
Al-Tawfiq, J. A., & Pittet, D. (2013). Improving hand hygiene compliance in healthcare settings using behavior change theories: Reflections. *Teaching and Learning in Medicine, 25,* 374–382.	4, 5	Al-Tawfiq (author) Pittet (author) "reflections" (title)
Chhapola, V., & Brar, R. (2015). Impact of an educational intervention on hand hygiene compliance and infection rate in a developing country neonatal intensive care unit. *International of Nursing Practice, 21,* 486–492.	1, 4, 8	Chhapola (author)

Citation	Chapter(s)	Search Terms (Limiters)
Articles to Search in CINAHL		
Chun, H., Kim, K., & Park, H. (2015). Effects of hand hygiene education and individual feedback on hand hygiene behavior, MRSA, acquisition rate, and MRSA colonization pressure among intensive care unit nurses. *International Journal of Nursing Practice, 21*, 709–715.	4, 6, 7	Chun (author) "individual feedback" (all fields)
Dyson, J., Lawton, R., Jackson, C., & Cheater, F. (2013). Development of a theory-based instrument to identify barriers and louvers to best hand hygiene practice among healthcare practitioners. *Implementation Science, 8*(111), 1–9.	4, 10	Dyson (author) Lawton (author) "barriers" (all fields)
Fakhry, M., Hannah, G. B., Anderson, O., Holmes, A., & Nathwain, D. (2012). Effectiveness of an audible reminder on hand hygiene adherence. *American Journal of Infection Control, 40*, 320–323.	4, 6, 7	"audible reminder" (title) "hand hygiene" (title)
Huis, A., Schoonhoven, L., Grol, R., Donders, R., Hulscher, M., & van Achterber, T. (2014). Impact of a team and leaders-directed strategy to improve nurses' adherence to hand hygiene guidelines: A cluster randomized trial. *International Journal of Nursing Studies, 50*, 464–474.	4, 7	Huis (author) Donders (author)
Jackson, C., Lowton, K., & Griffiths, P. (2014). Infection prevention as "a show": A qualitative study of nurses' infection prevention behaviours. *International Journal of Nursing Studies, 51*, 400–408.	4, 9, 14	Jackson (author) Lowton (author) "International Journal of Nursing Studies" (publication name)
Johnson, L., Jrueber, S., Schlotzhauer, C., Phillips, E., Bullock, P., Basnett, J., & Hahn-Cover, K. (2014). A multifactorial action plan improves hand hygiene adherence and significantly reduces central line-associated bloodstream infections. *American Journal of Infection Control, 42*, 1146–1151.	4	Johnson (author) "multifactorial action plan" (all fields)
Kingston, L., O'Connell, N. H., & Dunne, C. P. (2016). Hand hygiene-related clinical trials reported since 2010: A systematic review. *Journal of Hospital Infection, 92*, 309–320.	4, 12	Kingston (author) "systematic review" 2016 (publication date)
Mortell, M. (2012). Hand hygiene compliance: Is there a theory-practice-ethics gap? *Infection Control, 21*, 1011–1014.	3	Mortell (author) 2012 (publication date)

Citation	Chapter(s)	Search Terms (Limiters)
Articles to Search in CINAHL		
Salmon, S., & McLaws, M. (2015). Qualitative findings from focus group discussion on hand hygiene compliance among health care workers in Vietnam. *American Journal of Infection Control, 43*, 1086–1091.	1, 4, 9	Salmon (author) McLaws (author)
Whitby, M., & McLaws, M. (2007). Methodological difficulties in hand hygiene research. *Journal of Hospital Infection, 67*, 194–195.	4, 10	Whitby (author) "methodological difficulties" (title)
Obtain From JBI		
Nguyen, P. (2016). Hand hygiene: Alcohol-based solutions. The Joanna Briggs Institute.	12	

Citation	Chapter(s)	URLs
Sources From the Web		
National Cancer Institute	2	http://phrp.nihtraining.com/users/login.php
Bromwich, J. E. (2016, April 20). You've been washing your hands wrong. *New York Times.*	12	https://www.nytimes.com/2016/04/21/health/washing-hands.html?_r=0
Emotional Intelligence (EQ) Assessment	17	http://www.ihhp.com/free-eq-quiz/
The New Enneagram Test	17	http://9types.com/
World Health Organization	3	http://www.who.int/gpsc/5may/Hand_Hygiene_Why_How_and_When_Brochure.pdf?ua=1

Available in the Digital Resources		
Resource	**Chapter**	
Grid	4	Visit this text's accompanying digital resources to find links to these materials.
Poster guideline for making an EBP poster presentation	19	

REFERENCES

Rogers, E. M. (2003). *Diffusion of innovations* (5th ed.). New York, NY: Free Press.

Schmidt, N. A., & Brown, J. M. (2007). Use of the innovation–decision process teaching strategy to promote evidence-based practice. *Journal of Professional Nursing, 23*, 150–156.

ACKNOWLEDGMENTS

As with every endeavor, many individuals make accomplishing the goal a reality. We wish to begin by expressing our gratitude to the contributors who shared our vision to create a text that can excite undergraduate nurses about evidence-based practice. The efforts of Karen Stacy, Patti Reid, and Julie Ault to protect sacred writing times were instrumental in allowing us to meet deadlines. Without their help and understanding, writing sessions would not have been as productive as they were. Special thanks are in order for Jones & Bartlett Learning staff, especially Amanda Martin, Christina Freitas, and Alex Schab, who offered invaluable editorial assistance. We are grateful for the ways Jones & Bartlett has developed and marketed the book over the four editions, and we are delighted how the use of the book has surpassed our expectations. This success can be attributed to nursing faculty who are also committed to our vision of creating nurses who base their practices on evidence. Finally, we are indebted to our families, who afforded us the time to complete this book. They provided invaluable support throughout the process.

Introduction to Evidence-Based Practice

UNIT 1

Without evidence, clinical practice cannot advance scientifically.

At the end of this chapter, you will be able to:

< Define evidence-based practice (EBP)
< List sources of evidence for nursing practice
< Identify barriers to the adoption of EBP and pinpoint strategies to overcome them
< Explain how the process of diffusion facilitates moving evidence into nursing practice
< Define research
< Discuss the contribution of research to EBP
< Categorize types of research
< Distinguish between quantitative and qualitative research approaches

< Describe the sections found in research articles
< Describe the cycle of scientific development
< Identify historical occurrences that shaped the development of nursing as a science
< Identify factors that will continue to move nursing forward as a science
< Discuss what future trends may influence how nurses use evidence to improve the quality of patient care
< Identify five unethical studies involving the violation of the rights of human subjects

KEY TERMS

abstract
applied research
barriers
basic research
cycle of scientific
    development
deductive reasoning
descriptive research
discussion section
early adopters
empirical evidence
evidence-based practice
    (EBP)

evidence hierarchy
explanatory research
inductive reasoning
innovation
introduction
Jewish Chronic Disease
    Hospital study
laggards
list of references
methods section
model of diffusion of
    innovations
Nazi experiments

Nuremberg Code
predictive research
qualitative research
quantitative research
replication study
research
research utilization
results section
review of literature
theoretical framework
theory
Tuskegee study
Willowbrook studies

CHAPTER 1

What Is Evidence-Based Practice?

Nola A. Schmidt and Janet M. Brown

It is not uncommon for students to question the need to study a textbook such as this. To many students, it seems much more exciting and important to be with patients in various settings. It is often hard for beginning practitioners to appreciate the value of learning the research process and the importance of evidence in providing patient care. To appreciate the importance of *evidence*, imagine that a family member required nursing care. Would it not be much more desirable to have care based on evidence rather than on tradition, trial and error, or an educated guess? To be competent, a nurse must have the ability to provide care based on evidence. A journey through this textbook will assist you with developing your skills and talents for providing patients with care based on evidence so that the best possible outcomes can be achieved.

1.1 EBP: What Is It?

At the end of this section, you will be able to:

< Define evidence-based practice (EBP)
< List sources of evidence for nursing practice
< Identify barriers to the adoption of EBP and pinpoint strategies to overcome them
< Explain how the process of diffusion facilitates moving evidence into nursing practice

Overview of EBP

When examining the literature about *evidence-based practice (EBP)*, one will find a variety of definitions. Most definitions include three components: research-based information, clinical expertise, and patient preferences. Ingersoll's (2000) classic definition succinctly captures the essence of EBP, defining it as "the conscientious, explicit, and judicious use of theory-derived, research-based information in making decisions about care delivery to individuals or groups of patients and in consideration of individual needs and preferences" (p. 152). What does this mean? EBP is a process involving the examination and application of research findings or other reliable evidence that has been integrated with scientific theories. For nurses to participate in this process, they must use their critical thinking skills to review research publications and other sources of information. After the information is evaluated, nurses use their clinical decision-making skills to apply evidence to patient care. As in all nursing care, patient preferences and needs are the basis of care decisions and therefore essential to EBP.

EBP has its roots in medicine. Archie Cochrane, a British epidemiologist, admonished the medical profession for not critically examining evidence (Cochrane, 1971). He contended that individuals should pay only for health care based on scientific evidence (Melnyk & Fineout-Overholt, 2015), and he believed that random clinical trials were the "gold standard" for generating reliable and valid evidence. He suggested that rigorous, systematic reviews of research from a variety of disciplines be conducted to inform practice and policy making. As a result of his innovative idea, the Cochrane Center established a collaboration "to promote evidence-informed health decision-making by producing high-quality, relevant, accessible systematic reviews and other synthesized research evidence " (Cochrane Collaboration, 2017). Others built on Dr. Cochrane's philosophy, and the definition of EBP in medicine evolved to include clinical judgment and patient preferences (Sackett, Rosenberg, Gray, Haynes, & Richardson, 1996; Straus, Glasziou, Richardson, & Haynes, 2011).

During this time, nursing was heavily involved in trying to apply research findings to practice, a process known as *research utilization*. This process involves changing practice from the results of a single research study (Barnsteiner & Prevost, 2002). Nursing innovators recognized that shifting from this model to an EBP framework would be more likely to improve patient outcomes and provide more cost-effective methods of care (Ingersoll, 2000; Levin, Fineout-Overholt, Melnyk, Barnes, & Vetter, 2011; Melnyk, 1999; Schifalacqua, Mamula, & Mason, 2011). Why? Many nursing questions cannot be answered by a single study, and human conditions are not always amenable to clinical trials. Also, the research

CRITICAL THINKING EXERCISE 1-1

Look carefully at the steps in each EBP model cited in **Table 1-1**. Are you reminded of a similar process?

utilization process does not place value on the importance of clinical decision making, nor is it noted for being patient focused.

These nursing innovators recognized that the EBP framework allows for consideration of other sources of evidence relevant to nursing practice.

There are many different models for EBP. Three models that are especially well known in nursing are shown in **Table 1-1**. While each is unique, they have commonalities. For example, each one begins with a question or need for the identification of acquiring knowledge about a question. All involve appraisal of evidence and making a decision about how to use evidence. These models conclude by closing the loop through evaluation to determine that the practice change is actually meeting the expected outcomes.

Sources of Evidence

Over the years, a variety of sources of evidence has provided information for nursing practice. Although it would be nice to claim that all nursing practice is based on substantial and reliable evidence, this is not the case. Evidence derived from tradition, authority, trial and error, personal experiences, intuition, borrowed

TABLE 1-1   Models of EBP

Star Model of Knowledge Transformation	Iowa Model of EBP	Model of Diffusion of Innovations
1. Discovery research	1. Ask clinical question	1. Acquisition of knowledge
2. Evidence summary	2. Search literature	2. Persuasion
3. Translation to guidelines	3. Critically appraise evidence	3. Decision
4. Practice integration	4. Implement practice change	4. Implementation
5. Process, outcome evaluation	5. Evaluate	5. Confirmation
Stevens (2012)	Titler et al. (2001)	Rogers (2003)

evidence, and scientific research are all used to guide nursing practice. Just as you know from your own life, some sources are not as dependable as others.

Tradition has long been an accepted basis for information. Consider this: Why are vital signs taken routinely every 4 hours on patients who are clinically stable? The rationale for many nursing interventions commonly practiced is grounded in the phrase "This is the way we have always done it." Nurses can be so entrenched in practice traditions that they fail to ask questions that could lead to changes based on evidence. Consistent use of tradition as a basis for practice limits effective problem solving and fails to consider individual needs and preferences.

How often have you heard the phrase "Because I said so"? This is an example of authority. Various sources of authority, such as books, articles, web pages, and individuals and groups, are perceived as being meaningful sources of reliable information; yet, in reality, the information provided may be based in personal experience or tradition rather than scientific evidence. Authority has a place in nursing practice as long as nurses ascertain the legitimacy of the information provided.

Trial and error is another source of evidence. Although we all use this approach in our everyday problem solving, it is often not the preferred approach for delivering nursing care. Because trial and error is not based on a systematic scientific approach, patient outcomes may not be a direct result of the intervention. For example, in long-term care the treatment of decubitus ulcers is often based on this haphazard approach. Nurses frequently try a variety of approaches to heal ulcers. After some time, they settle on one approach that is more often than not effective. This approach can lead to reduced critical thinking and wasted time and resources.

Nurses often make decisions about patient care based on their personal experiences. Although previous experience can help to build confidence and hone skills, experiences are biased by perceptions and values that are frequently influenced by tradition, authority, and trial and error. Personal intuition has also been identified as a source of evidence. It is not always clear what is meant by intuition and how it contributes to nursing practice. Intuition is defined as "quick perception of truth without conscious attention or reasoning" (IA Users Club, Inc., 2015, p. 1). Whereas on very rare occasions a "gut feeling" may be reliable, most patients would prefer health care that is based on stronger evidence. Thus, intuition is not one of the most advantageous sources of evidence for driving patient care decisions because nurses are expected to use logical reasoning as critical thinkers and clinical decision makers.

Because of the holistic perspective used in nursing and the collaboration that occurs with other healthcare providers, it is not uncommon for nurses to borrow evidence from other disciplines. For example, pediatric nurses rely heavily on theories of development as a basis for nursing interventions. Borrowed evidence can be useful because it fills gaps that exist in nursing science and provides a basis on which to build new evidence; it can be a stronger type of evidence than are sources not based on theory and science. When nurses use borrowed evidence, it is important for them to consider the fit of the evidence with the nursing phenomenon.

Because nursing offers a unique perspective on patient care, nurses cannot rely solely on borrowed evidence and must build their own body of evidence through scientific research. Scientific research is considered to yield the best source of evidence. Nurses can use many different research methods to describe, explain, and predict phenomena that are central to nursing care. To have an EBP, whenever possible nurses must emphasize the use of *theory*-derived, research-based information over the use of evidence obtained through tradition, authority, trial and error, personal experience, and intuition.

Not all scientific research is equal. Some types of studies are designed in ways that yield results that nurses can use with confidence. For example, random controlled studies are considered more strongly designed than correlational or descriptive studies. When multiple studies have been conducted about a particular topic, the findings of the studies can be combined into a systematic review, which can be used with even more confidence. To rank evidence from lowest to highest, nurses refer to the *evidence hierarchy* (**Figure 1-1**). You will find the need to frequently refer to this figure as you learn about research designs and appraising evidence.

Adopting an Evidence-Based Practice

One would think that when there is compelling scientific evidence, findings would quickly and efficiently transition to practice. However, most often this is not the case. Many *barriers* complicate the integration of findings into practice. In fact, it can take as many as 200 years for an innovation to become a standard of care. Consider the history of controlling scurvy in the British Navy.

> In the early days of long sea voyages, scurvy killed more sailors than did warfare, accidents, and other causes. In 1601 an English sea captain, James Lancaster, conducted an experiment to evaluate the effectiveness of lemon juice in preventing scurvy. He commanded four ships that sailed from England on a voyage to India. Three teaspoonfuls of lemon juice were served every day to the sailors in one of his four ships. These men stayed healthy. The other three ships constituted Lancaster's "control group," as their sailors were not given any lemon juice. On the other three ships, by the halfway point in the journey, 110 out of 278 sailors had died from scurvy.
>
> The results were so clear that one would have expected the British Navy to promptly adopt citrus juice for scurvy prevention on all ships. But it did

KEY TERMS

theory: A set of concepts linked through propositions to explain a phenomenon

evidence hierarchy: A model showing how evidence can be categorized from strong to weak

barriers: Factors that limit or prevent change

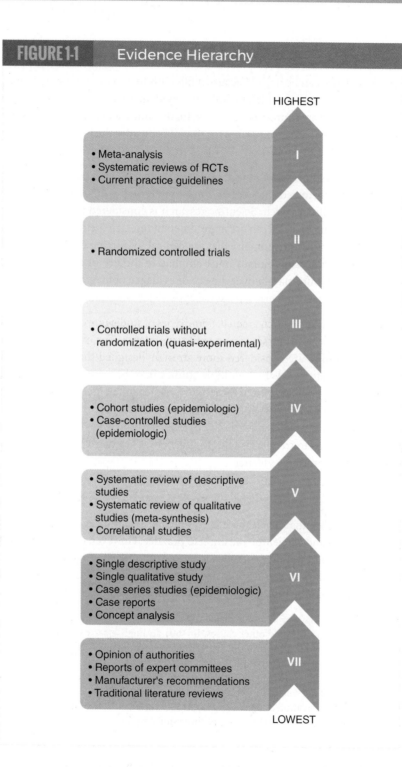

FIGURE 1-1   Evidence Hierarchy

not become accepted practice. In 1747, about 150 years later, James Lind, a British Navy physician who knew of Lancaster's results, carried out another experiment on the HMS *Salisbury*. To each scurvy patient on this ship, Lind prescribed either two oranges and one lemon, or one of five other supplements. The scurvy patients who got the citrus fruits were cured in a few days and were able to help Dr. Lind care for the other patients.

Certainly, with this further solid evidence of the ability of citrus fruits to combat scurvy, one would expect the British Navy to have quickly adopted this innovation for all ships' crews on long sea voyages. Yet it took another 48 years for this to become standard practice, and scurvy was finally wiped out.

Why were the authorities so slow to adopt the idea of citrus for scurvy prevention? Other competing remedies for scurvy were also being proposed, and each cure had its champions. For example, the highly respected Captain Cook reported that during his Pacific voyages there was no evidence that citrus fruits cured scurvy. In contrast, the experimental work by Dr. Lind, who was not a prominent figure in the field of naval medicine, did not get much attention. This leads one to wonder if the British Navy was typically hesitant to adopt new innovations. But, while it resisted scurvy prevention for years, other innovations, such as new ships and new guns, were readily accepted.

(Modified with the permission of Simon & Schuster Publishing Group from the Free Press edition of *Diffusion of Innovations*, 5th Edition, by Everett M. Rogers. Copyright ©1995, 2003 by Everett M. Rogers. Copyright © 1962, 1971, 1983 by The Free Press. All rights reserved.)

Even when the benefits and advantages of an *innovation* have been made evident, adoption can be slow to occur. In 2005, Pravikoff, Tanner, and Pierce conducted a large survey of registered nurses (RNs) from across the United States. Of the clinical nurses who responded to the survey, more than 54% were not familiar with the term *EBP*. The typical source of information for 67% of these nurses was a colleague. Alarmingly, 58% of the respondents had never used research articles to support clinical practice. Only 18% had ever used a hospital library. Additionally, 77% had never received instruction in the use of electronic resources. More recently, a survey conducted at a Magnet hospital found that 96% of nurses were aware that EBP was being implemented at their institution (White-Williams et al., 2013). Although this shows a significant improvement over 7 years, one must keep in mind that the inclusion of only a Magnet facility may present a bias because to earn Magnet Recognition, EBP must be inherent in the organization. This was confirmed by Warren et al. (2016), who compared perception of nurses who worked at Magnet facilities with those who did not. They found that nurses working at Magnet hospitals thought that their organizations were equipped to implement EBP. They also found that younger RNs who were newer to practice were more likely to have positive beliefs about EBP.

KEY TERM

innovation:
Something new or novel

CRITICAL THINKING EXERCISE 1-2

Consider your last clinical experience. How much was your practice based on scientific research? What other sources of evidence did you use? Divide a circle into sections (like a pie chart) to show how much influence each of the sources of evidence had on the patient care you provided.

Overcoming Barriers

Studies demonstrate that the reasons nurses do not draw on research are related to individual and organizational factors. Individual factors are those characteristics that are inherent to the nurse. Organizational factors are related to administration, resources, facilities, and culture of the system. Major barriers to nurses using research findings at the point of care are nurses not valuing research, nurses being resistant to change, and lack of time and resources to obtain evidence (Shivnan, 2011). In addition, the communication gap between researcher and clinician (Paris, Callahan, & Pierson, 2011), organizational culture, and the inability of individuals to evaluate nursing research have been identified as barriers by registered nurses (Majid et al., 2011; Melnyk, Fineout-Overholt, Gallagher-Ford, & Kaplan, 2012; Solomons & Spross, 2011; Van Patter Gale & Schaffer, 2009), clinical nurse specialists and educators (Malik, McKenna, & Plummer, 2016), nurse managers (Spieres, Lo, Hofmeyer, & Cummings, 2016), and chief nurse executives (Melnyk et al., 2016).

Strategies that do not overcome these barriers do little to promote EBP. To overcome barriers related to individual factors, strategies need to be aimed at instilling an appreciation for EBP, increasing knowledge, developing necessary skills, and changing behaviors. Strategies to overcome organizational barriers must be directed toward creating and maintaining an environment where EBP can flourish. Research has focused on strategies to overcome both individual and organizational factors to bring about change (Aitken et al., 2011; Fitzsimons & Cooper, 2012; Hauck, Winsett, & Kuric, 2013; Melnyk, Fineout-Overholt, Giggleman, & Cruz, 2010; Ogiehor-Enoma, Taqueban, & Anosike, 2010; Pennington, Moscatel, Dacar, & Johnson, 2010; Reicherter, Gordes, Glickman, & Hakim, 2013; Valente, 2010). Practical strategies for successfully overcoming these barriers are summarized in **Table 1-2**.

To overcome barriers to using research findings in practice, it can be helpful to use a model to assist in understanding how new ideas come to be accepted practice. The *model of diffusion of innovations* (Rogers, 2003) has been used in the nursing literature for this purpose (L'Esperance & Perry, 2016; Schmidt & Brown, 2007; Van Patter Gale & Schaffer, 2009). You are already familiar with the concept of diffusion. From studying chemistry you know that diffusion

KEY TERM

model of diffusion of innovations: Model to assist in understanding how new ideas come to be accepted practice

TABLE 1-2	Strategies for Overcoming Barriers to Adopting an EBP
Barrier	**Strategy**
Lack of time	Devote 15 minutes per day to reading evidence related to a clinical problem. Sign up for emails that offer summaries of research studies in your area of interest. Use a team approach to equitably distribute the workload among members. Bookmark websites that have clinical guidelines to promote faster retrieval of information. Evaluate available technologies (i.e., tablets) to create time-saving systems that allow quick and convenient retrieval of information at the bedside. Negotiate release time from patient care duties to collect, read, and share information about relevant clinical problems. Search for already established clinical guidelines because they provide synthesis of existing research.
Lack of value placed on research in practice	Make a list of reasons why healthcare providers should value research, and use this list as a springboard for discussions with colleagues. Invite nurse researchers to share why they are passionate about their work. When disagreements arise about a policy or protocol, find an article that supports your position and share it with others. When selecting a work environment, ask about the organizational commitment to EBP. Link measurement of quality indicators to EBP. Participate in EBP activities to demonstrate professionalism that can be rewarded through promotions or merit raises. Provide recognition during National Nurses Week for individuals involved in EBP projects.
Lack of knowledge about EBP and research	Take a course or attend a continuing education offering on EBP. Invite a faculty member to a unit meeting to discuss EBP. Consult with advanced practice nurses. Attend conferences where clinical research is presented and talk with presenters about their studies. Volunteer to serve on committees that set policies and protocols. Create a mentoring program to bring novice and experienced nurses together.
Lack of technological skills to find evidence	Consult with a librarian about how to access databases and retrieve articles. Learn to bookmark important websites that are sources of clinical guidelines. Commit to acquiring computer skills.

Barrier	Strategy
Lack of resources to access evidence	Write a proposal for funds to support access to online databases and journals.
	Collaborate with a nursing program for access to resources.
	Investigate funding possibilities from others (i.e., pharmaceutical companies, grants).
Lack of ability to read research	Organize a journal club where nurses meet regularly to discuss the evidence about a specific clinical problem.
	Write down questions about an article and ask an advanced practice nurse to read the article and assist in answering the questions.
	Clarify unfamiliar terms by looking them up in a dictionary or research textbook.
	Use one familiar critique format when reading research.
	Identify clinical problems and share them with nurse researchers.
	Participate in ongoing unit-based studies.
	Subscribe to journals that provide uncomplicated explanations of research studies.
Resistance to change	Listen to people's concerns about change.
	When considering an EBP project, select one that interests the staff, has a high priority, is likely to be successful, and has baseline data.
	Mobilize talented individuals to act as change agents.
	Create a means to reward individuals who provide leadership during change.
Lack of organizational support for EBP	Link organizational priorities with EBP to reduce cost and increase efficiency.
	Recruit administrators who value EBP.
	Form coalitions with other healthcare providers to increase the base of support for EBP.
	Use EBP to meet accreditation standards or gain recognition (i.e., Magnet Recognition).

involves the movement of molecules from areas of higher concentration to areas of lower concentration. In the same way, innovative nursing practices frequently begin in a small number of institutions and eventually spread or diffuse, becoming standard practice everywhere. The model includes four major concepts: innovation, communication, time, and social system. Rogers (2003) defines diffusion as "the process by which (1) an innovation (2) is communicated through certain channels (3) over time (4) among the members of a social system" (p. 11). An innovation is an idea, practice, or object that is perceived as new by an individual or other unit of adoption. Before adopting an innovation, individuals seek information about its advantages and disadvantages.

Initially, only a minimal number of individuals, known as *early adopters*, embrace the innovation. With time, early adopters who are opinion leaders, through their interpersonal networks, become instrumental as the diffusion progresses through the social system. Those individuals who are slow or who fail to adopt the innovation are known as *laggards*. In the scurvy example, it took about 200 years for the innovation to diffuse throughout the British Navy. You may also be surprised to see how long it has taken other things we take for granted to diffuse throughout American households (**Figure 1-2**).

KEY TERMS

early adopters:
Individuals who are the first to embrace an innovation

laggards:
Individuals who are slow or fail to adopt an innovation

FIGURE 1-2 Diffusion of Technological Innovations Over Time

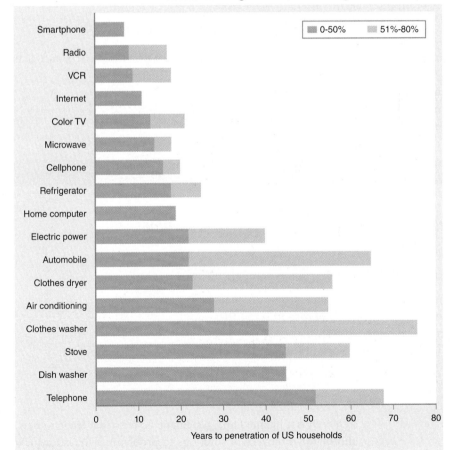

Courtesy of Asymco.

CRITICAL THINKING EXERCISE 1-3

In the scurvy example, identify communication channels and social system barriers to the adoption of citrus fruits as a treatment for scurvy. Now, consider how the model of diffusion of innovations could have been applied to this situation. How could the physicians have overcome the barriers you identified and convinced others to become early adopters so that citrus became accepted practice for the treatment of scurvy?

TEST YOUR KNOWLEDGE 1-1

1. Which of the following is not a component of the definition of EBP?
    a. Clinical expertise
    b. Nursing research
    c. Organizational culture
    d. Patient preferences
2. To promote EBP, which of the following strategies must be addressed? (Select all that apply.)
    a. Lack of commitment to EBP
    b. Lack of computer skills
    c. Lack of time
    d. Lack of value placed on research in practice

How did you do? 1. c; 2. a, b, c, d

1.2 What Is Nursing Research?

At the end of this section, you will be able to:

‹ Define research
‹ Discuss the contribution of research to EBP
‹ Categorize types of research
‹ Distinguish between quantitative and qualitative research approaches
‹ Describe the sections found in research articles

Research is a planned and systematic activity that leads to new knowledge and/or the discovery of solutions to problems or questions (Polit & Beck, 2016). Simply stated, research means to search again. But the search must be deliberate and organized as relevant questions are examined. It is essential that established steps be followed.

BOX 1-1 Steps of the Research Process

1. Identify the research question.
2. Conduct a review of the literature.
3. Identify a theoretical framework.
4. Select a research design.
5. Implement the study.
6. Analyze data.
7. Draw conclusions.
8. Disseminate findings.

Following a systematic approach (**Box 1-1**) is more likely to yield results that can be used with confidence. Through research, scientists aim to describe, explain, and predict phenomena. But isn't science supposed to prove that things are true? Sometimes you may hear or read the phrase "research proves"; however, the use of the word *prove* is inaccurate. Research findings *support* a particular approach or view because the possibility of error exists in every research study. This underscores why a planned, systematic approach is necessary and why *replication studies* are important.

Nurses use research to generate new knowledge or to validate and refine existing knowledge that directly or indirectly influences nursing practice. In nursing research, the phenomena of interest are persons, health, nursing, and environment. Nurses study patient outcomes, attitudes of nurses, effectiveness of administrative policy, and teaching strategies in nursing education. Nursing research contributes to the development and refinement of theory. But most important, as a baccalaureate-prepared nurse, you will use research as a foundation for EBP. Without research, nursing practice would be based on tradition, authority, trial and error, personal experiences, intuition, and borrowed evidence. This is why you must have the skills to read, evaluate, and apply nursing research so that as an early adopter you can be instrumental in moving an innovation to the point of care.

Types of Research

A variety of terms is used to describe the research conducted by scientists. Research can be categorized as *descriptive*, *explanatory*, or *predictive*; *basic* or *applied*; and *quantitative* or *qualitative*. These categories are not necessarily mutually exclusive. For example, a study may be descriptive, applied, and qualitative. Although this sounds complicated, when you understand the definitions, it will become clear.

KEY TERMS

research: Systematic study that leads to new knowledge and/or solutions to problems or questions

replication studies: Repeated studies to obtain similar results

descriptive research: A category of research that is concerned with providing accurate descriptions of phenomena

explanatory research: Research concerned with identifying relationships among phenomena

predictive research: Research that forecasts precise relationships between dimensions of phenomena or differences between groups

basic research: Research to gain knowledge for the sake of gaining knowledge; bench research

FYI

Research can be categorized as descriptive, explanatory, or predictive; basic or applied; and quantitative or qualitative. Nursing research concerns persons, health, nursing practice, and environment and can be used to generate new knowledge or to validate and refine existing knowledge that directly or indirectly influences nursing practice.

One way to classify research is by its aims. Descriptive research answers "What is it?" This category of research is concerned with providing accurate descriptions and can involve observation of a phenomenon in its natural setting. The goal of the explanatory category is to identify the relationships a phenomenon has with individuals, groups, situations, or events. Explanatory studies address why or how phenomena are related. Predictive research aims to forecast precise relationships between dimensions of phenomena or differences between groups. This category of research addresses when the phenomena will occur. **Table 1-3** provides an example of how these different types helped nurses to better understand the phenomenon of pain during chest tube removal.

Another way to classify research is to consider whether findings can be used to solve real-world problems. Basic research, sometimes known as bench research, seeks to gain knowledge for the sake of gaining that knowledge. This knowledge may or may not become applicable to practical issues or situations. It may be years before a discovery becomes useful when it is combined with other discoveries. For example, vitamin K was studied for the sake of learning more about its properties. Years later, the knowledge gained about its mechanism of action during coagulation formed the foundation for vitamin K becoming an accepted treatment for bleeding disorders. In contrast, the aim of applied research is to discover knowledge that will solve a clinical problem. The findings typically have immediate application to bring about changes in practice, education, or administration.

TABLE 1-3	An Example of Building Knowledge in Nursing Science: Pain and Chest Tube Removal (CTR)	
Study	**Aim of Research**	**Findings**
Gift, Bolgiano, & Cunningham (1991)	Describe	Individuals reported burning pain and pulling with CTR. Women reported pain more frequently than men did.
Puntillo (1994)	Describe	Compared CTR pain with endotracheal suctioning. Patients reported less pain with suctioning than with CTR. "Sharp" was the most frequent adjective for CTR pain.
Carson, Barton, Morrison, & Tribble (1994)	Predict	Patients were assigned to one of four groups for treatment with pain medications: IV morphine, IV morphine and subfascial lidocaine, IV morphine and subfascial normal saline solution, and subfascial lidocaine. There were no significant differences in pain alleviation.

Study	Aim of Research	Findings
Puntillo (1996)	Predict	Patients were assigned to either placebo normal saline interpleural injection or bupivacaine interpleural injection. There was no significant difference in pain reports.
Houston & Jesurum (1999)	Predict	Examined effect of Quick Release Technique (QRT), a form of relaxation using a breathing technique, during CTR. Patients were randomly assigned to either an analgesic-only group or an analgesic with QRT. Combination of QRT with analgesic was not more effective than was analgesic alone in reducing pain.
Puntillo & Ley (2004)	Predict	Patients were randomly assigned to one of four combinations of pharmacological and nonpharmacological interventions to reduce pain: 4 mg IV morphine with procedural information, 30 mg IV ketorolac and procedural information, 4 mg IV morphine with procedural and sensory information, and 30 mg IV ketorolac with procedural and sensory information. There were no significant differences among the groups regarding pain intensity, pain distress, or sedation levels.
Friesner, Curry, & Moddeman (2006)	Predict	A group of adults who had undergone coronary artery bypass used a slow deep-breathing relaxation exercise with opioid analgesia. Their pain ratings were compared to a group using opioids only. There was a significant reduction in pain ratings for the patients who used the breathing exercise combined with opioids.
Demir & Khorsbid (2010)	Predict	Cardiac patients were randomly assigned to a group that received ice and analgesia, a group that received warmth and analgesia, or a group that received only analgesia. Patients who received the application of ice reported significantly less pain than did patients from the other two groups.
Ertuğ & Ülker (2011)	Predict	Patients were randomly assigned to either an experimental group that received cold prior to CTR or a control group that had no intervention for pain management. Patients receiving cold reported significantly less pain than did those in the control group.
Pinheiro et al. (2015)	Predict	Patients were randomly assigned to either an experimental group that received 1% subcutaneous lidocaine or a control group that received a combination of inflammatory agents and opioids. There was no significant difference in pain reported by patients.

Note: CTR = chest tube removal.

CRITICAL THINKING EXERCISE 1-4

When you look at the word "quantitative," what root word do you see? Do you see that it comes from the word "quantity"? So, one knows that the focus will be on numbers.

Quantitative and *qualitative* are terms that are also used to distinguish among types of research. Philosophical approach, research questions, designs, and data all provide clues to assist you in differentiating between these two methods of classification. Sometimes, researchers even combine quantitative and qualitative methods in the same study.

Quantitative researchers views the world as objective. This implies that researchers can separate themselves from phenomena being studied. The focus is on collecting *empirical evidence*; in other words, evidence gathered through the five senses. Researchers quantify observations by using numbers to obtain precise measurements that can later be statistically analyzed.

Many quantitative studies test hypotheses. Some study designs typically associated with quantitative methods include descriptive survey, correlational, quasi-experimental, and experimental designs. For example, a nurse researcher may measure patient satisfaction with nursing care by having them complete a survey to rate their satisfaction, using a scale of 0–5.

In contrast, the premise of qualitative research is that the world is not objective. There can be multiple realities because the context of the situation is different for each person and can change with time. The emphasis is on verbal descriptions that explain human behaviors.

KEY TERMS

empirical evidence: Evidence that is verifiable by experience through the five senses or experiment

deductive reasoning: Thinking that moves from the general to the particular

In this type of research, the focus is on providing a detailed description of the meanings people give to their experiences. Some methods that are recognized as qualitative include phenomenology, grounded theory, ethnography, and historical. For example, a nurse researcher may measure patient satisfaction with nursing care by conducting individual interviews and summarizing common themes that patients expressed. **Table 1-4** provides a comparison of these two approaches.

Another important point about quantitative and qualitative approaches is that there are two styles of reasoning associated with them. *Deductive reasoning,*

CRITICAL THINKING EXERCISE 1-5

When you look for the root word in "qualitative," do you see the word "quality"? This shows that the emphasis is on words, rather than on numbers.

TABLE 1-4	Comparisons of Quantitative and Qualitative Approaches	
Attribute	**Quantitative**	**Qualitative**
Philosophical perspective	One reality that can be objectively viewed by the researcher	Multiple realities that are subjective, occurring within the context of the situation
Type of reasoning	Primarily deductive	Primarily inductive
Role of researcher	Controlled and structured	Participative and ongoing
Strategies	Control and manipulation of situations Analysis of numbers with statistical tests Larger number of subjects	Naturalistic; allows situations to unfold without interference Analysis of words to identify themes Smaller numbers of participants
Possible designs	Descriptive Survey Correlational Quasi-experimental Experimental	Phenomenological Ethnographic Grounded Theory Historical

primarily linked with quantitative research, is reasoning that moves from the general to the particular. For example, researchers use a theory to help them reason out a hunch. If the researcher believes that the position of the body affects circulation, then the researcher could deduce that blood pressure readings taken while lying down will be different from those measured while standing. In contrast, *inductive reasoning* involves reasoning that moves from the particular to the general and is associated with qualitative approaches. By using inductive reasoning, researchers can take particular ideas and express an overall general summary about the phenomenon (**Figure 1-3**).

What Makes Up a Research Article?

The development of EBP requires careful attention to research already published. Therefore, it is essential for nurses to identify research studies from among the many other types of articles included in the literature. The trick is knowing what sections are contained in a research article.

Typically, an *abstract* is the first section of a research article and is usually limited to 100–150 words. The purpose of the abstract is to provide an overview of the study, but the presence of an abstract does not necessarily mean that an

KEY TERMS

inductive reasoning: Thinking that moves from the particular to the general

abstract: The first section of a research article that provides an overview of the study

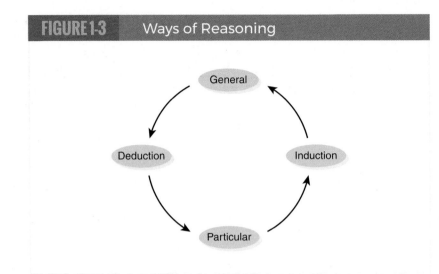

FIGURE 1-3   Ways of Reasoning

article is a research study. Because abstracts can frequently be found online, it is usually helpful to read them before printing or requesting a copy of the article. Careful attention to abstracts can avoid wasted time and effort retrieving articles that are not applicable to the clinical question.

The *introduction*, which follows the abstract, contains a statement of the problem and a purpose statement. The problem statement identifies the problem in a broad and general way. For example, a problem statement may read, "falls in hospitalized patients can increase length of stay." Authors usually provide background information and statistics about the problem to convince readers that the problem is significant. The background information provided should set the stage for the purpose statement, which describes what was examined in the study. For example, a purpose statement may read, "the purpose of this study was to examine the relationship between time of evening medication administration and time of falls." A good introduction convinces readers that the study was worthy of being conducted.

The third section is the *review of literature*. An unbiased, comprehensive, synthesized description of relevant, previously published studies should be presented. For each study included in the review, the purpose, sample, design, and significant findings are discussed. The review should focus on the most recent work in the field but may include older citations if they are considered to be landmark studies. A complete citation is provided for each article so that readers can retrieve the articles if desired. A well-written literature review concludes with a summary of what is known about the problem and identifies

KEY TERMS

introduction:
Part of a research article that states the problem and purpose

review of literature:
An unbiased, comprehensive, synthesized description of relevant previously published studies

gaps in the knowledge base to show readers how the study adds to existing knowledge.

The research article should include a discussion of the *theoretical framework*, which may be in a separate section or combined with the review of literature. A theoretical framework often describes the relationships among general concepts and provides linkages to what is being measured in the study. Authors frequently use a model or diagram to explain their theoretical framework.

A major portion of a research article is the *methods section*, which includes a discussion about study design, sample, and data collection. In most cases, authors explicitly describe the type of design they selected to answer the research question. In this section, it is important for the authors to describe the target population and explain how the sample was obtained. Procedures for collecting data, including the types of measures used, should also be outlined. Throughout this section, authors provide rationale for decisions made regarding how the study was implemented.

Readers frequently consider the *results section* to be the most difficult to understand. Here, authors describe the methods they used to analyze their data, and the characteristics of the sample are reported. In quantitative studies, data tables are frequently included for interpretation, and authors indicate which findings were significant and which were not. In qualitative studies, authors present themes that are supported by quotes from participants. After reading the results section, the reader should be confident that the researchers selected the appropriate analysis for the data collected.

The body of a research article concludes with a *discussion section*. Authors provide an interpretation of the results and discuss how the findings extend the body of knowledge. Results should be linked to the review of the literature and theoretical framework. The authors discuss the limitations of the study design and sometimes suggest possible solutions to address them in future studies. Implications for practice, research, and education are proposed. Often it is helpful to read this section after reading the abstract and introduction because it provides clarity by giving readers an idea of what is to come.

The article concludes with the *list of references* that are cited in the article. While styles vary, many journals adhere to the guidelines provided in the *Publication Manual of the American Psychological Association*. Because it is often helpful to refer to the original works listed in the reference section, it is wise for readers to obtain a copy of the entire article, including the reference list.

KEY TERMS

theoretical framework: The structure of a study that links the theory concepts to the study variables; a section of a research article that describes the theory used

methods section: Major portion of a research article that describes the study design, sample, and data collection

results section: Component of a research article that reports the methods used to analyze data and characteristics of the sample

discussion section: Portion of a research article where interpretation of the results and how the findings extend the body of knowledge are discussed

list of references: Publication information for each article cited in a research report

How Research Is Different from EBP

Research and EBP complement one another, but it is important to understand how they differ. Research is about generating new knowledge, and EBP is about applying new knowledge to practice. Research questions are often posed when a gap in the literature is discovered. For example, perhaps all of the studies about the effect of relaxation on anxiety have been done about adults. Because only adults have been studied, a gap in the literature exists about the effect of relaxation on anxiety in adolescents. In contrast, most EBP questions are raised while nurses are providing care to patients. Research is a scientific process that involves collecting and analyzing data from research subjects to evaluate the findings in light of the research question that is posed. While EBP also involves analysis of data, the data are about patients, and the analysis focuses on whether or not patient outcomes have improved (see **Table 1-5**).

TABLE 1-5	Comparison of Research and EBP

Research	EBP
Generates new knowledge	Applies new knowledge to point of care
Fills gap in literature	Based on evidence in literature
Research question	Clinical question
Subjects	Patients
Designed to describe a phenomenon, find a relationship, or test an intervention	Designed to change practice in clinical setting
Analysis of data	Analysis of data
Evaluates findings in light of research question	Evaluates practice change by measuring patient outcomes

 TEST YOUR KNOWLEDGE 1-2

True/False

1. When reading a quantitative research article, you would expect to see words being analyzed as data.
2. The purpose of research is to prove something is true.
3. It is possible for a descriptive, qualitative study to be applied to practice.

How did you do? 1. F; 2. F; 3. T

1.3 How Has Nursing Evolved as a Science?

At the end of this section, you will be able to:

‹ Describe the cycle of scientific development
‹ Identify historical occurrences that shaped the development of nursing as a science

Nursing has been described as both an art and a science. Historically, the emphasis was more on the art than the science. But as nursing has developed, the emphasis has shifted. We propose that nursing is the artful use of science to promote the health and well-being of individuals, families, and communities. Thus, nursing is based on scientific evidence that provides the framework for practice. The art of nursing is the blending of science with caring to create a therapeutic relationship in which holistic care is delivered. The profession of nursing is entering a new era in which the emphasis is on EBP, therefore reaffirming the importance of science in nursing.

Cycle of Scientific Development

To fully appreciate nursing as a science, an understanding of the history of research in nursing is necessary. Although a grasp of history is important, it can be confusing when one focuses on a list of events and dates to memorize. Instead, by focusing on the what and why of historical occurrences instead of the when, the evolution of nursing as a science will be more clear.

Nursing has developed in a similar fashion to other sciences. **Figure 1-4** depicts the *cycle of scientific development*. Scientists begin by developing grand theories to explain phenomena. A grand theory is a broad generalization that describes, explains, and predicts occurrences that take place around us. Research is then conducted to test these theories and to discover new knowledge. Conferences and publications result from the need to disseminate research findings. Findings are applied to patient care, resulting in changes in practice, and are used to refine established theories and propose new ones. This cycle repeats, building the science as new discoveries are made. Political and social factors are central to the cycle in that they channel research priorities, funding, and opportunities for dissemination of findings.

KEY TERM

cycle of scientific development: A model of the scientific process

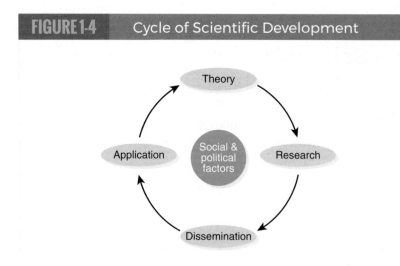

FIGURE 1-4   Cycle of Scientific Development

A Glimpse of the Past
Before 1900

Florence Nightingale is considered by most to be the first nurse researcher. One could say that, as an innovator, she was the first nurse to create an EBP. Through the systematic collection and analysis of data, she identified factors that contributed to the high morbidity and mortality rates of British soldiers during the Crimean War (1853–1856). Health reforms based on her evidence significantly reduced these rates. Her observations during the war led her to theorize that environmental factors were critical influences on the health of individuals. In 1859, she disseminated her ideas in *Notes on Nursing: What It Is, and What It Is Not* (1859/1946), which continues to be in print today. Even though Nightingale was an innovator in nursing research, 40 years passed before nursing research reemerged as relevant to nursing practice.

1900–1929

During the first quarter of the 20th century, the focus of nursing research was closely aligned with the social and political climate. Women were empowered by the suffragette movement; thus their interest in higher education increased. Nursing education became the focus of nursing research. The work of nursing leaders such as Lavinia Dock, Mary Adelaide Nutting, Isabel Hampton Robb, and Lillian Wald was instrumental in reforming nursing education. Similarly, the Goldmark Report (1923) identified many inadequacies in nursing educa-tion and recommended that advanced educational preparation for nurses was essential. As a result, Yale University School of Nursing became the first university-based nursing program in the United States. Also during this time, the first nursing doctoral program in education was started at Teachers College at Columbia University (1924). These events are important because aligning programs of nursing with universities provided the environment for the generation and dissemination of nursing research.

During this era, nursing was prominent in community health, addressing clinical problems such as pneumonia, infant mortality, and blindness. Because nursing research was still in its infancy, descriptive studies focusing on morbidity and mortality rates of these problems were typically conducted. The first nursing journal, *American Journal of Nursing*, was published (1900) and the American Nurses Association was established (1912). As a result, nursing was organized and promoted as a profession.

1930–1949

The time from 1930 to 1949 was influenced by the Great Depression, which was followed by World War II. During the Depression, families did not have money to provide a university education for their children. Consequently, university-based nursing education did not flourish, and nursing research did not advance. As a result of the war, the demand for nurses was so great that nursing education continued to take place primarily in hospital-based diploma programs because this was the quickest way to prepare individuals for the workforce. Nurses continued to focus their research on educational issues, and their studies began to be published in the *American Journal of Nursing*. At the close of this era, the Brown Report (1948) was published. Like the Goldmark Report published 25 years earlier, the Brown Report recommended that nurses be educated in university settings. These events illustrate how the social system can impede the diffusion of an innovation as accepted practice.

1950–1969

In the 1950s, significant events occurred that advanced the science of nursing. The innovation of moving nursing education into universities began to become accepted. Through the work of the Western Interstate Commission for Higher Education (1957), nursing research began to be incorporated into graduate curricula, which provided a structure for the advancement of nursing science. Several nursing research centers, including the Institute of Research and Service in Nursing Education at Teachers College (1953), the American Nurses Foundation (1955), the Walter Reed Institute of Research (1957), and the National League for Nursing Research for Studies Service (1959), were established. The availability of funds from government and private foundations increased awards for nursing research grants and predoctoral fellowships.

Also during the 1950s, the focus of nursing research shifted from nursing education to issues such as the role of the nurse in the healthcare setting and characteristics of the ideal nurse. Early nursing theories described the nurse–patient relationship (Peplau, 1952) and categorized nursing activity according to human needs (Henderson, 1966). To accommodate the growth of nursing science, journals were needed to disseminate findings. In response, *Nursing Research* (1952) and *Nursing Outlook* (1953) were published, and the *Cumulative Index to Nursing Literature* (CINL) became more prominent.

The scholarly work done by nurses during the 1960s propelled nursing science to a new level. Nursing's major organizations began to call for a shift to research that focused on clinical problems and clinical outcomes. Nurse researchers began to develop grand nursing theories in an attempt to explain the relationships among nursing, health, persons, and environment (King, 1964, 1968; Levine, 1967; Orem, 1971; Rogers, 1963; Roy, 1971). As in the evolution of any science, nursing began to conduct research to test these theories. Because of the volume of nursing scholarship, new avenues for dissemination of information became necessary. Conferences for the sole purpose of exposing nurses to theory and research were organized. For example, in 1965 the American Nurses Association began to sponsor nursing research conferences. Worldwide dissemination became possible with the addition of international journals, such as the *International Journal of Nursing Research* (1963), thus increasing the interest in nursing research.

1970–1989

The hallmark of the 1970s and 1980s was the increased focus on the application of nursing research. The Lysaught Report (1970) confirmed that research focusing on clinical problems was essential but that research on nursing education was still indicated. It was recommended that findings from studies on nursing education be used to improve nursing curricula. During this era, the number of nurses with earned doctorates significantly increased as did the availability of funding for research fellowships. The scholarship generated by these doctoral-prepared nurses increased the demand for additional journals. Journals, such as *Advances in Nursing Science* (1978), *Research in Nursing and Health* (1978), and *Western Journal of Nursing Research* (1979), contained nursing research reports and articles about theoretical and practice issues of nursing. In 1977, CINL expanded its scope to include allied health journals, thus changing its name to the *Cumulative Index to Nursing and Allied Health Literature* (CINAHL), which allowed individuals in other disciplines to be exposed to nursing research.

On the national scene, the ethical implications of research involving human subjects were given much attention. In 1973, the first regulations to protect human subjects were proposed by the Department of Health, Education, and Welfare. The formation of institutional review boards to approve all studies was an important result of this regulation. Work regarding ethics in research continued throughout the decade with publication of the Belmont Report (1979). This report identified ethical principles that are foundational for the ethical treatment of individuals participating in studies funded by the federal government. Because the focus of nursing research on clinical problems involving patients was growing, nursing research was held to the same standards as other clinical research. Thus, the protection of human subjects became an important issue for nurse researchers.

Despite the abundance of research produced during the 1960s and 1970s, little change occurred in practice. Because nurses recognized a gap between research and practice, the emphasis in the 1980s was on closing this gap. The term *research utilization* was coined to describe the application of nursing research to practice. Activities to move nursing science forward included the Conduct and Utilization of Research in Nursing Project. Through this project, current research findings were disseminated to practicing nurses, organizational changes were facilitated, and collaborative clinical research was supported.

The social and political climate of the 1980s included a major change in the financing of health care with the introduction of diagnosis-related groups (DRGs). As a result, significant changes in the way health care was reimbursed occurred. Nurse researchers began to respond to the social and political demand for cost containment by conducting studies on the cost-effectiveness of nursing care. Another important social and political influence on nursing research was the establishment of the National Center for Nursing Research (NCNR) at the National Institutes of Health (NIH) in 1986. This was significant because nursing was awarded a place among other sciences, such as medicine, for guaranteed federal funding.

Activities that took place in the 1980s are consistent with the maturing of nursing as a science. As the body of knowledge grew, specialty organizations popped up enabling individuals to share their expertise in various clinical areas. In addition, the demand for journals in which to publish research continued, and *Applied Nursing Research* (1988), *Scholarly Inquiry for Nursing Practice* (1987), *Nursing Science Quarterly* (1988), and *Annual Review of Nursing Research* (1983) were started. In 1984, the CINAHL database became electronic. As nursing researchers became more sophisticated in the use of research methods, they embraced approaches new to nursing, such as qualitative methods. New theories (Benner, 1984; Leininger, 1985; Watson, 1979) that used caring as an important concept were especially amenable to emerging research methods.

1990–1999

In the 1990s, organizations began setting research agendas compatible with the social and political climate. For example, public concerns about the inequities of healthcare delivery were at the forefront. Priorities for nursing research included access to health care, issues of diversity, patient outcomes, and the goals of Healthy People 2000. Because nursing research was gaining respect for its contributions to patient care, opportunities for interdisciplinary research became available. In 1993, the NCNR was promoted to full institute status within NIH and was renamed the National Institute of Nursing Research. This was significant because the change in status afforded a larger budget that enabled more nurses to conduct federally funded research. Furthermore, with increased funding, nurse researchers designed more complex studies and began to build programs of research by engaging in a series of studies on a single topic.

The knowledge explosion created by technological advances vastly influenced nursing research. Electronic databases provided rapid access for retrieval of nursing literature, and in 1995, CINAHL became accessible to individuals over the Internet. Through email, nursing researchers were able to communicate quickly with colleagues. Software programs to organize and analyze data became readily available, allowing researchers to run more sophisticated analyses. Practice guidelines, from organizations such as the Centers for Disease Control and Prevention, were easily obtained on the Internet. The *Online Journal of Knowledge Synthesis for Nursing* (1993) was the first journal to take advantage of this technology by offering its content in an electronic format.

In previous eras, the focus was on the application of findings from a single study to nursing practice. In the early to mid-1990s, the emphasis was on research utilization. The Iowa model of nursing utilization (Titler et al., 1994) and the Stetler model for research utilization (Stetler, 1994) were introduced to facilitate the movement of findings from one research study into nursing practice. In the late 1990s, it became apparent that multiple sources of evidence were desirable for making practice changes. Thus, EBP gained popularity over research utilization, and these models were adapted to fit with the EBP movement (Stetler, 2003; Titler et al., 2001).

2000–2009

In the new millennium, nursing research continued to be influenced by social and political factors. Healthcare reform in the United States, although considered a political priority, remained elusive throughout the decade. Although the H.R. 3962—Affordable Health Care for America Act—was passed, significant changes had yet to be implemented.

Globalization became an important influential factor during this decade. With the ease of retrieving information came the ability to share research findings internationally. Nurses were able to access articles about research conducted in a variety of other countries. Nurses in other countries became more equipped to conduct research as well. Sigma Theta Tau International significantly broadened its membership to include more chapters in other countries. Globalization also raised new concerns that provided nurses with opportunities for research.

During this decade, a renewed focus centered on patient safety and outcomes. The American Nurses Association was instrumental in creating the National Database of Nursing Quality Indicators (NDNQI). The purpose of this database is to collect and evaluate unit-specific nurse-sensitive data from hospitals in the United States. Participating facilities receive unit-level comparative data reports to use for quality improvement purposes. Refer to **Box 1-2** for a listing of the current NDNQI measures. Many of these measures are used by hospitals that have received Magnet Recognition for nursing excellence.

BOX 1-2   **2016 NDNQI Measures**

Staffing and Workforce Indicators

Hospital Readmission Rates

Psychiatric Physical/Sexual Assault Rate

Catheter-Associated Urinary Tract Infection Rate

Central Line–Associated Bloodstream Infection Rate

Patient Falls

Pressure Injury Prevalence

Nurse Turnover

Pediatric Pain Assessment

Pediatric Peripheral IV Infiltration Rate

Restraint Prevalence

RN Education/Specialty Certification

RN Survey

    Practice Environment Scale
    Job Satisfaction

Ventilator-Associated Pneumonia Rate

Data from Press Ganey National Database of Nursing Quality Indicators® (2016). *Nursing-Sensitive Quality Indicators.* Personal communication from steven.pauley@pressganey.com.

Another significant accomplishment during this time was the mapping of human genes. Conducted by the Human Genome Project (HGP), an international research effort to sequence and map all of the genes—together known as the genome—was completed in 2003. As a result, knowledge about genetics was integrated into nursing education. Genetic-related research became a high priority for nursing and other health professions.

Another challenge faced in the new millennium was a nursing shortage. Topics such as nurse–patient ratios and interventions to decrease length of stay became priorities for research. Other changes occurred in nursing education. The use of technology for distance learning became more prominent as a way to educate nurses. Additionally, the Doctor of Nursing Practice (DNP) degree was recommended as the minimal educational requirement for those entering advanced practice nursing. Nursing programs across the country began to offer DNP degrees. Nurses who are prepared at the doctoral level and practice in clinical settings can serve as leaders in EBP.

2010 to the Present

Despite the growth in nursing research and the focus on evidence-based practice, improvement of patient outcomes is lagging. Evidence shows that hospitals are not meeting core benchmarks in these areas. In a study by Mylnek et al. (2016), a third of hospitals failed to meet NDNQI performance metrics. Additionally, oversight of the NDNQI shifted from the ANA to Press Ganey. This change is congruent with the stronger emphasis that is being placed on benchmarking, using national data and a trend toward withholding reimbursement to organizations that do not meet these critical indicators. For example, there have been reductions in Medicaid reimbursement to organizations that have patient satisfaction scores below a certain cutoff. This trend highlights the need for nursing research about new interventions that improve patient outcomes and strategies for translating these findings into practice.

Since 2010, the Affordable Care for America Act has been passed, and changes to this act are on the horizon. Thus, nurses will be able to glean potential research questions as healthcare policy evolves. For example, nurses can study the impact of even shorter hospital stays on readmission rates. As care moves away from hospitals to alternative settings, research will be needed to determine the effects of these changes on patient outcomes.

Globalization continues to be an important social factor in health care. For example, globalization contributes to an increasing threat of pandemic. Outbreaks of Ebola and Zika provide challenges that may be addressed through nursing research. Nurses are in an excellent position to study ways to effectively prevent the spread of diseases and to contribute to the implementation of strategies to care for infected populations.

CRITICAL THINKING EXERCISE 1-6

Ten years from now, nursing students will study how historical occurrences have shaped the evolution of nursing as a science. Discuss four current events that will be considered to have influenced the development of nursing science.

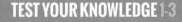

TEST YOUR KNOWLEDGE 1-3

True/False

1. Nursing research popular in the 1950s involved the study of nursing students.
2. Grand nursing theories were first introduced in the 1980s.
3. In the 1980s, DRGs were a driving force because they focused nursing research on cost-effectiveness.
4. Technological advances created a knowledge explosion that has vastly influenced nursing research.
5. Each historical era contributed to the development of nursing science.

How did you do? 1. T; 2. F; 3. T; 4. T; 5. T

The electronic medical record (EMR) is fast becoming standard in health care. Concerns about the protection of personal information are paramount. Additionally, linking EBP to EMRs will evolve. For example, when patient data are entered into the EMR, a message may appear suggesting practice guidelines based on the best evidence.

1.4 What Lies Ahead?

At the end of this section, you will be able to:

‹ Identify factors that will continue to move nursing forward as a science
‹ Discuss what future trends may influence how nurses use evidence to improve the quality of patient care

Factors similar to those that have propelled nursing research forward through history will continue to be influential into the future. In the 21st century, nursing research will grow in importance as EBP becomes more widely established and patient outcomes come under increased scrutiny. Nursing research agendas will continue to be driven by social and political influences.

The cycle of scientific development must continue in order to expand the body of nursing knowledge and to recognize nurses for their contributions to health care. Middle range and practice theories that are more useful in clinical settings need to be developed. Nursing research must include studies that replicate previous studies with different populations to confirm prior findings. Studies that demonstrate nursing's contribution to positive health outcomes will be especially important. A commitment to the continued preparation of nurses as scientists is vital to achieve excellence in nursing research. It will be increasingly important for nurses to advocate for monies and to draw on new funding sources. Interdisciplinary and international research will continue to be important as complex health problems are addressed. Technology will continue to offer new ways to communicate research findings to a broader audience, thereby improving diffusion of innovations. Research topics that are most likely to be priorities are listed in **Box 1-3**.

Nursing will continue to be challenged to bridge the gap between research and practice. EBP offers the greatest hope of moving research findings to the point of care. Nursing education must prepare nurses to appreciate the importance of basing patient care on evidence. Educators need to create innovative

---

BOX 1-3   Nursing Research Priorities

Bioterrorism

Chronic illness

Cultural and ethnic considerations

End-of-life/palliative care

Genetics

Gerontology

Healthcare delivery systems

Health disparities

Health promotion

HIV/AIDS

Management of pandemics/natural disasters

Mental health

Nursing informatics

Opioid epidemic

Patient outcomes/quality of care

Safe administration of medications

Symptom management

strategies that teach students to identify clinical problems, use technology to retrieve evidence, read and analyze research, weigh evidence, and implement change (Schmidt & Brown, 2007). Nurses must accept responsibility for creating their own EBP and collaborating with others to improve patient care.

Nurses who work in clinical settings and who are prepared at the doctoral level are especially well positioned to move EBP forward. Healthcare facilities are expected to embrace EBP to achieve Magnet Recognition. International collaborations, such as the Joanna Briggs Institute, are essential so that when best practices are identified they can easily be shared.

The Challenge

Make a commitment to be an innovator when it comes to EBP! You are already well on your way to having the knowledge and skills needed to overcome barriers that laggards often cite as reasons for not adopting EBP. As you study this text, don't go through the pages just to pass an exam. Learn the material so you can carry it with you throughout your career. To fulfill your commitment, with your next clinical assignment, adopt one or two of the strategies suggested in **Table 1-2**. Over the course of your career, your actions will convince laggards that EBP really does create excellence in patient care.

CRITICAL THINKING EXERCISE 1-7

Recall a question you encountered during your last clinical experience. How might you have answered that question using an EBP approach?

TEST YOUR KNOWLEDGE 1-4

1. How can nurses who use EBP best be described?
   a. As change agents
   b. As early adopters
   c. As innovators
   d. As laggards

True/False

2. As the cycle of science continues, more middle range and practice theories will emerge that will be useful in clinical settings.

How did you do? 1. b; 2. T

1.5 Keeping It Ethical

At the end of this section, you will be able to:

< Identify five unethical studies involving the violation of the rights of human subjects

Scientific research has made significant contributions to the good of society and the health of individuals, but these contributions have not come without cost. In the past, studies have been conducted without regard for the rights of human subjects. It is surprising to learn that even after national and international guidelines were established, unethical scientific research continued. Four major studies involved the violation of the rights of human subjects: (1) the Nazi experiments, (2) the Tuskegee study, (3) the Jewish Chronic Disease Hospital study, and (4) the Willowbrook studies. In addition, falsification and fabrication of data by the "Red Wine Researcher" provide another example of misconduct.

During World War II, physicians conducted medical studies on prisoners in Nazi concentration camps (NIH Office of Extramural Research, 2011). Most of the *Nazi experiments* were aimed at determining the limits of human endurance and learning ways to treat medical problems faced by the German armed forces. For example, physicians exposed prisoners of war to mustard gas, made them drink seawater, and exposed them to high-altitude experiments. People were frozen or nearly frozen to death so that physicians could study the body's response to hypothermia. The researchers infected prisoners with diseases so that they could follow the natural course of disease processes. Physicians also continued Hitler's genocide program by sterilizing Jewish, Polish, and Russian prisoners through X-ray and castration. The War Crimes Tribunal at Nuremberg indicted 23 physicians, many of whom were leading members of the German medical community. They were found guilty for their willing participation in conducting "crimes against humanity." Seven physicians were sentenced to death, and the remaining 16 were imprisoned. As a result, the *Nuremberg Code*, a section in the written verdict, outlined what constitutes acceptable medical research and forms the basis of international codes of ethical conduct. The experiments conducted were so horrific that debate continues about whether the findings from these Nazi studies, or other unethical studies, should be published or even used (Luna, 1997; McDonald, 1985; Miller & Rosenstein, 2002), and publishers must decide whether or not they will abide by guidelines outlined in the Declaration of Helsinki (Angelski, Fernandez, Weijer, & Gao, 2012).

In the 1930s, the *Tuskegee study* was initiated to examine the natural course of untreated syphilis (NIH Office of Extramural Research, 2011). In this study conducted by the U.S. Public Health Service, black men from Tuskegee,

KEY TERMS

Nazi experiments: An example of unethical research using human subjects during World War II

Nuremberg Code: Ethical code of conduct for research that uses human subjects

Tuskegee study: An unethical study about syphilis in which subjects were denied treatment so that the effects of the disease could be studied

Alabama, were recruited to participate. Informed consent was not obtained, and many of the volunteers were led to believe that procedures, such as spinal taps, were free special medical care. Three hundred ninety-nine men with syphilis were compared to 201 men who did not have syphilis. Within 6 years, it was apparent that many more of the infected men had complications compared with the uninfected men, and by 10 years, the death rate was twice as high in the infected men as compared with the uninfected men. Even when penicillin was found to be effective for the treatment of syphilis in the 1940s, the study continued until 1972, and subjects were neither informed about nor offered treatment with penicillin.

FYI

In the past, research was conducted with human subjects who were not fully informed of the purpose and/or methods of the study. Today, studies must be reviewed to ensure that human subjects are protected.

In 1963, the *Jewish Chronic Disease Hospital study* began and involved the injection of foreign, live cancer cells into hospitalized patients with chronic diseases (NIH Office of Extramural Research, 2011). The purpose of the study was to examine whether the body's inability to reject cancer cells was due to cancer or the presence of a debilitating chronic illness. Because earlier studies indicated that injected cancer cells were rejected, researchers hypothesized that debilitated patients would reject the cancer cells at a substantially slower rate than healthy participants did. When discussing the study with potential subjects, researchers failed to inform them about the injection of cancer cells because researchers did not want to frighten them. Although researchers obtained oral consent, they did not document the consent, claiming the documentation was unnecessary because it was a standard of care to perform much more dangerous procedures without consent forms. Researchers also failed to inform physicians caring for the patients about the study. At a review conducted by the Board of Regents of the State University of New York, researchers were found guilty of scientific misconduct, including fraud and deceit.

Also in the 1960s, a series of studies was conducted to observe the natural course of infectious hepatitis by deliberately infecting children admitted to the Willowbrook State School, an institution for children with mental disabilities (NIH Office of Extramural Research, 2011). During the *Willowbrook studies*, administrators claimed overcrowded conditions and stopped admitting patients; however, children could be admitted to the facility if they participated in the hepatitis program. Because at that time facilities to care for children with mental disabilities were few, many parents found they were unable to

KEY TERMS

Jewish Chronic Disease Hospital study: Unethical study involving injection of cancer cells into subjects without their consent

Willowbrook studies: An unethical study involving coercion of parents to allow their children to participate in the study in exchange for admission to a long-term care facility

CRITICAL THINKING EXERCISE 1-8

Do you think that the findings from unethical studies should be published? Why or why not?

obtain care for their children and fell victim to being coerced to allow their children to participate in the study.

Unfortunately, ethical violations are not a thing of the past. In 2008, a 3-year investigation was launched into claims of scientific misconduct at the University of Connecticut (Callaway, 2012). Dr. Das studied the beneficial health effects of red wine and other foods on cardiac health and longevity. He was found guilty of falsifying data on more than two dozen papers and grant applications. This type of behavior creates public distrust of research findings and can also inhibit researchers' ability to recruit subjects.

TEST YOUR KNOWLEDGE 1-5

Match the following.

1. Nazi medical experiments
2. Tuskegee study
3. Jewish Chronic Disease Hospital study
4. Willowbrook studies
5. "Red Wine Researcher"

a. Infected subjects with cancer cells
b. Coerced parents to allow children into study
c. Exposed subjects to cold
d. Falsified and fabricated data
e. Failed to treat subjects with penicillin

How did you do? 1. c; 2. e; 3. a; 4. b; 5. d

RAPID REVIEW

» EBP involves: (1) practice grounded in research evidence integrated with theory, (2) clinician expertise, and (3) patient preferences.

» Tradition, authority, trial and error, personal experiences, intuition, borrowed evidence, and scientific research are sources of evidence.

» Individual and organizational barriers can prevent adoption of EBP.

» Innovations are adopted by the diffusion of the innovation over time through communication channels among the members of a social system.

» Research is a planned and systematic activity that leads to new knowledge and/or the discovery of solutions to problems or questions.

» Scientific research offers the best evidence for nursing practice.

» Nurses use the evidence hierarchy to rank evidence from strongest to weakest.

» Research can be categorized as descriptive, explanatory, or predictive; basic or applied; and quantitative or qualitative.

» By analyzing words, qualitative research focuses on the meanings individuals give to their experiences. Quantitative research views the world as objective and focuses on obtaining precise measurements that are later analyzed.

» Most research articles include an abstract, introduction, review of literature, theoretical framework, and methods, results, and discussion sections, and they conclude with a list of references.

» The cycle of scientific development involves theory, research, dissemination, and application. Social and political factors are central to the cycle.

» The cycle of scientific development can be seen operating in each historical era.

» Social and political factors will continue to influence nursing research.

» For nurses to use EBP to improve patient care, they must be committed to being early adopters of innovations.

» NDNQI is a national database that involves measurement and reporting of nursing-sensitive outcomes.

» Four studies are recognized for their gross violation of human rights: Nazi medical experiments, the Tuskegee study, the Jewish Chronic Disease Hospital study, and the Willowbrook studies. A fifth study, known as the "red wine researcher," involved falsification or fabrication of data.

Apply What You Have Learned

Sign into a nursing database for nursing literature (i.e., CINAHL, Nursing and Allied Health Database, PubMed). For this chapter, you will need to obtain the following two articles:

» Chhapola, V., & Brar, R. (2015). Impact of an educational intervention on hand hygiene compliance and infection rate in a developing country neonatal intensive care unit. *International Journal of Nursing Practice, 21,* 486–492.

» Salmon, S., & McLaws, M. (2015). Qualitative findings from focus group discussion on hand hygiene compliance among healthcare workers in Vietnam. *American Journal of Infection Control, 43,* 1086–1091.

Identify the various sections of each of these articles. Look for similarities and differences between the quantitative and qualitative articles. After you have done that, you may want to share these articles with nurses during your next clinical experience and consider ways the recommendations can be incorporated into practice.

REFERENCES

Aitken, L. M., Hackwood, B., Crouch, S., Clayton, S., West, N., Carney, D., & Jack, L. (2011). Creating an environment to implement and sustain evidence based practice: A developmental process. *Australian Critical Care, 24*, 244–254.

American Nurses Association. (2010). National Database of Nursing Quality Indicators: Guidelines for data collection on the American Nurses Association's National Quality Forum endorsed measures: Nursing Care Hours per Patient Day, Skill Mix, Falls, Falls with Injury. Retrieved from http://www.k-hen.com/Portals/16/Topics/Falls/ANAsNQFspecs.pdf

Angelski, C., Fernandez, C. V., Weijer, C., & Gao, J. (2012). The publication of ethically uncertain research: Attitudes and practices of journal editors. *BMC Medical Ethics, 13*(4), 1–6.

Barnsteiner, J., & Prevost, S. (2002). How to implement evidence-based practice. Some tried and true pointers. *Reflections on Nursing Leadership, 28*(2), 18–21.

Benner, P. (1984). *From novice to expert: Excellence and power in clinical nursing practice.* Menlo Park, CA: Addison-Wesley.

Callaway, E. (2012). Red-Wine Researcher implicated in data misconduct case. *Scientific American.* Retrieved from http://www.scientificamerican.com/article/red-wine-researcher-implicated-misconduct/

Carson, M. M., Barton, D. M., Morrison, L. G., & Tribble, C. G. (1994). Managing pain during mediastinal chest tube removal. *Heart & Lung, 23*, 500–505.

Cochrane, A. L. (1971). *Effectiveness and efficiency. Random reflections on health services.* Abingdon, Berks, United Kingdom: Nuffield Provincial Hospitals Trust.

Cochrane Collaboration. (2017). About us. Retrieved 6/22/17 from http://www.cochrane.org/about-us/our-vision-mission-and-principles

Dedui, H. (2012). When will smartphones reach saturation in the United States? Retrieved from http://www.asymco.com/2012/04/11/when-will-smartphones-reach-saturation-in-the-us/

Demir, Y., & Khorsbid, L. (2010). The effect of cold application in combination with standard analgesic administration on pain and anxiety during chest tube removal: A single blinded, randomized, double-controlled study. *Pain Management Nursing, 22*(3), 186–196.

Ertuğ, N., & Ülker, S. (2011). The effect of cold application on pain due to chest tube removal. *Journal of Clinical Nursing, 21*, 784–790.

Fitzsimons, E., & Cooper, J. (2012). Embedding a culture of evidence-based practice. *Nursing Management, 19*(7), 14–19.

Flanagan, J. M., Carroll, D. L., & Hamilton, G. A. (2010). The long-term lived experience of patients with implantable cardioverter defibrillators. *MEDSURG Nursing, 19*, 113–119.

Friesner, S. A., Curry, D. M., & Moddeman, G. R. (2006). Comparison of two pain-management strategies during chest tube removal: Relaxation exercise with opioids and opioids alone. *Heart & Lung, 35*(4), 269–276.

Gift, A. G., Bolgiano, C. S., & Cunningham, J. (1991). Sensations during chest tube removal. *Heart & Lung, 20*, 131–137.

Hauck, S., Winsett, R. P., & Kuric, J. (2013). Leadership facilitation strategies to establish evidence-based practice in an acute care hospital. *Journal of Advanced Nursing, 69*(3), 664–674.

Henderson, V. (1966). *The nature of nursing*. New York, NY: Macmillan.

Houston, S., & Jesurum, J. (1999). The quick relaxation technique: Effect on pain associated with chest tube removal. *Applied Nursing Research, 12*, 196–205.

IA Users Club, Inc. (2015). *FunkAndWagnalls.com*. Retrieved 6/22/17 from http://www.funkandwagnalls.com/?search=intuition

Ingersoll, G. L. (2000). Evidence-based nursing: What it is and what it isn't. *Nursing Outlook, 48*, 151–152.

King, I. M. (1964). Nursing theory: Problems and prospects. *Nursing Science, 1*, 394–403.

King, I. M. (1968). A conceptual frame of reference for nursing. *Nursing Research, 17*(1), 27–31.

Leininger, M. (1985). Transcultural care diversity and universality: A theory of nursing. *Nursing and Health Care, 6*, 209–212.

L'Esperance, S. T., & Perry, D. J. (2016). Assessing advantages and barriers to telemedicine adoption in the practice setting: A MyCare Team[TM] exemplar. *Journal of the American Association of Nursing Practitioners, 28*, 311–319.

Levin, R. F., Fineout-Overholt, E., Melnyk, B. M., Barnes, M., & Vetter, M. J. (2011). Fostering evidence-based practice to improve nurse and cost outcomes in a community health setting: A pilot test of the advancing research and clinical practice through close collaboration model. *Nursing Administration Quarterly, 35*(1), 21–33.

Levine, M. E. (1967). The four conservation principles of nursing. *Nursing Forum, 6*, 45–59.

Luna, F. (1997). Vulnerable populations and morally tainted experiments. *Bioethics, 11*, 256–264.

Majid, S., Foo, S., Luyt, B., Xue, Z., Yin-Leng, T., Yun-Ke, C., & Mokhtar, I. A. (2011). Adopting evidence-based practice in clinical decision making: Nurses' perceptions, knowledge and barriers. *Journal of the Medical Library Association, 99*(3), 229–236.

Malik, G., McKenna, L., & Plummer, V. (2016). Facilitators and barriers to evidence-based practice: Perceptions of nurse educators, clinical coaches and nurse specialists from a descriptive study. *Contemporary Nurse, 52*, 544–554.

McDonald, A. (1985). Ethics and editors: When should unethical research be published? *Canadian Medical Association Journal, 133*, 803–805.

Melnyk, B. M. (1999). Building a case for evidence-based practice: Inhalers vs. nebulizers. *Pediatric Nursing, 25*(1), 102–104.

Melnyk, B. M., & Fineout-Overholt, E. (2015). Making the case for evidence-based practice. In B. M. Melnyk & E. Fineout-Overholt (Eds.), *Evidence-based practice in nursing and healthcare: A guide to best practice* (3rd ed.) (pp. 3–23). Philadelphia, PA: Lippincott Williams & Wilkins.

Melnyk, B. M., Fineout-Overholt, E., Gallagher-Ford, L., & Kaplan, L. (2012). The state of evidence-based practice in U.S. nurses: Critical implications for nurse leaders and education. *Journal of Nursing Administration, 42*(9), 410–417.

Melnyk, B. M., Fineout-Overholt, E., Giggleman, M., & Cruz, R. (2010). Correlates among cognitive beliefs, EBP implementation, organizational culture, cohesion and job satisfaction in evidence-based practice mentors from a community hospital system. *Nursing Outlook, 58*(6), 301–308.

Melnyk, B. M., Gallagher-Ford, L., Thomas, B. K., Troseth, M., Wyngarden, K., & Szalacha, L. (2016). A study of chief nurse executives indicates low prioritization of evidence-based practice and shortcomings in hospital performance metrics across the United States. *Worldviews on Evidence-Based Nursing, 13*(1), 6–14.

Miller, F. G., & Rosenstein, D. L. (2002). Reporting of ethical issues in publications of medical research. *The Lancet, 360*, 1326–1328.

Nightingale, F. (1946). *Notes on nursing: What it is, and what it is not.* London, England: Harrison. (Original work published 1859)

NIH Office of Extramural Research. (2011). *Protecting human research participants.* Retrieved from http://phrp.nihtraining.com/users/PHRP.pdf

Ogiehor-Enoma, G., Taqueban, L., & Anosike, A. (2010). 6 steps for transforming organizational EBP culture. *Nursing Management, 41*(5), 14–17.

Orem, D. E. (1971). *Nursing: Concepts of practice.* New York, NY: McGraw-Hill.

Paris, W., Callahan, M. B., & Pierson, M. (2011). Academic and clinical research collaboration: Part 3: Challenges for the clinician and researcher . . . third in a series of four articles. *Nephrology News & Issues, 25*(1), 31–33.

Pennington, K., Moscatel, S., Dacar, S., & Johnson, C. (2010). EBP partnerships: Building bridges between education and practice. *Nursing Management, 41*(4), 19–21.

Peplau, H. E. (1952). *Interpersonal relations in nursing: A conceptual frame of reference for psychodynamic nursing.* New York, NY: Putnam.

Pinheiro, V. F. O., Costa, J. M. V., Cascudo, M. M., Pinheiro, E. Q., Fernandez, M. A. F., & Araujo, I. B. (2015). Analgesic efficacy of lidocaine and multimodal analgesia for chest tube removal: A randomized trial study. *Revista Latino-Americana de Enfermagem, 23*(6), 1000–1006.

Pipe, T. B., Kelly, A., LeBrun, G., Schmidt, D., Atherton, P., & Robinson, C. (2008). A prospective descriptive study exploring hope, spiritual well-being, and quality of life in hospitalized patients. *MEDSURG Nursing, 17*, 247–257.

Polit, D. F., & Beck, C. T. (2016). *Nursing research: Generating and assessing evidence for nursing practice* (10th ed.). Philadelphia, PA: Lippincott Williams & Wilkins.

Pravikoff, D. S., Tanner, A. B., & Pierce, S. T. (2005). Readiness of U.S. nurses for evidence-based practice. *American Journal of Nursing, 105*(9), 40–51.

Puntillo, K. A. (1994). Dimensions of procedural pain and its analgesic management in critically ill surgical patients. *American Journal of Critical Care, 3*, 116–122.

Puntillo, K. A. (1996). Effects of interpleural bupivacaine on pleural chest tube removal pain: A randomized control trial. *American Journal of Critical Care, 5*, 102–108.

Puntillo, K., & Ley, S. J. (2004). Appropriately timed analgesics: Control pain due to chest tube removal. *American Journal of Critical Care, 13*, 292–301.

Reicherter, E. A., Gordes, K. L., Glickman, L. B., & Hakim, E. W. (2013). Creating disseminator champions for evidence-based practice in health professions education: An educational case report. *Nurse Education Today, 33*, 751–756.

Rogers, E. M. (2003). *Diffusion of innovations* (5th ed.). New York, NY: Free Press.

Rogers, M. E. (1963). Some comments on the theoretical basis of nursing practice. *Nursing Science, 1*(1), 11–13, 60–61.

Roy, C. (1971). Adaptation: A basis for nursing practice. *Nursing Outlook, 19*, 254–257.

Sackett, D. L., Rosenberg, W. M. C., Gray, J. A. M., Haynes, R. B., & Richardson, W. S. (1996). Evidence based medicine: What it is and what it isn't. *British Medical Journal, 312*, 71–72.

Schifalacqua, M. M., Mamula, J., & Mason, R. (2011). Return on investment imperative: The cost of care calculator for an evidence-based practice program. *Nursing Administration Quarterly, 35*(1), 15–20.

Schmidt, N. A., & Brown, J. M. (2007). Use of the innovation-decision process teaching strategy to promote evidence based practice. *Journal of Professional Nursing, 23*, 150–156.

Shivnan, J. C. (2011). How do you support your staff? Promote EBP. *Nursing Management, 42*(2), 12–14.

Solomons, N. M., & Spross, J. A. (2011). Evidence-based practice barriers and facilitators from a continuous quality improvement perspective: An integrative review. *Journal of Nursing Management, 19*, 109–120.

Spieres, J. A., Lo, E., Hofmeyer, A., & Cummings, G. G. (2016). Nurse leaders' perceptions of influence of organizational restructuring on evidence-informed decision-making. *Nursing Research, 29*, 64–81.

Stetler, C. B. (1994). Refinement of the Stetler/Marram model for application of research findings to practice. *Nursing Outlook, 42*, 15–25.

Stetler, C. B. (2003). Role of the organization in translating research into evidence-based practice. *Outcomes Management, 7*, 97–105.

Stevens, K. R. (2012). Star model of EBP: Knowledge transformation. Academic Center for Evidence-Based Practice. Retrieved from http://www.acestar.uthscsa.edu /acestar-model.asp

Straus, S. E., Glasziou, P., Richardson, W. S., & Haynes, R. B. (2011). *Evidence-based medicine. How to practice and teach EBM* (4th ed.). Edinburgh, Scotland: Churchill Livingstone.

Titler, M. G., Kleiber, C., Steelman, V., Goode, C., Rakel, B., Barry-Walker, J., . . . Buckwalter, K. (1994). Infusing research into practice to promote quality care. *Nursing Research, 43*, 307–313.

Titler, M. G., Kleiber, C., Steelman, V. J., Rakel, B. A., Budreau, G., Everett, L. Q., . . . Goode, C. J. (2001). The Iowa model of evidence-based practice to promote quality care. *Critical Care Nursing Clinics of North America, 13*, 497–509.

Valente, S. M. (2010). Three practical approaches to EBP. *Nursing Management, 41*(3), 10–13.

Van Patter Gale, B., & Schaffer, M. A. (2009). Organizational readiness for evidence-based practice. *Journal of Nursing Administration, 39*(2), 91–97.

Warren, J. I., McLaughlin, M., Bardsley, J., Eich, J., Esche, C. A., Kropkowski, L., & Risch, S. (2016). The strengths and challenges of implementing EBP in healthcare systems. *Worldviews on Evidence-Based Nursing, 13*(1), 15–24.

Watson, J. (1979). Nursing: The philosophy and science of caring. Boston, MA: Little, Brown.

White-Williams, C., Patrician, P., Fazeli, P., Degges, M. A., Graham, S., Andison, M., . . . McCaleb, K. A. (2013). Use, knowledge, and attitudes toward evidence-based practice among nursing staff. *Journal of Continuing Education in Nursing, 44*(6), 246–254.

At the end of this chapter, you will be able to:

- Discuss contributions to evidence-based practice (EBP) that nurses practicing in various roles have made
- Examine organizational strategies that facilitate EBP
- Describe regional resources that foster collaborative EBP
- Identify national resources committed to EBP
- List international organizations that are committed to the promotion of EBP
- Discuss international and national initiatives designed to promote ethical conduct
- Describe the rights that must be protected and the three ethical principles that must be upheld when conducting research
- Explain the composition and functions of institutional review boards (IRBs) at the organizational level
- Discuss the nurse's role as patient advocate in research situations

KEY TERMS

autonomous
Belmont Report
beneficence
Declaration of Helsinki
exempt
expedited review
full review
human rights
individual nurse level

informed consent
institutional review
  boards
international level
justice
minimal risk
model of EBP levels
  of collaboration
national level

obligations
organizational level
regional level
research imperative
respect for persons
therapeutic imperative
translational research
  model

CHAPTER 2

Using Evidence Through Collaboration to Promote Excellence in Nursing Practice

Emily Griffin and Marita G. Titler

2.1 The Five Levels of Collaboration

At the end of this section, you will be able to:

‹ Discuss contributions to EBP that nurses practicing in various roles have made
‹ Examine organizational strategies that facilitate EBP
‹ Describe regional resources that foster collaborative EBP
‹ Identify national resources committed to EBP
‹ List international organizations that are committed to the promotion of EBP

In the late 1800s, Florence Nightingale followed many of the principles of evidence-based practice (EBP). Principles of EBP have been present for many years; however, until recently this process was not called EBP, nor was EBP fully acknowledged as having an important impact on patient care. Development of a culture of EBP is underway in nursing through collaborative efforts by nurses and healthcare organizations, as well as by regional, national, and international entities. Collaboration is critical for success with EBP, and **Figure 2-1** illustrates the *model of EBP levels of collaboration*. Nurses need to understand how they can maximize their collaborative efforts at all five levels.

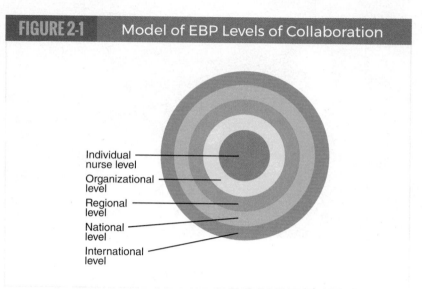

FIGURE 2-1 Model of EBP Levels of Collaboration

Individual nurse level
Organizational level
Regional level
National level
International level

FYI

A culture of EBP has emerged in nursing through collaborative efforts by nurses and healthcare organizations, as well as by regional, national, and international entities. Nurses need to collaborate at these five levels.

In the model, the five levels are intertwined with one another. An international entity can be a resource for staff nurses, and nurses can reciprocate and contribute to EBP nationally and internationally. Nurses or organizations may use regional-level resources to help move EBP projects forward. In return, nurses or organizations assist regional or national resources to advance EBP. For example, a staff nurse may use the Joanna Briggs Institute to find evidence to support an EBP project. When the project is complete, the staff nurse disseminates her work by publishing the project and presenting at an annual Sigma Theta Tau International (STTI) EBP conference. At the conference, the nurse educates other nurses so that best practices can be adopted at their organizations.

KEY TERMS

model of EBP levels of collaboration: A model explaining how five levels are intertwined to contribute to EBP

individual nurse level: Practice changes that can be implemented by an individual nurse

Individual Nurse Level

At the *individual nurse level*, nurses play an integral role in advancing EBP. Although it takes a team approach to be successful with EBP, each nurse has a unique set of skills to contribute that helps to advance EBP. Identifying clinical issues, education approaches, and implementation strategies is an example of contributions that nurses can make to the team. Nurses can assume various roles for the team, such as project leader, opinion leader, and mentor.

Staff nurses are an important link between research and the point of care. They are clinical experts and know how to access unit resources. Staff nurses can contribute by problem solving, collaborating with the team, and acting as change champions. Essential for implementation, staff nurses are often the adopters of the EBP change. They can be designated as group leaders to help with planning and troubleshooting during the implementation phase (Cullen & Adams, 2012).

Because staff nurses are integral to EBP, many organizations provide performance criteria for promoting best practices. For example, performance criteria for staff nurses may include critical thinking, continual questioning of practice, participating in making EBP practice changes, serving as leaders of change in their site of care delivery, and participating in evaluating evidence-based changes in practice (Titler, 2014; see **Box 2-1**).

Nurse managers are also essential to EBP. Their aim is to "get their units on board" with practice changes. They help to set unit expectations by discussing projects with staff and other healthcare providers. Managers facilitate progress by rewarding nurses involved in EBP and assisting noncompliant nurses to improve their performances. The commitment of nurse managers makes a significant impact on patient outcomes and is crucial to the success of EBP projects (Cullen, Dawson, Hanrahan, & Dole, 2014).

Advanced practice nurses (APNs) are EBP experts who facilitate appraisal and synthesis of the literature for the purpose of improving nursing practice. They often are mentors and are thus important to the advancement of EBP in the clinical setting (Shirey, 2006). They help with problem solving, planning, leading, and coaching. As clinical experts, APNs are ideally positioned to be opinion leaders and change champions. Opinion leaders are experts in their fields who facilitate adoption of an innovation through modeling and peer influence. Their sphere of influence is broad, usually encompassing several units or departments (Doumit, Gattellari, Grimshaw, & O'Brien, 2007). Change champions are also experts in their fields and facilitate change through persistence. They often work with a core group of nurses who are also working toward making EBP changes. To promote consistent practice changes, this core group of nurses should include nurses across different shifts.

Nurse executives are responsible for establishing the culture for EBP. They create a culture in which making evidence-based decisions and changing practice are valued. It is important for nursing leaders to create a vision that includes EBP and to identify methods to sustain this vision. This can include celebrating successes or providing individual recognition during public forums (Cullen & Adams, 2012). Shirey (2006) states that nurse leaders are expected to work to maximize the capabilities of the staff and to partner with key professional organizations with goals to advance EBP.

FYI

APNs are ideally positioned to be opinion leaders and change champions. To promote and facilitate consistent practice changes, this core group of nurses should include nurses across different shifts.

BOX 2-1   Sample EBP Performance Criteria for Nursing Roles

Staff Nurse (RN)

» Questions current practices
» Participates in implementing changes in practice based on evidence
» Participates as a member of an EBP project team
» Reads evidence related to practice
» Participates in quality improvement (QI) initiatives
» Suggests resolutions for clinical issues based on evidence

Nurse Manager (NM)

» Creates a microsystem that fosters critical thinking
» Challenges staff to seek out evidence to resolve clinical issues and improve care
» Role models EBP
» Uses evidence to guide operations and management decisions
» Uses performance criteria about EBP in evaluation of staff

Advanced Practice Nurse (APN)

» Serves as coach and mentor in EBP
» Facilitates locating evidence
» Synthesizes evidence for practice
» Uses evidence to write/modify practice standards
» Role models use of evidence in practice
» Facilitates system changes to support use of EBP

Nurse Executive

» Ensures that governance reflects EBP if initiated in councils and committees
» Assigns accountability for EBP
» Ensures explicit articulation of organizational and department commitment to EBP
» Modifies mission and vision to include EBP language
» Provides resources to support EBP by direct care providers
» Articulates value of EBP to chief executive officer and governing board
» Role models EBP in administrative decision making
» Hires and retains NMs and APNs with knowledge and skills in EBP
» Provides learning environment for EBP
» Uses evidence in leadership decisions

Data from Titler, M. (2014). Developing an evidence-based practice. In G. LoBiondo-Wood & J. Haber (Eds.), *Nursing research: Methods and critical appraisal for evidence-based practice* (8th ed., pp. 418–440). St. Louis, MO: Mosby Elsevier.

Table 2-1 provides examples of performance criteria that may be expected at the individual nurse level (Titler, 2014). It is important to remember that each nurse is part of a team that is moving EBP forward. Specific advantages of teamwork include division of workload, comprehensive problem solving, building "buy-in," and expanding expertise. Overall, teamwork builds a more comprehensive plan for EBP.

Organizational Level

National initiatives and accrediting bodies support EBP and urge healthcare systems to base patient care on evidence. At the *organizational level*, healthcare systems are finding increased interest from nurses who want to practice from a research base, need time to explore EBP, and desire to develop excellence in the profession. "The goal of achieving excellence requires development of an organizational capacity, culture, and vision for evidence-based practice" (Cullen, Greiner, Greiner, Bombei, & Comried, 2005, p. 127).

Healthcare organizations with a vision of providing excellence in nursing need an infrastructure that accommodates EBP. As organizations restructure to focus on EBP, they embrace a culture of EBP. This culture sets a tone so that nurses know what is valued within the organization. One method for developing this culture is adding value statements about EBP to organizational mission or vision statements. For example, at the University of Iowa (UI) Hospitals and Clinics, the mission statement is "provide safe high-quality patient care based on a strong commitment to clinical expertise, education, evidence-based practice, research, shared governance, leadership and collaboration with multidisciplinary team members" (UI Hospitals and Clinics, 2013). This statement outlines expectations for nursing care at this organization.

Other factors that build a culture for EBP include setting performance expectations for individual nurses, integrating EBP into governance structures, and providing recognition and rewards for involvement in EBP. To help build organizational capacity for EBP, it is recommended that responsibility be designated to at least one committee (Cullen et al., 2005). One recommendation is to create four committees: an EBP steering committee, an EBP committee, a specialty focus team, and a nursing policy and procedure committee. The EBP steering committee oversees the other three committees, allocates the resources, and provides support and direction for the work involved with adopting EBP (Hudson, 2005).

At the organizational level, the focus is not only on developing a capacity for EBP to take place but also on facilitating the adoption of individual EBP protocols. As social systems, organizations can facilitate or impede change. The *translational research model* (**Figure 2-2**), which is based on Rogers's model of diffusion of innovations (Rogers, 2003), provides specific strategies that organizations can use to improve adoption of an evidence-based innovation (Titler, 2014; Titler & Everett, 2001). Components of this model

> **FYI**
>
> Librarians are important resources for EBP, making them critical partners. They are experts in searching databases, such as the *Cumulative Index to Nursing and Allied Health Literature* (CINAHL) and PubMed, and many healthcare librarians specialize in searching for evidence in nursing and medicine.

> **KEY TERMS**
>
> **organizational level:** When nurses in an organization effect practice changes
>
> **translational research model:** A model that provides specific strategies organizations can use to improve adoption of an evidence-based innovation

FIGURE 2-2   Translational Research Model

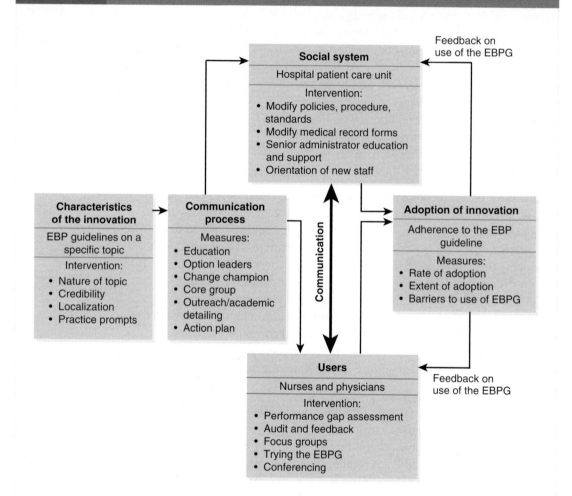

Titler, M. G., & Everett, L. Q. (2001). Translating research into practice: Considerations for clinical care investigators. *Critical Care Nursing Clinics of North America, 13*(4), 587–604. Reproduced with permission from Maria G. Titler, PhD, RN, FAAN; for permission to use and/or reproduce the model, please contact Dr. Titler.

describe how characteristics of the innovation, communication process, social system, and users lead to the adoption of innovations. Organizational characteristics that influence the use of EBP include expectations that policies are evidence-based, access to clinical researchers, authority to change practice, and support from peers, administrators, and other disciplines (Titler & Everett, 2001).

As social systems, organizations can use four specific interventions described in this model to promote excellence in nursing and move EBP forward. These interventions include modifying policies and standards, modifying medical record forms, ensuring senior administrators are educated and provide support, and orienting new staff members.

The first intervention is for organizations to include EBP within policies and standards (Titler & Everett, 2001). Policies should be based on evidence. For example, the UI Hospitals and Clinics developed a schema for rating the type of evidence for each statement within a policy. To indicate the type of evidence available, each statement is assigned an R, N, E, or L, which stands for research article, national guideline, expert opinion, or literature review, respectively. At the end of the policy, full citations are provided for each piece of evidence cited in the policy. Staff nurses, nurse managers, and APNs serve on committees to develop policies and procedures and collaborate to see them implemented.

Modifying medical record forms or electronic documentation, the second intervention, is an excellent way to help integrate evidence into care (Titler & Everett, 2001). Reassessment of pain after an intervention is an example of a recommended best practice that practitioners might not always follow. As a way to increase compliance with this standard of care, a medical record form or electronic documentation field could be modified to include a place for nurses to document pain reassessment. Similarly, a clinical reminder can be set up within some computerized documentation systems to prompt nurses to reassess patient pain levels.

The third intervention recommended involves supporting education of senior administrators (Titler & Everett, 2001). It is important for leaders to receive frequent updates on EBP activities within the organization. Updates could be given through email or as a narrative summary or through rounds with a project team. It is essential for senior administrators to develop the vision and the organizational culture, and they need to be kept up-to-date with changes that are being made. Keeping nurse leaders updated enhances the EBP culture while keeping the organization accountable.

The fourth intervention that a social system can implement involves orienting new staff and travel staff (Titler & Everett, 2001). The orientation should send a message that EBP is valued at the organization. New staff members should be made aware of how policies and standards are developed in the organization so they can participate in the process.

It is imperative to find a model that is clear to those using the model and that matches the organization's values. Many models continue to be developed and adapted to fit an organization. For example, Schaffer, Sandau, and Diedrick

(2013) reviewed several models, such as the ACE Star Model of Knowledge Transformation and the Iowa Model of EBP, that can be used within an organization to facilitate EBP.

Regional Level

At the *regional level*, collaboration is very important for the advancement of EBP. Using the skills of a local librarian, collaborating with a local program of nursing, and using resources from regional centers of excellence are examples of using regional collaboration.

It is critical for nurses to partner with a local librarian when trying to find evidence. Many healthcare librarians specialize in searching for evidence in nursing and medicine. Librarians are an important resource for EBP because they are experts in searching databases, such as CINAHL, PubMed, and Ovid (DiCenso, 2003). At the University of Iowa, the health sciences library has a program called "housecalls" in which librarians call on individual researchers in their offices to facilitate a literature search.

Programs of nursing are another regional resource available for collaboration. The expertise of faculty can help nurses find, synthesize, and appraise the evidence. Some hospital systems match staff nurses with students or professors to appraise literature. Nursing professors can join organizational committees such as research committees, evidence-based planning committees, or quality outcomes committees.

Quality improvement committees or programs provide another opportunity for collaboration. These committees might be groups from within or outside the hospital setting. For instance, a unit-based committee might be formed to address infection rates. Examples of groups operating outside the hospital setting are a workgroup for fall prevention and a childhood obesity task force. Communities continue to develop and expand these types of workgroups, which often include nurses, public health employees, community members, parents, and other involved individuals. Okihiro, Pillen, Ancog, Inda, and Sehgal (2013) reported about a community collaborative project to improve childhood obesity. They used the chronic care model and its adaptation, the obesity care model, to guide the collaboration among primary healthcare, community-based, and public health approaches to support self-management. Evidence-based strategies included changing clinic personnel to include a dietician and pediatric clinical

KEY TERM

regional level: When nurses from a large geographic area collaborate to change practice

CRITICAL THINKING EXERCISE 2-1

Consider the facilities where you have been for clinical experiences. Which facilities appear to have embraced EBP? Why do you think that is the case? How are individual nurses involved?

| TABLE 2-1 | Regional Resource Centers of Excellence |

Regional Resource Center	Region	Website
University of North Carolina at Chapel Hill	Eastern	http://www.shepscenter.unc.edu/programs-projects/evidence-based-practice-center/
Arizona State University at Tempe	Western	http://libguides.asu.edu/health/HealthEBP
University of Iowa Hospitals and Clinics at Iowa City	Midwestern	http://www.nursing.uiowa.edu/excellence/evidence-based-practice-guidelines
University of Texas at San Antonio	Southern	http://www.acestar.uthscsa.edu/acestar-model.asp

psychologist. The dietician met with children during their wellness visits. The authors also aligned the electronic medical record with obesity management best practice guidelines. The Department of Pediatrics and university provided research resources, infrastructure for training, and salary support. This EBP project shows how regional resources can be maximized to improve patient outcomes.

Shirey (2006) identified four EBP regional resource centers of excellence (see **Table 2-1**). These regional centers provide resources for nurses and organizations incorporating best practices. Resources include toolkits, intensive training programs, conferences, and specific guidelines that are available for purchase. Most of these centers of excellence provide experts who are available by phone and email to answer questions and guide nurses and organizations through the EBP process.

National Level

On the *national level*, several entities have made considerable contributions to nursing research and EBP. The Agency for Healthcare Research and Quality (AHRQ; http://www.ahrq.gov) launched an initiative in 1997 to establish EBP centers around the United States. These centers review scientific literature about specific topics and publish technology assessments and evidence reports. The National Guideline Clearinghouse (NGC) is another initiative of AHRQ that maintains a comprehensive database of EBP guidelines. The NGC website (http://www.guideline.gov/) provides abstracts of practice guidelines and access to full-text publications. The National Institute of Nursing Research (NINR) has also significantly contributed to the development of nursing research.

KEY TERM

national level: Collaboration among nurses throughout the country to effect practice changes

NINR is a federal agency that allocates funds for clinical and basic research and research training (NINR, n.d.). Funded areas of research are based on social and political factors involving health and illness across the life span. Nursing research generated as a result of NINR funding is disseminated for the purpose of improving patient outcomes.

Specialty nursing societies, such as the Oncology Nursing Society (ONS) and Association of Women's Health, Obstetric and Neonatal Nurses (AWHONN), are other examples of national organizations that facilitate the generation, dissemination, and use of new knowledge. ONS has an EBP area on its website (https://www.ons.org/practice-resources/pep) that provides information for starting an EBP project, topic reviews, and a toolkit with more resources. AWHONN regularly publishes EBP guidelines in its journal and on the website (http://www.awhonn.org/). The American Society of PeriAnesthesia Nurses provides position statements, standards of care, and forums in which to post questions and discussions to encourage collaboration (see http://www.aspan.org/).

The National Nursing Practice Network (NNPN; http://www.nnpnetwork.org) is committed to the promotion and implementation of EBP through a collaborative model designed to encourage shared learning and participation. The mission of the NNPN is to foster exceptional healthcare outcomes, advance professional nursing practice through application of evidence, support nursing leadership development for EBP, and increase understanding of mechanisms and strategies that foster the use of evidence. The vision of the NNPN is to be a national exemplar of nursing practice excellence, innovation, translation science, and promotion of EBP.

The American Nurses Credentialing Center (ANCC) has developed the Magnet Recognition Program to recognize healthcare organizations that provide nursing excellence. This program includes 14 forces of magnetism that are criteria for organizations to become nationally recognized as Magnet Recognition Program healthcare facilities. Initiatives involving nursing research and EBP must be present to earn Magnet Recognition. For example, the organization must be able to demonstrate a culture that embraces EBP and nursing research. Structures and processes such as committees, resources, and release time for research endeavors must be evident. Nurses in direct care are expected to be involved in EBP, quality assurance, and nursing research. This national recognition has increased awareness about the importance of EBP at the individual nurse and organizational levels (ANCC, 2013).

National associations, such as the American Heart Association (AHA) and the American Diabetes Association (ADA), continue to expand to provide patients and healthcare professionals with evidence-based guidelines and clinic practice recommendations. Many of these associations or foundations have a disease-specific focus. Other examples of national associations or foundations include the Crohn's and Colitis Foundation of America, the American Lung Association, and the Asthma and Allergy Foundation.

Healthcare professionals can also find national evidence-based point-of-care resources such as DynaMed and UpToDate. A part of EBSCO, DynaMed (http://www.dynamed.com/home/about) is a company that provides the CINAHL database, which offers clinical references for nurses, physicians, pharmacists, physical therapists, and other healthcare professionals. UpToDate (http://www.uptodate.com/home/about-us), a Wolters Kluwer Health product, also provides point-of-care solutions for the healthcare industry. The Institute of Medicine brief report discusses the importance of decision support and point-of-care tools (Smith, Saunders, Stuckhardt, & McGinnis, 2012). The authors of the report suggest that these tools be developed, accessible, and evidence-based through research organizations, advocacy organizations, and professional specialty societies, as well as emphasized within education programs. National collaboration continues to expand, and nurses can use these evidence-based recommendations at the point of care.

International Level

Efforts to enhance EBP are also conducted at the *international level*. Dr. Archie Cochrane (1971) criticized the medical profession for not providing systematic reviews of evidence from existing studies. In response to this criticism, the Cochrane Center was established 20 years later in Oxford, England. One year after that, the Cochrane Collaboration was established. This international not-for-profit organization is dedicated to making up-to-date, accurate healthcare information available worldwide (see http://www.cochrane.org). The purpose of this establishment is to offer healthcare providers current systematic reviews of medical interventions and treatments. These summary reports are essential because mass media and the Internet provide an abundance of information, making it difficult for practitioners to stay current.

Sigma Theta Tau International (STTI) is a leader in the development and dissemination of knowledge to improve nursing practice (see http://www.nursingsociety.org). This organization has published a position statement on evidence-based nursing and strives to provide nurses with the most current comprehensive resources to assist them with translating evidence into nursing research, education, administration, policy, and practice. STTI presents awards to honor nurses who have demonstrated excellence in research and EBP. For example, the Founder's Award is given for excellence in research. Several specific research awards for research dissemination in nursing and research utilization are also given.

KEY TERM

international level: Changes that result from collaboration among nurses from different countries

The Joanna Briggs Institute is an international research and development unit of the Royal Adelaide Hospital, which is located in Adelaide, South Australia (see http://www.joannabriggs.org). The institute was established in 1995 and became fully operational in 1996. It aims to improve the effectiveness of nursing practice and healthcare outcomes. Some initiatives include conducting systematic reviews, collaborating with expert researchers to facilitate development of practice information sheets, and designing, promoting, and delivering short courses about EBP.

TEST YOUR KNOWLEDGE 2-1

Match the following entities to the corresponding level of collaboration they provide:

1. APN
2. Joanna Briggs Institute
3. Policy committee
4. AHRQ
5. Librarian
6. NINR
7. Staff nurse

a. Individual nurse level
b. Organizational level
c. Regional level
d. National level
e. International level

How did you do? 1. a; 2. e; 3. b; 4. d; 5. c; 6. d; 7. a

2.2 Keeping It Ethical

At the end of this section, you will be able to:

< Discuss international and national initiatives designed to promote ethical conduct
< Describe the rights that must be protected and the three ethical principles that must be upheld when conducting research
< Explain the composition and functions of IRBs at the organizational level
< Discuss the nurse's role as patient advocate in research situations

Ethical research exists because international, national, organizational, and individual factors are in place to protect the rights of individuals. Without these factors, scientific studies that violate human rights, such as the Nazi experiments, could proceed unchecked. Many factors of ethical research, which evolved in response to unethical scientific conduct, are aimed at protecting human rights. *Human rights* are "freedoms, to which all humans are entitled, often held to include the right to life and liberty, freedom of thought and expression, and equality before the law" (Human rights, 2007). Rights cannot be claimed unless they are justified in the eyes of another individual or group of individuals (Haber & LoBiondo, 2014). When individuals have rights, others have *obligations*; that is, they are required to act in particular ways. This means that when nursing research is being conducted, subjects participating in studies have rights, and all nurses are obligated to protect those rights.

International and National Factors: Guidelines for Conducting Ethical Research

One of the earliest international responses to unethical scientific conduct was the Nuremberg Code. This code was contained in the written verdict at the trial of the German Nazi physicians accused of torturing prisoners during medical experiments. Writers of the Nuremberg Code (**Box 2-2**) identified that voluntary consent was absolutely necessary for participation in research. Research that avoided harm, produced results that benefited society, and allowed participants to withdraw at will was deemed ethical. The Nuremberg Code became the standard for other codes of conduct.

Another example of an international standard is the *Declaration of Helsinki*, which was adopted by the World Medical Association (WMA) in 1964. Last amended in 2013, the declaration provides guidelines for physicians conducting biomedical research (WMA, 2013). *Informed consent* is considered to be the hallmark requirement for the conduct of ethical research (National Cancer Institute, n.d.). The 32 articles and two clarifications included in the document address issues such as protecting the health of all patients, obtaining informed consent, and conducting research with the aim of benefiting science and society (WMA, 2013). The Declaration of Helsinki offers more specific detail about what constitutes ethical scientific research than does the Nuremberg Code.

Like the WMA, the American Nurses Association (ANA) was ahead of the federal government in establishing codes of scientific conduct. In 1968, *The Nurse in Research: ANA Guidelines on Ethical Values* was approved by the ANA board of directors (Haber & LoBiondo, 2014). ANA established the Commission on Nursing Research, whose report emphasized the rights of human subjects in three ways: (1) right to freedom from harm, (2) right to privacy and dignity, and (3) right to anonymity. ANA (1985) published six ethical guidelines for nurses (**Table 2-2**). As a result of these guidelines, all nurses are charged with

BOX 2-2	Articles of the Nuremberg Code

1. The voluntary consent of the human subject is absolutely essential.
2. The experiment should be such as to yield fruitful results for the good of society, unprocurable by other methods or means of study, and not random and unnecessary in nature.
3. The experiment should be so designed and based on the results of animal experimentation and a knowledge of the natural history of the disease or other problem under study that the anticipated results will justify the performance of the experiment.
4. The experiment should be so conducted as to avoid all unnecessary physical and mental suffering and injury.
5. No experiment should be conducted where there is an a priori reason to believe that death or disabling injury will occur; except, perhaps, in those experiments where the experimental physicians also serve as subjects.
6. The degree of risk to be taken should never exceed that determined by the humanitarian importance of the problem to be solved by the experiment.
7. Proper preparations should be made and adequate facilities provided to protect the experimental subject against even remote possibilities of injury, disability, or death.
8. The experiment should be conducted only by scientifically qualified persons. The highest degree of skill and care should be required through all stages of the experiment of those who conduct or engage in the experiment.
9. During the course of the experiment the human subject should be at liberty to bring the experiment to an end if he has reached the physical or mental state where continuation of the experiment seemed to him to be impossible.
10. During the course of the experiment the scientist in charge must be prepared to terminate the experiment at any stage, if he has probably [sic] cause to believe, in the exercise of the good faith, superior skill and careful judgment required of him that a continuation of the experiment is likely to result in injury, disability, or death to the experimental subject.

Office for Human Research Protections. (1993). Appendix 6 (pp. 7–8). In *IRB guidebook*. Retrieved from https://archive.hhs.gov/ohrp/irb/irb_appendices.htm#j5

the responsibility of protecting the rights of all subjects in their care. Similar guidelines have also been created by professional nursing organizations (Ketefian, Bays, Draucker, Herrick, & Lee, 2002).

Not until the 1970s were federal guidelines about the ethical treatment of human subjects formulated (National Cancer Institute, n.d.). In 1973, the Department of Health, Education, and Welfare published the first set of proposed regulations about the protection of human rights. One of the most important regulations to emerge was the mandated implementation of *institutional review boards* to review and approve all studies. The National Commission for the Protection of Human Subjects of Biomedical and Behavioral Research was established in 1974 when the National Research Act was passed. One of the first charges to the commission was to identify basic ethical principles that are foundational to the conduct of ethical scientific research involving human

KEY TERM

institutional review boards: Committees that review research proposals to determine whether research is ethical

TABLE 2-2	ANA Guidelines for Protecting the Rights of Human Subjects

Rights/guidelines	Obligations
Right to Self-Determination	Employers must inform nurses in writing if participating as a subject in research is a condition of employment. Potential subjects must be advised of risks and benefits of participation.
Right to Freedom from Risk or Harm	Nurses must ensure freedom from harm. Researchers must monitor vulnerable or captive subjects to reduce potential risk of injury.
Scope of Application	All nurses must ensure that all human subjects enjoy protection of their rights.
Responsibilities to Support Knowledge Development	All nurses must support the development of scientific knowledge.
Informed Consent	Nurses must ensure that informed consent from potential subjects (or legal guardians) protects right to self-determination.
Participation on IRB	Nurses should support inclusion of nurses on IRB. Nurses have an obligation to serve on IRB.

Modified from American Nurses Association. (1985). *Guidelines for nurses in clinical and other research*. Kansas City, MO: Author.

subjects. The commission was also charged with developing guidelines to ensure that medical research was conducted in a manner consistent with the principles the commission identified. The result was the *Belmont Report*, issued in 1979. In the report, three major principles were identified: (1) respect for persons, (2) beneficence, and (3) justice. These same principles provide the foundation for present codes of conduct in many disciplines that conduct research with human subjects.

Respect for Persons

In the Belmont Report (U.S. Department of Health, Education, and Welfare, 1979), *respect for persons* is based on two ethical convictions. The first conviction is that individuals should be treated as *autonomous*; that is, having the ability to make decisions. An autonomous person can deliberate about personal goals and act in accordance with those goals. Nurses are obligated to show respect for the autonomy of others. When they elicit and act upon the opinions of

KEY TERMS

Belmont Report: A report outlining three major principles (respect for persons, beneficence, and justice) foundational for the conduct of ethical research with human subjects

respect for persons: Principle that individuals should be treated as autonomous and that those with diminished autonomy are entitled to protection

others, nurses are fulfilling their obligations. The second conviction related to the ethical principle of respect for persons is the recognition that persons with diminished autonomy are entitled to protection. Individuals with diminished autonomy, often referred to as vulnerable, include children, individuals with mental disabilities, and prisoners. Some past research studies have violated this right. During the Nazi experiments, individuals were not allowed to refuse participation. In the Jewish Chronic Disease Hospital study, subjects were not able to make deliberate decisions because the information about the injection of cancer cells was not shared. Researchers conducting the Willowbrook studies did not allow parents free choice; rather, researchers allowed admission to the facility in return for enrolling children in the study.

Beneficence

Beneficence is the principle of doing good. In the Belmont Report, two rules were formulated: (1) to do no harm, and (2) to maximize possible benefits and minimize possible harm (U.S. Department of Health, Education, and Welfare, 1979). Individuals may face risk of harm while participating in research because in order to learn what is harmful, subjects risk being harmed. Therefore, researchers are obligated to identify and reduce possible risks as much as possible. Furthermore, the risks must be justified in light of the possible benefits that may result from the research. The principle of beneficence was not upheld in a number of earlier studies. In the Willowbrook studies, injection of live hepatitis virus created a monumental risk for harm that was not justified by the researchers' rationale that children were at risk for infection because they were institutionalized. Furthermore, learning about the natural course of the disease was not an outcome that could be justified by the high risk for harm. Individuals were also harmed in the Tuskegee studies. Men with syphilis were not offered penicillin even when it was known that penicillin was an effective treatment.

Justice

The principle of *justice* is concerned with equity or fairness in the distribution of burdens and benefits. In this third principle identified in the Belmont Report, the main consideration is that individuals ought to be treated equally

KEY TERMS

autonomous: Having the ability to make decisions

beneficence: The principle of doing good

justice: The principle of equity or fairness in the distribution of burdens and benefits

CRITICAL THINKING EXERCISE 2-2

Which vulnerable groups of individuals were targeted in the Jewish Chronic Disease Hospital study and the Willowbrook studies? Can you think of other groups of individuals who may be at risk for unjust selection?

(U.S. Department of Health, Education, and Welfare, 1979). Nurses and other healthcare providers are obligated to ensure that some groups of subjects, such as ethnic minorities or institutionalized individuals, are not selected for studies because they are easily available or in compromised positions. Individuals cannot be denied treatment because they decline to participate in research. Subjects cannot receive less than the standard of care. Furthermore, outcomes of publicly funded research need to be reported. Unfair treatment of individuals has been a problem in past studies. In the Tuskegee study, black men were singled out and were not provided standard care. In the Jewish Chronic Disease Hospital study and the Willowbrook studies, vulnerable subjects were targeted.

Organizational Factors: The IRB

There are also mechanisms in place for the protection of human subjects at the organizational level. The primary mechanism is the IRB. Although the structure and functions of IRBs are federally mandated, organizations are held accountable. Hospitals, nursing homes, and universities commonly have established IRBs because these organizations typically have employees conducting research. Organizations without established IRBs or organizations with established IRBs that do not hold researchers accountable for upholding ethical standards are not eligible for federal funds to conduct research. Furthermore, conducting research without IRB approval is illegal. In 1991, a statutory framework was enacted, and these laws resulted in standards set forth in the Code of Federal Regulations 45 C.F.R. 46 (National Cancer Institute, n.d.). IRBs do not review research involving animals, food and drug testing, and other kinds of research not involving human subjects. Components and areas of concern that are reviewed by the IRB are listed in **Table 2-3**.

Federal guidelines stipulate membership of the IRB (National Cancer Institute, n.d.; U.S. Department of Health, Education, and Welfare, 1979). The organization that establishes the IRB appoints or invites members to participate. Members are selected because they have knowledge of and experience working with people of vulnerable populations, because the major purpose of the IRB is to protect the rights of vulnerable populations. Members must also have knowledge of the research process and the ethical and legal regulations of research. IRBs must have a minimum of five members. Members' expertise must vary because all members cannot practice in the same discipline. At least one member of the IRB must be employed in a scientific area; at least one member, often a clergy member residing in the community, must be employed in a nonscientific area. At least one member must have no affiliation with the organization and no family member affiliated with the organization. Membership must include both men and women. When conflicts of interest arise, conflicted

TABLE 2-3	Components and Areas of Concern Appraised by IRBs

Component	Areas of Concern
Risk/benefit analysis	Are possible risks and benefits identified, evaluated, and described? Are risks greater than minimal risk? Have attempts been made to minimize risks? Will the risk/benefit ratio be reassessed as the study progresses? Are subjects receiving less than the standard of care?
Informed consent	Does the study involve vulnerable subjects? Is the language appropriate for the subjects? Who will explain the study to potential subjects? Do subjects need to be reinformed about the purpose of the study periodically? Is a waiver of consent justified?
Selection of subjects	Does the burden of participating in research fall (most likely) on those who will benefit from the findings? Does the research require using the proposed population? Are there groups of people who will be more susceptible to risk? Have vulnerable subjects been overprotected?
Privacy and confidentiality	Does the research involve intrusion? How will information be kept private? Should permission be sought for records? Should documentation of consent be waived to protect confidentiality? Are procedures compliant with Health Insurance Portability and Accountability Act (HIPAA) rules?
Monitoring and observation	How will data be recorded and maintained? Who will have access to the data? Can information be provided to the IRB should unexpected results be discovered?
Additional safeguards	Are recruitment procedures designed to ensure that informed consent is given freely? Does the nature of the disease or behavioral issue permit free consent?
Incentives for participation	Are offered incentives reasonable? Should the IRB monitor subject recruitment to ensure that coercion is not a problem?
Continuing review	Are the actual risks and benefits as anticipated? Has any subject been seriously harmed? Have any unforeseen accidents or problems occurred?

Data from IRB Guidebook/HHS.

members must not participate in the review. For example, when a researcher who is a member of the IRB submits a proposal, that researcher is excused from the deliberations about that specific study. Each IRB has a chairperson who is accountable for leading the IRB and who can make decisions about how applications are reviewed.

There are two kinds of review: full and expedited. A *full review* is necessary when a proposed research study involves vulnerable populations or when risks are not minimal. A proposal might be eligible for an *expedited review* when the research study poses minimal risk to human subjects (U.S. Department of Health, Education, and Welfare, 1979). *Minimal risk* means that the probability and magnitude of harm or discomfort anticipated in the research are not greater in and of themselves than those ordinarily encountered in daily life or during the performance of routine physical or psychological examinations or tests.

Prior to the review meeting, members of the IRB read the proposals in need of a full review, and then convene to discuss whether each study's protocols meet the requirements of the Code of Federal Regulations (**Box 2-3**). Members vote on whether or not to approve each study and might make recommendations for changes to researchers. Proposals of studies qualifying for expedited review are read by the chairperson of the IRB, who confirms that expedited review is appropriate and determines whether the standards of the Code of Federal Regulations are being met.

Examples of research qualifying for expedited review include the following:

» Collecting hair and nail clippings
» Collecting excreta and external secretions
» Recording data on subjects 18 years or older using noninvasive routine clinical procedures
» Making voice recordings
» Studying existing documents, data, records, and specimens

KEY TERMS

full review: A type of review by an institutional review board that requires all members of the board to participate; an IRB conducts a full review if there is potential risk to human subjects

expedited review: A type of review by an institutional review board that can occur quickly; an IRB may conduct an expedited review if there is minimal risk to human subjects

minimal risk: The probability and magnitude of harm from participating in a research study are not greater than those encountered in daily life

| **BOX 2-3** | Key Points of the Code of Federal Regulations |

1. Risks to subjects are minimized.
2. The risks to subjects are reasonable in relation to anticipated benefits.
3. The selection of subjects is equitable.
4. Informed consent must be sought from potential subjects or their legal guardians.
5. Informed consent must be properly documented.
6. When appropriate, research plans monitor data collection to ensure subject safety.
7. When appropriate, privacy of subjects and confidentiality of data are maintained.
8. Safeguards must be in place when subjects are vulnerable to coercion.

Data from National Cancer Institute (n.d.).

| **BOX 2-4** | Six Categories of Exempt Research |

1. Research conducted in established or commonly accepted educational settings, involving normal educational practices.
2. Research involving the use of educational tests (i.e., cognitive, diagnostic, aptitude, achievement), survey procedures, interview procedures, or observation of public behavior, unless:
   a. Information obtained is recorded in such a manner that human participants can be identified, directly or through identifiers linked to them.
   b. Any disclosure of the human participant's responses outside the research could reasonably place the participant at risk of criminal or civil liability or be damaging to the participant's financial standing, employability, or reputation.
3. Research involving the use of educational tests (i.e., cognitive, diagnostic, aptitude, achievement), survey procedures, interview procedures, or observation of public behavior that is not exempt under item (2) of this list, if:
   a. The participants are elected or appointed public officials or candidates for public office.
   b. Federal statute(s) require(s) without exception that the confidentiality of the personally identifiable information be maintained throughout the research and thereafter.
4. Research involving the collection or study of existing data, documents, records, pathological specimens, or diagnostic specimens, if these sources are publicly available or the information is recorded by the researcher in such a manner that participants cannot be identified, directly or through identifiers linked to them.
5. Research and demonstration projects conducted by or subject to the approval of federal department or agency heads and designed to study, evaluate, or otherwise examine public health benefit or service programs.
6. Taste and food-quality evaluation and consumer acceptance studies.

Data from National Cancer Institute (n.d.).

KEY TERM

exempt: Certain studies may be low enough risk not to require consent from individuals

Certain low-risk studies can be considered *exempt* from obtaining consent from individuals. These studies still need IRB approval. There are six exempt categories of research (**Box 2-4**). These exemptions do not apply to prisoners, pregnant women, fetuses, newborns, and most children (National Cancer Institute, n.d.). Researchers should never assume that their proposals qualify for exempt status, but rather they must follow the policies specified by their organizations. Most policies require that another person, usually the IRB chairperson, review proposals to ensure that they qualify for exempt status.

It is becoming more common for IRBs to require EBP projects to be reviewed, especially when personal data (e.g., demographic information or patient outcomes) are to be collected. Because interest in EBP is growing, data from such projects are being shared at conferences and in publications. Sometimes nurses do not consider the possibility of publicly sharing their findings until the end of a project, but at this point, it may be unethical to present findings, especially if personal data were collected without consent.

CRITICAL THINKING EXERCISE 2-3

A physician comes to the unit and states that she is working in the lab and needs some blood to run a lab test for her research study. The physician asks the nurse to assist with drawing some blood. The physician and nurse enter the room of one of the physician's patients. Without a parent present, the physician asks the 17-year-old patient if she can draw the patient's blood. The adolescent seems reluctant but agrees to the procedure. The physician and nurse draw the blood, and the physician leaves the unit without documenting the procedure. The nurse feels uncomfortable and talks with the charge nurse about the situation. Which ethical principles are violated in this situation? How did the nurse fail to act as a patient advocate? What should the nurse have done to protect the rights of the adolescent? What should the charge nurse recommend?

Therefore, it is wise for nurses who are initiating EBP projects to obtain IRB approval prior to implementing data collection even when they do not anticipate sharing findings publicly.

In many organizations, other factors ensure that research is ethical. Many hospitals also have nursing research committees that review research proposals. These committees are usually composed of staff nurses, nurse managers, APNs, and the director of nursing research if there is such a person in the organization.

Individual Factors: Nurses as Patient Advocates

Individual nurses are accountable for ensuring that the rights of subjects are protected. ANA has charged nurses to be patient advocates. Thus, nurses must be familiar with international, national, and organizational standards to be effective in their role as patient advocate. Nurses must be able to distinguish between advocacy and science. Nurses have both a duty to care and duty to advance nursing knowledge. This means that the *research imperative* must be weighed against the *therapeutic imperative*. When there is doubt, the therapeutic imperative must take precedence over the research imperative. Nurses can act as patient advocates in a variety of ways. Nurses should be certain that subjects receive treatment that meets the standard of care and that subjects choose freely to participate in research. Ensuring that HIPAA guidelines are followed when data are collected advocates for the privacy of patients and confidentiality of information. When subjects express the desire to withdraw from a study, nurses can assist by contacting the researcher. If nurses observe unethical behaviors, they should report these violations to the chairperson of the IRB at their institution. Nurses can also contribute by participating on IRBs and nursing research committees.

It is imperative that nurses recognize that IRB approval does not guarantee that ethical dilemmas will not arise. Unanticipated events can lead to unethical

KEY TERMS

research imperative: An ethical rule stating that nurses should advance the body of knowledge

therapeutic imperative: An ethical rule stating that nurses should perform actions that benefit the patient

conduct, whether intentional or unintentional. Nurses must use their own ethical frameworks to judge whether their actions, or the actions of others, are in the best interest of patients and nursing science.

TEST YOUR KNOWLEDGE 2-2

True/False

1. Informed consent is the hallmark of the Declaration of Helsinki.

2. The Belmont Report identified four ethical principles: respect for persons, nonmaleficence, beneficence, and justice.

3. IRB approval must be obtained for studies involving animals, foods, or drugs.

4. A qualitative study of adults that only involves tape recording interviews would likely receive an expedited review.

5. When there is a conflict, the therapeutic imperative takes precedence over the research imperative.

How did you do? 1. T; 2. F; 3. F; 4. T; 5. T

RAPID REVIEW

» The model of EBP collaboration has five levels: individual nurse level, organizational level, regional level, national level, and international level.

» Nurses, in a variety of roles, contribute to creating EBP. They can identify clinical problems, participate in EBP changes, serve as change agents or opinion leaders, and establish a vision for the organization.

» Organizational factors that build a culture for EBP include setting performance expectations for individual nurses, integrating EBP into governance structures, and providing recognition and rewards for involvement in EBP.

» Interventions that social systems can use to promote excellence in nursing and move EBP forward include modifying policies and standards, modifying medical record forms, educating senior administrators and garnering their support, and orienting new staff members.

» Regional interventions include using skills of a local librarian, collaborating with a local program of nursing, and using resources from regional centers.

» Many national and international entities have made considerable contributions to nursing research and EBP.

» The Nuremberg Code and the Declaration of Helsinki are international guidelines aimed at protecting the rights of human subjects.

» Federal laws have been enacted to protect subjects who participate in research. National organizations have created codes of conduct for researchers.

» The Belmont Report identified three ethical principles for guiding research: respect for persons, beneficence, and justice.

» IRBs are federally mandated organizational structures that review research proposals to ensure that the rights of human subjects are protected. Nursing research committees can also be involved in the protection of human subjects.

» Nurses are expected to act as patient advocates by ensuring that their patients' rights are upheld. Nurses are also expected to facilitate the development of scientific knowledge in nursing.

Apply What You Have Learned

The National Cancer Institute offers a free web-based course about protecting the rights of human subjects. Many researchers complete this tutorial as a requirement for obtaining federal funds. Visit the National Cancer Institute website at http://phrp.nihtraining.com/users /login.php. Sign in, take the tutorial, and print your certificate. Successfully completing the tutorial means that you can qualify to be a research assistant over the next 2 years!

REFERENCES

American Nurses Association. (1985). *Guidelines for nurses in clinical and other research.* Kansas City, MO: American Nurses Association.

American Nurses Credentialing Center. (2013). Magnet Recognition Program Model. Retrieved 6/23/17 from http://www.nursecredentialing.org/Magnet/ProgramOver view/New-Magnet-Model

Cochrane, A. L. (1971). *Effectiveness and efficiency. Random reflections on health services.* Abingdon, Berks, United Kingdom: Nuffield Provincial Hospitals Trust.

Cullen, L., & Adams, S. (2012). Planning for implementation of evidence-based practice. *Journal of Nursing Administration, 42*(4), 222–230.

Cullen, L., Dawson, C. J., Hanrahan, K., & Dole, N. (2014). Evidence-based practice: Strategies for nursing leaders. In D. Huber (Ed.), *Leadership and nursing care management* (5th ed., pp. 274–290). St. Louis, MO: Elsevier Saunders.

Cullen, L., Greiner, J., Greiner, J., Bombei, C., & Comried, L. (2005). Excellence in evidence-based practice: Organizational and unit exemplars. *Critical Care Nursing Clinics of North America, 17*, 127–142.

DiCenso, A. (2003). Evidence-based nursing practice: How to get there from here. *Nursing Leadership, 16*(4), 20–26.

Doumit, G., Gattellari, M., Grimshaw, J., & O'Brien, M. A. (2007). Local opinion leaders: Effects on professional practice and health care outcomes. *Cochrane Database of Systematic Reviews, 1*, CD000125. doi:10.1002/14651858.CD000125.pub3

Haber, J., & LoBiondo-Wood, G. (2014). Legal and ethical issues. In G. LoBiondo-Wood & J. Haber (Eds.), *Nursing research: Methods and critical appraisal for evidence-based practice* (8th ed., pp. 254–272). St. Louis, MO: Mosby.

Hudson, K. (2005). From research to practice on the Magnet pathway. *Nursing Management, 36*(3), 33–37.

Human rights. (2007). In *American heritage dictionary of the English language* (4th ed.). Boston, MA: Houghton Mifflin.

Ketefian, S., Bays, C., Draucker, C., Herrick, L., & Lee, R. K. (2002). *Guidelines for scientific integrity* (2nd ed.). Wheat Ridge, CO: Midwest Nursing Research Society.

National Cancer Institute. (n.d.). *Human participant protections education for research teams*. Retrieved 6/23/17 from http://phrp.nihtraining.com/users/login.php

National Institute of Nursing Research. (n.d.). *Changing practice, changing lives: 10 landmark nursing research studies*. Retrieved 6/23/17 from http://www.ninr.nih.gov/sites/www.ninr.nih.gov/files/10-landmark-nursing-research-studies.pdf

Office for Human Research Protections. (1993). *IRB guidebook*. Retrieved 6/23/17 from https://archive.hhs.gov/ohrp/irb/irb_appendices.htm#j5

Okihiro, M., Pillen, M., Ancog, C., Inda, C., & Sehgal, V. (2013). Implementing the obesity care model at a community health center in Hawaii to address childhood obesity. *Journal of Health Care for the Poor and Underserved, 24*(2), 1–11.

Rogers, E. (2003). *Diffusion of innovations* (5th ed.). New York, NY: Free Press.

Schaffer, M., Sandau, K., & Diedrick, L. (2013). Evidence-based practice models for organizational change: Overview and practical applications. *Journal of Advanced Nursing, 69*(5), 1197–1209.

Shirey, M. (2006). Evidence-based practice: How nurse leaders can facilitate innovation. *Nursing Administration Quarterly, 30*, 252–265.

Smith, M., Saunders, R., Stuckhardt, L., & McGinnis, J. M. (Eds.). (2012, September). *Best care at lower cost: The path to continuously learning health care in America* (Institute of Medicine Brief Report, pp. 1–4). Washington, DC: National Academies Press.

Titler, M. (2014). Developing an evidence-based practice. In G. LoBiondo-Wood & J. Haber (Eds.), *Nursing research: Methods and critical appraisal for evidence-based practice* (8th ed., pp. 418–440). St. Louis, MO: Mosby Elsevier.

Titler, M., & Everett, L. (2001). Translating research into practice: Considerations for critical care investigators. *Critical Care Nursing Clinics of North America, 13*, 587–604.

University of Iowa Hospitals and Clinics. (2017). Nursing mission and vision. Retrieved 6/23/17 from https://uihc.org/nursing-mission-and-vision

U.S. Department of Health, Education, and Welfare. (1979). *The Belmont Report: Ethical principles and guidelines for the protection of human subjects of research*. Retrieved 6/23/17 from http://www.hhs.gov/ohrp/humansubjects/guidance/belmont.html

World Medical Association. (2013). World Medical Association declaration of Helsinki: Ethical principles for medical research involving human subjects. Retrieved 6/23/17 from https://www.wma.net/policies-post/wma-declaration-of-helsinki-ethical-principles-for-medical-research-involving-human-subjects/

Acquisition of Knowledge

UNIT 2

Questioning the efficacy of practice lends itself to the discovery of innovations.

At the end of this chapter, you will be able to:

- Discuss ways research problems are identified
- Describe relationships among the purpose statement, the research problems, and the research question
- Differentiate among associative, causal, simple, complex, nondirectional, directional, null, and research hypotheses
- Use criteria to appraise research questions

- Identify independent and dependent variables
- Define mediators, moderators, and confounding variables
- Compare the purposes of research questions and evidence-based practice (EBP) questions
- Describe the PICOT method
- Discuss ethical issues associated with the development of research and EBP questions

KEY TERMS

associative relationship	generalize	problem statement
case studies	hypotheses	purpose statement
causal relationship	hypothesis testing	replication
complex hypothesis	independent variable	research hypothesis
confounding variables	mediators	research problem
covary	moderators	research question
dependent variable	nondirectional hypothesis	research topic
directional hypothesis	null hypothesis	simple hypothesis
empirical testing	PICOT model	statistical hypothesis
extraneous variables	pilot	systematic reviews

CHAPTER 3

Identifying Research Questions

Susie Adams

3.1 How Clinical Problems Guide Research Questions

At the end of this section, you will be able to:

‹ Discuss ways research problems are identified
‹ Describe relationships among the purpose statement, the research problems, and the research question

The primary goals for conducting nursing research are to generate new knowledge that has wide application to promote positive health outcomes for a particular patient population, enhance the overall quality and cost-effectiveness of care, improve the healthcare delivery system, and validate the credibility of the nursing profession through evidence-based practice (EBP). Determining what problems to study, framing research questions, and developing research hypotheses are often the most challenging aspects of the research process. Where does one begin?

Identifying Nursing Research Problems

An infinite number of nursing problems merit investigation. The challenge is to narrow the focus of problems so they are clinically relevant and can be answered through empirical testing. **Figure 3-1** shows the logical flow for narrowing a nursing research problem. A *research problem* is an area of concern when

FIGURE 3-1   Narrowing the Research Question

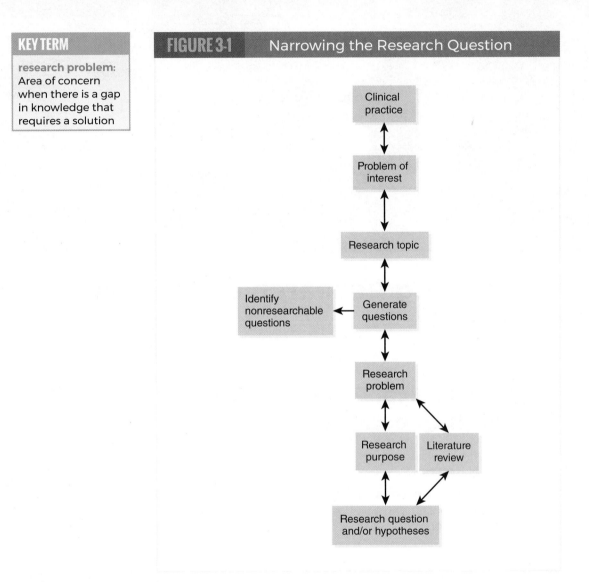

there is a gap in knowledge that requires a solution that
can be described, explained, or predicted to improve
nursing practice (Norwood, 2000). Research problems are
identified through a variety of sources: personal clinical
experience, professional literature, current nursing theories, previous research, and national initiatives. Nursing,
like all healthcare professions, is constantly seeking ways
to improve clinical outcomes and promote health across
the life span.

Clinical Experience

Experience most often leads nurses to question whether there is a better approach to a clinical procedure or situation. Clinical curiosity and a desire to improve patient care can be the most important motivators to begin further inquiry that ultimately shapes research studies. Discussions with nursing colleagues regarding their clinical experiences and practice approaches can identify mutual clinical problems. Such discussions may stimulate shared interest for inquiry into best practice approaches for a specific clinical problem.

Professional Literature

Consulting the professional literature is another way to identify research problems. Journal clubs provide an approach to investigate clinical problems identified at the practice level. Internet search engines and databases such as Google Scholar (http://scholar.google.com/), PubMed (http://www.ncbi.nlm.nih.gov/pmc/), and PsycINFO (http://www.apa.org/pubs/databases/psycinfo/index.aspx) provide access to scholarly literature across many disciplines and sources including books, abstracts, articles, and dissertations. Refinement of Internet search skills to extract relevant professional literature can be learned through online tutorials and formal classes and can be assisted by public or university research librarians. Reading, sharing, and discussing clinical articles from professional journals typically lead to further inquiry into the clinical research literature.

Previous Research

Identifying and reading research articles on particular clinical problems help nurses to understand the current knowledge about the topic. Reading research articles also reveals gaps about what is known or has not been tested or adequately evaluated. For example, there is a gap when nurses are not using a new clinical approach or intervention yielding better clinical results than the traditional intervention does. A gap would also exist if there have been only one or two *case studies* reported in the literature. A gap may become apparent when the study design, method, measures, and outcomes apply to a small or limited sample. Traditionally, new interventions are tested with a small number of subjects in *pilot* studies before testing with larger samples. These types of studies begin to fill knowledge gaps. Whether this same intervention will result in a positive outcome in a more culturally diverse population, different age group, or different geographic sample merits investigation. This type of research is called *replication* studies. Finding that multiple studies have obtained similar positive results increases the extent to which one can *generalize* or apply findings to a wider population.

KEY TERMS

case studies: A description of a single or novel event; a unique methodology used in qualitative research that may also be considered a design or strategy for data collection

pilot: A small study to test a new intervention with a small number of subjects before testing with larger samples; adopting an innovation on a trial basis

replication: Repeated studies to obtain similar results

generalize: Applying findings from a sample to a wider population

With the proliferation of professional journals across disciplines, it is no longer feasible to read all the published information on any given healthcare topic. A search of the literature about a narrowly focused clinical problem may yield dozens of relevant articles. Articles presenting a synthesis of several articles about a clinical topic, called *systematic reviews*, usually make gaps in the literature more apparent.

Current Nursing Theories

The earliest nursing theories, called grand theories, organized knowledge and explained phenomena about the nature and goals of nursing related to four key elements: the person or recipient of care; the environment, including both internal and external conditions; health, reflecting the degree of wellness or illness of the person; and nursing, reflecting the actions and characteristics of the person giving care. These grand theories each provide a set of concepts, definitions, relationships, assumptions, and propositions that articulate a systematic view of phenomena with the intent of describing, explaining, and/or predicting interactions and outcomes. Peplau's (1952) interpersonal relations theory, Orem's (2001) self-care deficit theory, Roy's (1970) adaptation model, Rogers's (1980) science of unitary beings, Newman's (1986) theory of health as expanding consciousness, and Parse's (1981, 1992) theory of human becoming are all examples of grand nursing theories with general concepts and propositions that broadly describe nursing.

Developing studies that empirically test a specific nursing theory is challenging, and most grand nursing theories or models have few studies that validate major theoretical concepts. For example, Peplau's (1952) interpersonal relations theory has been widely cited in clinical papers; yet, only a few studies actually explore and test nurse–patient relationship factors derived from this theory (Forchuk, 1994, 1995; Forchuk & Reynolds, 2001). These types of studies are more likely to be initiated by experienced researchers who are well versed in theory construction and the measurement of concepts. However, beginning researchers may have opportunities to participate as members of a research team engaged in testing a nursing theory, thereby gaining valuable conceptual knowledge and pragmatic research skills as they develop their own programs of research.

Middle range theories are narrower in scope and provide a bridge from grand theories to a testable theory with a limited number of variables that describe, explain, and predict outcomes of interest in nursing practice. Middle range theories can have diverse testable applications that contribute to a growing body of EBP. Kolcaba's (1994) theory of holistic comfort is one example of a middle range theory that has generated testing in a variety of clinical settings. Kolcaba's theory posits basic assumptions that human beings (1) have holistic responses to complex stimuli, (2) desire comfort as a holistic outcome that is relevant to nursing care, and (3) strive to meet, or have met, basic comfort needs. Kolcaba (1992, 1994) described three states of comfort (relief, ease, and transcendence) within four contexts of care (physical, psychospiritual, social, and environmental). Koehn (2000) applied Kolcaba's theory to comfort within a labor and delivery setting. Kolcaba and DiMarco (2005) applied the theory on pediatric inpatient units. March and McCormack (2009) have most recently modified Kolcaba's theory, to apply institution-wide, to guide nursing care and evaluate patient outcomes on overall comfort and satisfaction with nursing care. Other well-known middle range nursing theories include Mercer's (1986) maternal role attainment theory, Pender's (1997) theory of health promotion, and Resnick's theory of self-efficacy (Resnick & Nigg, 2003). Angelo G. Gonzalo maintains a useful website on nursing theorists at http://nursingtheories.weebly.com/.

National Initiatives

A number of U.S. government agencies routinely identify major health problems and establish national research priorities. These include the U.S. Surgeon General's Office (http://surgeongeneral.gov/) and the National Institutes of Health (http://www.nih.gov/) and their member institutes (https://www.nih.gov/institutes-nih), such as the National Institute of Nursing Research (http://www.ninr.nih.gov/) and the National Institute of Mental Health (http://www.nimh.nih.gov/index.shtml/).

The U.S. Department of Health and Human Services (USDHHS) convenes the Secretary's Advisory Committee on National Health Promotion and Disease Prevention Objectives for 2020 (Advisory Committee) to produce recommendations regarding the development and implementation of Healthy People 2020. The 12 members on the Advisory Committee are nationally known experts in public health who, together with its subcommittees, produce recommendations for the Healthy People guidelines and implementation (https://www.healthypeople.gov/). The web portal not only outlines the 10-year priorities to improve the health and health care of the nation but also maintains database information accessible to health services researchers.

The Agency for Healthcare Research and Quality (AHRQ) works to improve delivery and coordination of primary care services to meet the need for high-quality, safe, effective, and efficient clinical prevention and chronic disease care (http://www.ahrq.gov/). Ongoing initiatives by AHRQ include healthcare data collection, cost and utilization statistics and reports, EBP guidelines clearinghouse, and information portals for the public, policymakers, healthcare providers, and researchers. Recent AHRQ initiatives have directed funding for patient-centered outcomes research (PCOR). With the January 2014 implementation of the Affordable Health Care for America Act, AHRQ will continue to gather information on healthcare outcomes and costs and be an important source of determining integrated models of healthcare delivery across the United States.

National research agendas identify areas of health concerns with significant implications for the general public, such as access to affordable health care, childhood obesity, oral health in children, health disparities in minority populations, cardiovascular disease in women, mental health and substance use disorders, genomics, disease prevention, and integration of primary care and behavioral health services. Collectively, national agencies identify areas with high priority for federal research funding to evaluate both prevention and intervention healthcare strategies. Nursing research studies derived from such national research agendas typically have greater opportunities for federal funding.

Narrowing the Problem of Interest

A clinical problem of interest is sometimes called the *research topic*. Because clinical problems tend to be quite broad in scope, it is essential to narrow the scope to design studies that are manageable. When narrowing clinical problems, it is important to consider several factors. Having a strong interest and passion for a clinical problem is vital because even a pilot study requires the investment of considerable time and effort. Sustained motivation is needed to see a study through to completion. The problem selected for the study needs to be of clinical significance so it adds to the body of nursing knowledge. Consideration should be given to whether the problem affects a large number of people; whether the outcomes will improve the care or quality of life for individuals, families, or groups; and whether findings will be applicable in a practice environment. Additional considerations include feasibility in terms of time, research expertise, available resources, access to subjects, and ethical considerations for research subjects.

When developing research questions about clinical problems, one must consider whether the problem can be answered by the research process of empirical testing. Some questions are inherently philosophical in nature and cannot be answered by a research study. Questions that pose a moral choice are questions for philosophical inquiry and public policy deliberation. For example, stem cell research is a current clinical topic that may offer new solutions to a broad range of genetically linked disorders. The question, "Should stem cell research be limited to current strains, and should access to fetal stem cells be prohibited?" poses an ethical and philosophical question. However, reframing the question as "What are the attitudes of patients with Parkinson's disease and their family members toward research that could involve stem cells injected into brain tissue to generate myelinated neurons to reduce Parkinsonian tremors?" makes it empirically testable. Research questions must always be framed in a manner that can be empirically tested within ethical boundaries.

KEY TERM

research topic: A clinical problem of interest

Even when questions can be framed for empirical testing, one must further consider whether the question can be answered by existing knowledge or through basic problem-solving skills. For example, "Can stem cells be safely transplanted via injection into human bone marrow to treat leukemia?" is an EBP question that can be answered through consulting current literature (Laughlin & Lazarus, 2003). At an earlier time, this posed a researchable question, but that question has subsequently been answered. It is critical to investigate current literature because it would be a waste of resources to conduct research when knowledge already exists. Some questions may be answered through basic problem solving. For example, the question "What is the best method to reduce fall risks among elderly clients served by a home healthcare agency?" could be addressed through a continuous quality improvement process. Initial and periodic fall risk assessments could be developed and compared with ongoing monitoring to track falls. Questions included in the fall risk assessment might be modified as data are obtained about client medications, cognitive function, and home conditions associated with falls and how to reduce these risks.

Problem Solving, Nursing Process, and Research Process

It is helpful to recognize the similarities and differences among the problem-solving process, nursing process, and research process. All three use abstract, critical thinking, and complex reasoning to identify new information, discover relationships, and make predictions about phenomena (Gray, Grove, & Sutherland, 2017). All involve the scientific method of observation, data collection, problem identification, implementation of a solution, and evaluation of results. These processes are iterative; that is, continual refinement of knowledge occurs as the process is repeated.

Primary differences among the problem-solving process, nursing process, and research process are in their foci, purposes, and outcomes (Gray et al., 2017). The focus of the problem-solving process is on a specific goal in a particular setting for the purpose of generating the best solution to achieve the goal. The focus of the nursing process is on a specific patient care problem using assessment, nursing diagnosis, planning, implementation, and evaluation. The goal of the nursing process is to plan and direct care for a particular patient, family, or group of patients. The outcome is the improvement of health for a particular patient or family. In contrast, the research process has a broad focus drawing on knowledge from nursing and other disciplines. Rigorous application of scientific methods is used, and findings are disseminated through presentations and publications. The purpose of the research process is to generate new knowledge that has wide application to promote positive health outcomes for a

KEY TERMS

problem statement: A formal statement describing the problem addressed in the study

purpose statement: A statement indicating the aim of the study

research question: An interrogatory statement describing the variables and population of the research study

particular patient population, enhance the overall quality and cost-effectiveness of care, and improve the healthcare delivery system.

Developing Problem Statements

Problem statements are derived from a research problem that has been identified as a situation that is unsatisfactory and requires further description, explanation, or a solution (Norwood, 2000). The *problem statement* formally identifies what problem is being addressed in the study. A problem statement must include the scope of the research problem, the specific population of interest, the independent and dependent variables, and the goal or question the study intends to answer (Gillis & Jackson, 2002). Additionally, the problem statement should implicitly or explicitly indicate that the proposed study is ethical, feasible, and of significant interest to nursing (Nieswiadomy, 2012). **Box 3-1** contains criteria nurses can use to evaluate problem statements. The research purpose and research questions logically flow from problem statements. The *purpose statement* is derived from the problem statement and indicates the aim of the study. The *research question* flows from the problem statement and study purpose, and often it is the interrogatory form of the problem statement. Examples illustrating the differences among the problem statement, the purpose of a study, and the research question are presented in **Box 3-2**.

Some researchers use the problem statement and research question interchangeably. The difference is the use of a declarative or an interrogatory sentence. The research problem when stated in the interrogative form is called the research question. Other researchers frame the problem statement in a broader manner that generates several research questions, as in the example in Box 3-1. Not all research studies include both a formal problem statement and a research question, but the research question can be implied from the problem statement.

BOX 3-1	Criteria for Evaluating Problem Statements

1. Problem (or purpose) statement is clear and concise.
2. Problem statement is written as a declarative statement or a formal question (interrogatory).
3. Population of interest is clearly described.
4. Independent and dependent variables are identified.
5. Empirical data can be derived for the variables in the population of interest.
6. Indication that study is ethical.
7. Indication that study is feasible.
8. Indication that study is clinically significant and relevant to nursing practice.

| BOX 3-2 | Examples of Problem Statements, Purpose Statements, and Research Questions |

Problem statement: The use of alcohol by college freshmen contributes to alcohol-related injuries and emergency department visits at a state university.

Purpose statement: To determine if brief screening and nursing intervention for alcohol use during freshmen orientation reduces self-reported alcohol use, alcohol-related injuries, and emergency department visits among college freshmen at a state university.

Research question 1: Is there a difference in self-reported alcohol use between college freshmen who receive brief screening and nursing intervention for alcohol use during fall orientation and the previous class of freshmen students who did not receive brief screening and nursing intervention?

Research question 2: Is there a difference in alcohol-related injuries and emergency department visits between college freshmen who receive brief screening and nursing intervention for alcohol use during fall orientation and the previous class of freshmen students who did not receive brief screening and nursing intervention?

TEST YOUR KNOWLEDGE 3-1

1. Which of the following can be used to identify researchable problems? (Select all that apply.)
   a. Current nursing theories
   b. Personal clinical experiences
   c. Philosophical questions
   d. National initiatives
2. In an article, a nurse reads the following statement: This study aims to examine the effect of guided imagery on postoperative pain in adults. This statement is an example of a:
   a. problem statement.
   b. research question.
   c. purpose statement.
   d. hypothesis.

How did you do? 1. a, b, d; 2. c

3.2 Developing Hypotheses

At the end of this section, you will be able to:

< Differentiate among associative, causal, simple, complex, nondirectional, directional, null, and research hypotheses
< Use criteria to appraise research questions
< Identify independent and dependent variables
< Define mediators, moderators, and confounding variables

hypotheses:
Formal statements
of the expected
or predicted
relationship among
two or more
variables

associative
relationship: A
type of relationship
such that when one
variable changes,
the other variable
changes

covary: When
change in
one variable is
associated with
change in another
variable

Study *hypotheses* are formal statements regarding the expected or predicted relationship between two or more variables in a specific population. They are derived from either the problem statement or the research question. Some studies do not have formally stated hypotheses; yet, the hypothesis can be implied from the research question. Hypotheses include independent and dependent variables that are directly linked to the problem statement and research question; predict the relationship between the independent and dependent variables in a specific population; and define the variables in a manner so that empirical data can be gathered to test the predicted relationship between variables. Additionally, hypotheses need to be ethical, feasible, and relevant to nursing research practice. Criteria to evaluate hypotheses are outlined in **Box 3-3**.

Types of Hypotheses

Hypotheses can be categorized in four broad ways: (1) associative versus causal, (2) simple versus complex, (3) nondirectional versus directional, and (4) null versus research. Hypotheses can fit into more than one category. For example, a researcher can state a simple, directional research hypothesis. Sometimes multiple independent and dependent variables can be included in a hypothesis.

Associative Versus Causal Hypotheses

Relationships identified in hypotheses are either associative or causal. Variables that have an *associative relationship* (**Figure 3-2A**) occur or exist together in the real world so that when one variable changes, the other variable changes. In an associative relationship, the two variables may change, or *covary*. When

---

BOX 3-3   Criteria for Evaluating Hypotheses and Research Questions

1. Does the study have an explicit hypothesis (or hypotheses)? Or does the study present a research question(s)?
2. Hypotheses are written in concise, present-tense, declarative statements that are directly linked to the study problem.
3. For studies with an identified theoretical framework, each hypothesis is derived from the framework.
4. Each hypothesis clearly identifies the population and at least two variables that can be measured and empirically tested.
5. Each hypothesis will state one directional relationship between two variables, or a rationale will be stated for a nondirectional hypothesis.
6. For studies that present research questions (rather than hypotheses), the research questions are concise, clear, and specific.
7. Studies with research questions meet similar criteria to studies testing hypotheses with a clearly identified population, measurable variables, and theoretical framework.

FIGURE 3-2   Associative and Causal Relationships

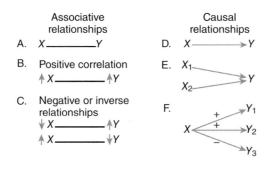

two variables covary in the same direction, a positive (**Figure 3-2B**) correlation results. For example, as people age, measures of blood pressure increase normally. There is a positive correlation between age and blood pressure. When variables vary in opposite directions, they are known as negative or inverse relationships (**Figure 3-2C**). The degree to which variables change may or may not be equal or proportional. This is different from a *causal relationship* in which one variable, the independent variable, is thought to cause or determine the presence of the other variable, the dependent variable (**Figure 3-2D**). One must be cautious not to misinterpret an associative relationship as one that is causal because association does not equal causation.

Simple Versus Complex Hypotheses

A *simple hypothesis* states or describes the relationship, associative or causal, between two variables. A simple associative hypothesis would state that variable X is related to variable Y (Figure 3-2A). A simple causal hypothesis would state that one independent variable is causally related to one dependent variable (Figure 3-2D). A *complex hypothesis* predicts the relationships, either associative or causal, among three or more variables. For example, multiple independent variables may act in a causal relationship to produce one or more dependent variables (**Figure 3-2E**). One independent variable may act in a causal fashion to produce multiple dependent variables (**Figure 3-2F**). Similar statements and illustrations could be made for associative relationships among three or more variables.

Nondirectional Versus Directional Hypotheses

Sometimes researchers have hunches about the direction that variables may take. Other times they may not. A *nondirectional hypothesis* is one that states that a relationship exists between two variables, but it does not predict the direction or nature of the relationship (Figure 3-2A). When no clear direction between the variables has been identified in clinical practice, natural observation of phenomena, relevant nursing theories, or existing clinical or research literature, then no clear prediction can be hypothesized. Nondirectional hypotheses are commonly used in exploratory and descriptive studies. Common nondirectional descriptors include terms such as *associated, correlated,* or *related*. When a nondirectional hypothesis is used, a rationale is included in the problem statement explaining why a directional relationship cannot be predicted between the variables. In contrast, a *directional hypothesis* states the nature or direction of the relationship between two or more variables (Figure 3-2B–F). This type of hypothesis is based on nursing theories, observed phenomena, clinical experience, and existing clinical and research literature. Directional hypotheses are used to predict relationships between two or more variables. Common directional descriptors include terms such as *increase, decrease, less, more, smaller,* and *greater*. Directional hypotheses can also be categorized as associative or causal, simple or complex.

Null Hypotheses Versus Research Hypotheses

The fourth category of hypotheses includes the *null hypothesis* (H_0), which is also commonly called the *statistical hypothesis*. The null hypothesis states that there is no relationship between two variables, and statistical testing is used to either accept or reject this statement. Conversely, the *research hypothesis* (H_1) states that a relationship exists between two or more variables. These relationships can be described and categorized as associative or causal, simple or complex, nondirectional or directional. *Hypothesis testing*

CRITICAL THINKING EXERCISE 3-1

A common problem in the newborn nursery is that infants undergoing circumcision show decreases in body temperature following the procedure. A nurse researcher is interested in studying the effect of a warming tray on the body temperature of infants undergoing circumcisions. Write a research question, associative hypothesis, directional hypothesis, and null hypothesis that would be appropriate for this study.

TABLE 3-1	Examples of Hypotheses for the Research Question: What Is the Relationship Between Self-esteem and Adherence to a Diabetic Diet in Adolescents with Type 1 Diabetes?

Type of Hypothesis	Hypothesis Statement
Associative	There is a relationship between the amount of self-esteem and adherence to a diabetic diet in adolescents with type 1 diabetes.
Causal	Increased amounts of self-esteem increase adherence to a diabetic diet in adolescents with type 1 diabetes.
Simple	Increased amounts of self-esteem increase adherence to a diabetic diet in adolescents with type 1 diabetes.
Complex	Increased amounts of self-esteem increase adherence to a diabetic diet and insulin administration in adolescents with type 1 diabetes.
Nondirectional	There is an association between the amount of self-esteem and adherence to a diabetic diet in adolescents with type 1 diabetes.
Directional	Increased amounts of self-esteem increase adherence to a diabetic diet in adolescents with type 1 diabetes.
Null	There is no relationship between the amount of self-esteem and adherence to a diabetic diet in adolescents with type 1 diabetes.
Research	Increased amounts of self-esteem increase adherence to a diabetic diet in adolescents with type 1 diabetes.

or *empirical testing* involves the collection of objectively measurable data that are gathered through the five senses to confirm or refute a hypothesis. **Table 3-1** offers examples of how hypotheses can be worded.

What Is a Variable?

To understand hypothesis testing, it is important to understand the nature of variables. Variables may be phenomena that can be directly measured, such as pulse rate, blood pressure, respiratory rate, red blood cell count, antibody titer, thyroid stimulating hormone, or salivary cortisol level. Variables may also be qualities, properties, or characteristics of people, groups, or objects; for example, sociodemographic characteristics, intelligence, social support, and self-esteem. Because these qualities, properties, and characteristics are not directly observable, they are measured indirectly using questionnaires and scales. Variables may also be derived from abstract concepts such as depression, anxiety, grieving, and quality of life,

KEY TERMS

hypothesis testing: Collection of objectively measurable data that are gathered through the five senses to confirm or refute a hypothesis; empirical testing; a test for construct validity

empirical testing: Collection of objectively measurable data that are gathered through the five senses to confirm or refute a hypothesis; hypothesis testing

which require some indirect type of measurement. There is an entire body of research dedicated to the development and testing of variables used to measure such abstract concepts. The Beck Depression Inventory (Beck, Ward, Mendelson, Mock, & Erbaugh, 1961), the Hamilton Anxiety Scale (Hamilton, 1959), and the Holmes and Rahe Social Readjustment Rating Scale (Holmes & Rahe, 1967) are several examples of ways to measure variables associated with abstract concepts.

Regardless of whether a variable is one that can be directly measured or requires some form of indirect measurement, variables are also categorized as independent, dependent, and confounding variables. The *independent variable*, commonly labeled the X variable, is the variable that influences the dependent variable or outcome. In experimental studies it is the intervention or treatment that is manipulated by the researcher. The *dependent variable*, commonly labeled the Y variable, is the variable or outcome that is influenced by the independent variable.

Mediators and *moderators* are intervening variables that affect the association between an independent variable and a dependent or outcome variable. A mediator is an intervening variable that is necessary to complete a cause-effect link between an independent and dependent variable. Mediators account for how or why two variables are strongly associated. There may be a single mediating variable or a series of sequential mediating variables between the independent and dependent variables (Bennett, 2000; Kraus et al., 2010). For example, an exercise program for older adults that evaluates a number of physical activity outcomes would need to consider a variety of mediating variables such as social support, perceived physical competence, or behavior change strategies. A moderator is an interaction variable that affects the direction and/or strength of the relationship between the independent variable and the outcome variable. In the example of an exercise program for older adults on physical activity outcomes, gender is a modifier that explains differences if the effects were greater for men than for women. This is typically recognized as an interaction between gender and the exercise program (Bauman, Sallis, Dzewaltowski, & Owen, 2002). See **Figure 3-3**.

Confounding variables, or *extraneous variables*, commonly labeled Z, are factors that distort or interfere with the relationship between the independent and dependent variables. The confounding variable predicts the outcome variable, but it is also associated with the independent variable. Sometimes a confounding variable is known before a study begins; other times a confounding variable is identified while the study is being conducted or after the study is completed. If a confounding variable is known in advance, the researcher may try to use strategies to minimize or eliminate the effect of these variables.

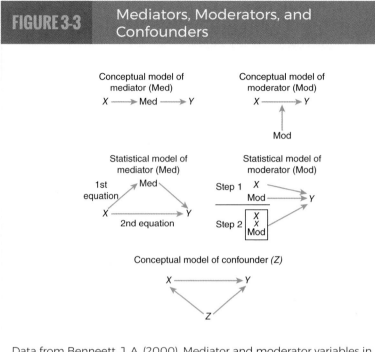

FIGURE 3-3 Mediators, Moderators, and Confounders

Conceptual model of mediator (Med)

$X \longrightarrow \text{Med} \longrightarrow Y$

Conceptual model of moderator (Mod)

$X \longrightarrow Y$

Mod

Statistical model of mediator (Med)

1st equation   Med
$X \longrightarrow Y$
2nd equation

Statistical model of moderator (Mod)

Step 1   X
Mod $\longrightarrow$ Y

Step 2 | X |
         | X |
         | Mod |

Conceptual model of confounder (Z)

$X \longrightarrow Y$

Z

Data from Benneett, J. A. (2000). Mediator and moderator variables in nursing research: Conceptual and statistical differences. *Research in Nursing and Health, 23*, 415–420.

Another way to control for confounding variables is to use specific statistical tests to adjust for their effects. Using the example of the exercise program for older adults on physical activity outcomes, age may confound the relationship between the exercise program and program outcomes. Older people may be less physically active, which is associated with the outcome, and older people may be less likely to engage in a physical exercise program, which is associated with the intervention or independent variable. The confounder influences the association between the exercise program and the physical activity outcomes, thus distorting the actual strength of the effects (Bauman et al., 2002).

Symbols are used to express the relationships between independent and dependent variables and mediators, moderators, or confounders. The direction of the "causal arrows" is important. If the intervention or independent variable "causes" the confounder (the causal direction X→Z), this represents a mediator. In contrast, a confounder acts on the independent variable (Z→X) and/or the dependent variable (Z→Y). A mediator does not act on the variable, but rather acts on the relationship between the independent and dependent variables (see Figure 3-3).

TEST YOUR KNOWLEDGE 3-2

Indicate which of the following terms best describes hypotheses 1–3 below:

    a. associative

    b. causal

    c. simple

    d. complex

    e. directional

    f. nondirectional

    g. null

    h. research

    i. research question

1. Age, number of medical diagnoses, and number of medications affect the incidence of falls in older adults.

2. There is no relationship between seatbelt use and head injury in auto accidents.

3. Does consuming one glass of red wine daily reduce the incidence of heart disease in middle-aged men?

4. Hypothesis: Scores on the Beck Depression Inventory will be lower in women who take yoga classes than in women who do not. What is the independent variable?

    a. Score on Beck Depression Inventory

    b. Yoga ability

    c. Women

    d. Type of participation in yoga

How did you do? 1. b, d, f, h; 2. c, g; 3. i; 4. d

3.3 Formulating EBP Questions

At the end of this section, you will be able to:

‹ Compare the purposes of research questions and EBP questions

‹ Describe the PICOT method

Although research and EBP both involve questions, their purposes are quite different. The primary purpose of nursing research is to generate new knowledge, and the purpose of EBP is to make decisions about patient care based on the best current evidence gathered from a systematic problem-solving approach. EBP incorporates a systematic search for evidence and a critical appraisal of the findings with clinical expertise and the patient's and family's values and preferences to provide the best patient care (Melnyk & Fineout-Overholt, 2014). Clinical curiosity motivates nurses and other healthcare providers to identify choices available for a particular patient to determine the best course of treatment. Given the burgeoning amount of new healthcare products, drugs, procedures, alternative medicine approaches, and the emerging information on risks, benefits, and efficacy of these products, procedures, and interventions, healthcare providers will be continually required to judiciously find the right evidence to make informed treatment care decisions in a time-efficient manner. In EBP, questions are generated in a manner slightly different from how research questions are generated. One widely used model in EBP is the *PICOT model*. Clinical questions for specific patient problems are identified so that healthcare providers can find clinically relevant information using Internet search engines and databases (Higgins & Green, 2011). The mnemonic PICOT stands for the following five components:

> **KEY TERM**
>
> **PICOT model:** A model in EBP used to formulate EBP questions; the acronym stands for patient population, intervention of interest, comparison of interest, outcome of interest, and time frame used to formulate EBP

P = Patient population or patient condition of interest
I = Intervention of interest
C = Comparison of interest
O = Outcome of interest
T = Time (this element is not always included)

The patient population or patient condition needs to be carefully delineated so that the search for evidence yields relevant information and prevents retrieval of too broad or off-target information. During information retrieval, it is important to keep in mind that findings may not be generalizable to a specific patient. For example, a teaching strategy that is successful with children may not be successful with adolescents.

In the PICOT model, the intervention of interest requires similar delineation to yield focused, relevant information. When conducting a literature search, consider the main intervention or treatment, diagnostic test, procedure, or exposure. Also consider any factors that may influence the prognosis such as age, gender, ethnicity, coexisting conditions, and exposures to risk factors such as cigarette smoke, asbestos, or other toxins.

> **FYI**
>
> Nurses must consider patient preferences when making practice decisions, as well as take limited resources into consideration by selecting questions that are broad in scope and that can be completed. Priority should be given to studies that have the potential to generate significant contributions to patient outcomes.

The comparison of interest can be a comparison with another intervention or treatment. The intervention of interest can also be compared to the standard of care. It is best to select the main alternative to the proposed intervention. For example, is the issue about whether to implement a new treatment for sacral decubital ulcers in immobile elderly nursing home patients? An approach to answer this question would be to compare the patient outcomes with the new treatment and the usual standard of care.

> **FYI**
>
> The primary purpose of nursing research is to generate new knowledge, and the purpose of EBP is to make decisions about patient care based on the best current evidence gathered through a systematic problem-solving approach.

The outcome of interest is the desired accomplishment, measurement, or improvement as a result of the selected intervention or treatment approach. It is important to identify clear outcome measures to evaluate the efficacy of the intervention with the identified comparison. In the previous example, the outcome of decubital healing could be determined by measuring diameter and depth of ulcer, type and amount of drainage, formation of new tissue, and ulcer closure. Specifying the desired outcome measures further refines the literature search. Once the components of the PICOT question have been identified, a statement can be written. **Box 3-4** includes a resource for developing EBP questions using the PICOT model. For example, this template can be used to develop a PICOT question about ways to improve hand hygiene compliance by nurses:

In _____nurses_____(P), how does _____education_____ (I) compared to _____current practice_____ (C) affect_____ hand hygiene compliance_____(O) within _____2 months_____ (T)?

BOX 3-4 Resource for Developing EBP Questions Using the PICOT Model

American Association of Ambulatory Care Nurses provides a resource for developing a PICOT question (https://www.aaacn.org/sites/default/files/documents/misc-docs/1e_PICOT_Questions_template.pdf). Be sure to check out the link to the PICOT and Search Query Worksheet.

CRITICAL THINKING EXERCISE 3-2

Consider how you would describe a group of patients similar to your specific patient. Include important patient characteristics, primary problem or disease, and any coexisting conditions. If age, gender, race, ethnicity, or other characteristics are relevant to the diagnosis or treatment, then those factors also need to be included.

TEST YOUR KNOWLEDGE 3-3

True/False

1. There are no differences between research questions and EBP questions.
2. The PICOT model is useful when considering EBP questions.
3. The standard of care or alternate interventions can be used as comparisons of interest in the PICOT model.

How did you do? 1. F; 2. T; 3. T

3.4 Keeping It Ethical

At the end of this section, you will be able to:

‹ Discuss ethical issues associated with the development of research and EBP questions

Although there are not very many ethical issues involved with the development of research and EBP questions, the issues that exist are important. First and foremost, nurses must be certain that research questions posed can be answered while respecting the rights of human subjects. For example, it would be unethical to leave wounds untreated to determine how much time it takes for a stage IV ulcer to develop because that intervention is less than the standard of care. Nurses must also keep in mind that EBP is not based solely on evidence. Regardless of answers that are found to questions, nurses must consider patient preferences when making practice decisions.

Researchers must also be aware that resources are limited. Problems that are broad in scope should be selected. Priority should be given to studies that have the potential to generate significant contributions to patient outcomes. It is also important to address questions that can be seen through to completion. Selecting problems that are of interest makes it easier for one to invest the time, energy, and resources necessary to finish a study. Nurses need to recognize the difference between ethical questions and researchable questions. Although ethical questions do not lend themselves to research methods, discussion about them can make important contributions to nursing knowledge.

TEST YOUR KNOWLEDGE 3-4

1. Which ethical issues are associated with the development of research questions? (Select all that apply.)

   a. Limited resources
   b. Respecting human rights
   c. Interests of the researcher
   d. Patient preferences

How did you do? 1. a, b, c, d

Apply What You Have Learned

So that you can better understand EBP, throughout the remainder of the text you will be guided through a series of exercises designed to involve you in the EBP process. The clinical problem used in this exercise is hand hygiene. You will search for articles on your own; however, there will be instructions within this text's digital resources. As you progress through the process, you will critique the evidence and decide which best practice to recommend. You will also design a policy and evaluate outcomes. By actively engaging in this exercise, you will be well prepared to be a leader who successfully moves evidence to the point of care.

Imagine you are assigned to an EBP committee in a hospital. The committee has been charged with determining best practices for improving hand hygiene compliance. To become familiar with the magnitude of this problem, read the following article:

»   Mortell, M. (2012). Hand hygiene compliance: Is there a theory-practice-ethics gap? *Infection Control, 21*, 1011–1014.

After reading this article, think about your ethical obligation to patients regarding hand hygiene and best practices. View the World Health Organization (WHO) recommendations about hand hygiene at http://www.who.int/gpsc/5may/Hand_Hygiene_Why_How_and_When _Brochure.pdf?ua=1.

Next, formulate possible PICOT questions for this clinical problem.

RAPID REVIEW

»   Identifying clinical practice and research questions is a critical skill for nurses and health-care providers.

»   A research problem is an area of concern where there is a gap in knowledge. These are identified through personal clinical experience, professional literature, current practice theories, previous research, and national initiatives.

»   To narrow the problem of interest, it is best to select a problem that is of interest, can be answered by empirical testing, has not already been answered, or cannot be answered through basic problem-solving skills.

»   Problem statements identify what the study is about, while purpose statements indicate why the study is being conducted.

» Research questions are interrogatory statements that flow from the problem statement.

» Hypotheses are formal statements regarding the expected or predicted relationships between two or more variables in a specific population. Hypotheses can be associative, causal, simple, complex, nondirectional, directional, null, and research.

» Variables can be measured directly or indirectly.

» The independent variable, X, influences the dependent variable, Y, or outcome. In experimental studies, the intervention is the independent variable.

» The dependent variable is the outcome that is influenced by the independent variable.

» Mediators, moderators, and confounding variables are factors that interfere with relationships between independent and dependent variables.

» The purpose of research questions is to generate new knowledge, while the purpose of EBP questions is to make decisions about patient care.

» The PICOT model is commonly used to formulate EBP questions. PICOT stands for patient population, intervention of interest, comparison of interest, outcome of interest, and time.

» Ethical considerations associated with research questions involve formulating questions that are answered by studies that respect the rights of human subjects, are feasible, and are of interest.

REFERENCES

Bauman, A. E., Sallis, J. F., Dzewaltowski, D. A., & Owen, N. (2002). Toward a better understanding of the influences on physical activity: The role of determinants, correlates, causal variables, mediators, moderators, and confounders. *American Journal of Preventive Medicine, 23*(2S), 5–14.

Beck, A. T., Ward, C. H., Mendelson, M., Mock, J., & Erbaugh, J. (1961). An inventory for measuring depression. *Archives of General Psychiatry, 4*, 461–571.

Bennett, J. A. (2000). Mediator and moderator variables in nursing research: Conceptual and statistical differences. *Research in Nursing and Health, 23*, 415–420.

Forchuk, C. (1994). The orientation phase of the nurse–client relationship: Testing Peplau's theory. *Journal of Advanced Nursing, 20*(3), 532–537.

Forchuk, C. (1995). Development of nurse–client relationships: What helps. *Journal of American Psychiatric Nurses Association, 1*(5), 146–151.

Forchuk, C., & Reynolds, W. (2001). Clients' reflections on relationships with nurses: Comparisons from Canada and Scotland. *Journal of Psychiatric and Mental Health Nursing, 8*(1), 45–51.

Gillis, A., & Jackson, W. (2002). *Research for nurses: Methods and interpretation.* Philadelphia, PA: Davis.

Gray, J., Grove, S. K., & Sutherland, S. (2017). Burns and Grove's the practice of nursing research: Appraisal, synthesis and generation of evidence (8th ed.). Philadelphia, PA: Elsevier.

Hamilton, M. (1959). The assessment of anxiety states by rating. *British Journal of Medical Psychology, 32*(1), 50–55.

Higgins, J. P. T., & Green, S. (Eds.). (2011, March). *Cochrane handbook for systematic reviews of interventions* (Version 5.1.0). Cochrane Collaboration. Retrieved from http://www.cochrane-handbook.org

Holmes, T. H., & Rahe, R. H. (1967). Holmes-Rahe social readjustment rating scale. *Journal of Psychometric Research, 11*, 213–218.

Koehn, M. L. (2000). Alternative and complementary therapies for labor and birth: An application of Kolcaba's theory of holistic comfort. *Holistic Nursing Practice, 15*(1), 66–77.

Kolcaba, K. Y. (1992). Holistic comfort: Operationalizing the construct as a nurse-sensitive outcome. *Advanced Nursing Science, 15*(1), 1–10.

Kolcaba, K. Y. (1994). A theory of holistic comfort for nursing. *Journal of Advanced Nursing, 19*, 1178–1184.

Kolcaba, K. Y., & DiMarco, M. A. (2005). Comfort theory and its application to pediatric nursing. *Pediatric Nursing, 31*(3), 187–194.

Krause, M. R., Serlin, R. C., Ward, S. E., Rony, R. Y. Z., Ezenwa, M. O., & Naab, F. (2010). Testing mediation in nursing research: Beyond Baron and Kenny. *Nursing Research, 59*, 288–294.

Laughlin, M. J., & Lazarus, H. M. (2003). *Allogeneic stem cell transplantation: Clinical research and practice: Current clinical oncology.* Totowa, NJ: Humana Press.

March, A., & McCormack, D. (2009). Nursing theory–directed healthcare: Modifying Kolcaba's comfort theory as an institution-wide approach. *Holistic Nursing Practice, 23*(2), 75–80.

Melnyk, B. M., & Fineout-Overholt, E. (2014). *Evidence-based practice in nursing and healthcare: A guide to best practice* (3rd ed.). Philadelphia, PA: Lippincott Williams & Wilkins.

Mercer, R. T. (1986). Predictors of maternal role attainment at one year postbirth. *Western Journal of Nursing Research, 8*(1), 9–32.

Newman, M. A. (1986). *Health as expanding consciousness.* St. Louis, MO: Mosby.

Nieswiadomy, R. M. (2012). *Foundations of nursing research* (6th ed.). Upper Saddle River, NJ: Prentice Hall.

Norwood, S. L. (2000). *Research strategies for advanced practice nurses.* Upper Saddle River, NJ: Prentice Hall.

Orem, D. E. (2001). *Nursing: Concepts of practice* (6th ed.). St. Louis, MO: Mosby.

Parse, R. R. (1981). *Man-living-health: A theory of nursing.* New York, NY: Wiley.

Parse, R. R. (1992). Human becoming: Parse's theory of nursing. *Nursing Science Quarterly, 5*, 35–42.

Pender, N. J. (1997). Health promotion: An emerging science for self-care and professional care. *Quality Nursing, 3*(5), 449–454.

Peplau, H. E. (1952). *Interpersonal relations in nursing.* New York, NY: Putnam.

Resnick, B., & Nigg, C. (2003). Testing a theoretical model of exercise behavior for older adults. *Nursing Research, 52*(2), 80–88.

Rogers, M. (1980). Nursing: A science of unitary man. In J. P. Riehl & C. Roy (Eds.), *Conceptual models for nursing practice* (2nd ed., pp. 329–337). New York, NY: Appleton-Century-Crofts.

Roy, C. (1970). Adaptation: A conceptual framework for nursing. *Nursing Outlook, 18*, 42–45.

At the end of this chapter, you will be able to:

< Explain why performing a quality literature review is an essential skill for nursing students, researchers, and nurses

< Differentiate between searching for evidence and literature in lay and professional sources

< Explain the scientific literature publication cycle

< Differentiate between primary and secondary sources

< Identify different types of articles found in the literature

< Characterize the four major types of reviews

< Identify and use a variety of sources, both within and outside of the field of nursing, as appropriate

< Explain how the sources are structured

< Distinguish between the different sources' content, in both topic or subject matter and in format

< Perform various types of searches using basic and advanced source tools and search techniques

< List four databases where scholarly literature of disciplines is indexed

< Consider the ethical presentation and application of evidence

KEY TERMS

Boolean operators
call number
CINAHL
citation chasing
controlled vocabularies
electronic indexes
exploding
grey literature
indexes
integrative review
interlibrary loan
journal
keyword
magazine

meta-analyses
narrative reviews
nesting
peer review
periodical
plagiarism
popular literature
positional operators
precision
primary sources
print index
qualification
recall
record

scholarly literature
scientific literature
    publication cycle
search field
secondary sources
stopwords
subject headings
subject searching
systematic reviews
trade literature
truncation
wildcards

CHAPTER 4

Finding Sources of Evidence

Patricia Mileham

4.1 Purpose of Finding Evidence

At the end of this section, you will be able to:

‹ Explain why performing a quality literature review is an essential skill for nursing students, researchers, and nurses

‹ Differentiate between searching for evidence and literature in lay and professional sources

Most often, your first introduction to the literature review is tied to writing an academic paper. The focus of your papers as an undergraduate student is usually one of gathering information on a topic and perhaps sharing a resulting opinion about the findings. The literature review provides a consideration of what has been studied previously. For researchers, the literature review identifies gaps in the current research, highlights areas of needed change, increases awareness about practice, and helps sharpen and focus a research question. Because of the increasing emphasis on evidence-based practice (EBP), nurses must develop abilities to perform literature reviews to increase knowledge about a specific topic and provide the basis for an informed, professional opinion to champion EBP in clinical settings.

Knowing how to search for, access, and evaluate information is as important to your successful practice tomorrow as it is to earning a good grade on an academic paper today. In an insightful editorial directed to nursing faculty, Christie, Hamill, and Power (2012) specifically detailed the contextual support students should be provided in learning about research: "The educator has a key role in supporting and guiding

FYI

Research questions and practice considerations must be based on informed, ethical opinions resulting from consideration of evidence that is currently available. This requires a detailed review of the literature.

students in: the nature of research-evidence (authority), the type of research required in clinical practice (relevance), the potential power of research to transform, and improve practice (utility)" (p. 2792).

Lander (2005) further details the ties between research and EBP by delineating competencies nursing students should possess to complete this connection themselves:

> They need to know what sources of information are reliable and credible and how to gain access to them. They need some specific skills that enable them to comprehend designs and specific design issues. They need to know how to differentiate poor quality from good quality reports of studies, systematic reviews, and clinical guidelines. They need an approach for assessing the value of an intervention for clinical practice. Above all, they need access to computers and technical resources. (p. 300)

These are competencies needed to perform quality literature reviews, not just an academic exercise left behind when your diploma is in hand.

Whether you are performing a literature review for the 1st, 15th, or 50th time, consider it a part of your practice worth doing well every time. Just as patients are assessed before treatment recommendations are made, literature reviews are assessments of topics before the research or practice continues. Whether the literature review is part of an EBP proposal in your workplace, a research question in your graduate studies, or an academic paper as an undergraduate, the process is the same. Depending on the situation, search complexity and access to resources may be different; however, the procedural steps and attention to quality work remain the same. This is because the desired outcome stays the same: Research questions or practice considerations must be based on informed, ethical opinions resulting from consideration of evidence that is currently available.

With ever-increasing amounts of information available via the Internet and the proliferation of journal and monograph materials, skilled literature review practices have never been more necessary. Although it is well known that anyone can publish anything on the Internet, today's more sophisticated tools, such as wikis and blogs, increase the challenge of evaluating the validity of information. Information of all types travels rapidly from source to source. This results in mixing hoaxes, urban legends, and other types of misinformation along with accurate and reliable information. Nurses face this situation not only as information consumers but also as patient advocates. Patients are bombarded with information as well. Their desire to be knowledgeable about their illnesses and health care often makes them even more vulnerable to misinformation. Most patients do not have the knowledge base nurses have to evaluate information and make informed decisions. As Gilmour, Scott, and Huntington (2008) note:

> Nurses in our study were concerned about the quality of Internet health information, judged by criteria such as the use of research-based evidence, evidence of peer review, named authors and currency of information. Their evaluative practices were in sharp contrast to the findings by Fox (2006) that 75% of public health information-seeker respondents (n = 2928) checked the source and date only sometimes at best. (p. 27)

Books such as *The Patient Safety Perspective: Health Information and Resources Online and in Print* (Burt, 2013), *The Knowledgeable Patient: Communication and Participation in Health* (Hill & Cochrane Collection, 2011), *Health Technology Literacy: A Transdisciplinary Framework for Consumer-Oriented Practice* (Jordan-Marsh, 2011), and *Surviving Health Care: A Manual for Patients and Their Families* (Kimbrough Kushner, 2010) provide nurses with an insightful understanding of the structure and use of healthcare resources available on the Internet. Resources such as these position nurses to assist patients with obtaining accurate information.

Nurses have an ethical responsibility to skillfully use all tools and resources available. Not everything is, or will ever be, available electronically. Nurses should be aware of and use print materials that are still current and viable. Conversely, because not all electronic resources based on print resources are comprehensive and some contain older or archival information, research questions can take reviewers back to older print journals or *indexes*.

Many reputable government, organizational, and educational resources are available on the Internet (sites that are free and accessible to all), such as Valparaiso University Christopher Center Library's Nursing Libguide: Evidence-Based Practice Resource (http://libguides.valpo.edu/content .php?pid=42078&sid=337662) and the University of Washington Health Sciences Library's Evidence-Based Practice LibGuide (http://guides.lib.uw.edu /friendly.php?s=hsl/ebp). There are also many restricted resources, such as literature databases (often paid for by a school or hospital) and resources within organizational sites available only to members. These restricted resources usually contain professional literature that has been compiled, sorted, indexed, and made available. Content in these resources is written for professional colleagues, not for the lay person or the consumer. It is not unreasonable to expect nurses to be well versed in both the professional and lay perspectives, using professional resources to keep current about practice while also helping patients as consumers of health care.

Access to academic, health sciences, or hospital library resources is vital to quality literature review. Because each library and database has its own best

KEY TERM

indexes: A listing of electronic or print resources

practice procedures, initial time spent orienting with an expert about these systems is worthwhile. Just as nursing faculty are subject content experts, librarians are searching and system experts.

TEST YOUR KNOWLEDGE 4-1

1. Learning to perform a quality literature review is essential for which of the following reasons? (Select all that apply.)

   a. Lays the foundation for writing quality undergraduate academic papers
   b. Identifies gaps in current research
   c. Provides the basis for making best practice decisions
   d. Develops skills necessary for lifelong learning

True/False

2. All sources retrieved from the Internet are applicable to EBP.

3. Access to computers and technical resources is critical to link research to EBP.

4. Librarians are searching and system experts.

5. All useful resources on the Web are free and accessible to all.

How did you do? 1. a, b, c, d; 2. F; 3. T; 4. T; 5. F

4.2 Types of Evidence

At the end of this section, you will be able to:

‹ Explain the scientific literature publication cycle
‹ Differentiate between primary and secondary sources
‹ Identify different types of articles found in the literature
‹ Characterize the four major types of reviews

Not all information is created equal, nor is it presented in the same manner. Being able to identify various types of information and sources is fundamental to starting a successful literature review search.

KEY TERM

scientific literature publication cycle: A model describing how research becomes disseminated in publications

Scientific Literature Publication Cycle

It is helpful first to consider the *scientific literature publication cycle* to make searching easier (University of Washington Libraries, 1999). As shown in **Figure 4-1**, the cycle generally begins with the idea and the research itself, which is available only informally through raw data reports, grant proposals,

FIGURE 4-1	The Scientific Publication Cycle

1 Develop and discuss ideas to begin preliminary research through raw data reports, grant proposals, and conference papers.

2 Researchers prepare findings and presentations for the publication of a professional, scholarly paper.

3 Papers are accepted by editors of scholarly journals and indexed in literature indexes and databases.

4 Papers move into a less professional publication format, such as reviews or magazines. They are summarized or compiled with other like-topic papers to be searched for by a general audience.

5 The most noteworthy information from the paper may be cited in textbooks or reference materials.

and perhaps as-yet-unpublished conference papers. At the next point, when researchers are confident in the findings and their presentations, information is prepared for dissemination as professional, scholarly papers. Papers judged to be of high quality about studies using sound research methods are accepted by editors of scholarly journals and indexed in literature indexes and databases so that others may find them when conducting literature searches. After this point, papers, or information contained within them, move into a more generalized publication format where they may be summarized or compiled with other like-topic papers. They are typically published in reviews or magazines directed toward a wider, less professionally focused audience. Finally, if findings are considered noteworthy, they may be cited in textbooks or reference materials, such as encyclopedias or bibliographies.

Keeping the scientific literature publication cycle in mind, you might now realize that when looking for the most current, authoritative information on a topic, you should be checking the published, scholarly literature. If the goal is to compare evidence, systematic reviews are a useful way to locate similar topics quickly. By keeping in mind the publication dates of the studies contained in the systematic review, you can complete the search by searching for evidence published during time spans not covered by the systematic review.

Making Sense of Types of Evidence in the Literature

Evidence in the literature can be categorized in a variety of ways. Nurses find that understanding the terms associated with these categories is helpful when making decisions about evidence. Evidence can be categorized as: (1) primary or secondary, (2) peer reviewed or not peer reviewed, and (3) scholarly, trade, or popular.

Primary and Secondary Sources

Primary sources present original information by the person or people responsible for creating it. Paintings, speeches, diary entries, autobiographies, and interviews are some common examples. In the world of research, however, primary sources are the journal articles, book chapters, dissertations, or conference proceedings written by the people involved in the original research. Primary sources always provide full references to other works cited within the paper. *Secondary sources* are the resulting commentaries, summaries, reviews, or interpretations of primary sources. Always written after primary sources are presented, and often written by those not involved in the original work, secondary sources can provide new insights or historical perspectives not previously available. Some common secondary sources are textbooks, systematic reviews, biographies, and general magazines. Secondary sources often do not cite the work of others.

For example, an original research paper on Internet use by patients with diabetes was published in the scholarly journal *Nursing Research*. This publication of the paper is considered to be a primary source. Several weeks later, *Newsweek* published a more general article about the effect of the Internet on patient education. In this article, results from the original paper published in *Nursing Research* were mentioned along with a short quote. This article constitutes a secondary source about the original research conducted. Sometimes it is important to eliminate secondary sources because of the bias inherent when someone other than the original researcher provides the information. When creating EBP, nurses should always read primary sources and draw their own conclusions.

Peer-Reviewed and Refereed Sources

Research and empirical papers published as primary sources in scholarly literature undergo rigorous evaluation by experts and editors, which is known as *peer review* or refereed judging. Subject significance, methods, and conclusions

KEY TERMS

primary sources: Original information presented by the person or people responsible for creating it

secondary sources: Commentaries, summaries, reviews, or interpretations of primary sources; often written by those not involved in the original work

peer review: When experts and editors rigorously evaluate a manuscript submitted for publication

are judged by peer reviewers. When papers meet established criteria, they are accepted for publication. This process is designed to ensure high quality of published works and enables readers who are not experts about the topic to have confidence in what is being presented.

Scholarly, Trade, and Popular Literature Categories

Distinguishing between different types of information categories can help determine the type of information contained within them. There are generally three broad categories: *scholarly*, *trade*, and *popular literature*. Scholarly works are written and edited by professionals in the discipline for other colleagues. They are the vehicles for publication of original research, focus on narrow topics within the discipline, and are often filled with discipline-specific vocabulary. For example, the *Journal of Nursing Scholarship*, published by Sigma Theta Tau International, is a scholarly journal. Trade publications are also written for professionals within a discipline but are written with a more casual tone. They contain information related to professional development, products, practices, or trends in the discipline. *American Journal of Nursing* and *RN Magazine* are examples of trade publications. Popular literature is written to inform or entertain the general public. The writing level is very basic, and graphics often get as much space as the text. For example, *Prevention* is a source of information about health that is written for the general public.

Periodicals, Journals, and Magazines

Few terms used in libraries cause more confusion than these three: *periodicals*, *journals*, and *magazines*. Although some people use these terms as synonyms, it is best to understand the differences between these terms and to use them correctly. *Periodical* is the broadest term of the three and indicates a resource that is published periodically, usually on a set schedule. In many libraries, *periodical* is the term used to designate these types of publications as a collection. Both journals and magazines are designated as periodicals. *Journal* is the term used to indicate resources of a scholarly or professional nature. *Magazine* indicates a resource targeted for the general reading audience, most often in the popular works category. When you have difficulty distinguishing among these three types of resources, a quick consultation with a librarian or a search of a library website for information about this topic can be helpful.

Understanding Types of Reviews

Before the electronic information age, researchers developed ways to keep up-to-date by creating early forms of reviews to summarize information. Because of the increased volume of information being made available as a result of

KEY TERMS

scholarly literature: Works written and edited by professionals in the discipline for other colleagues

trade literature: Works written for professionals in a discipline using a more casual tone than used in scholarly literature

popular literature: Works written to inform or entertain the general public

periodical: A resource that is published on a set schedule

journal: A scholarly or professional resource

magazine: A resource targeted to the general reading audience

information technology, there is some cause for concern. Hawker, Payne, Kerr, Hardey, and Powell (2002) make the concern clear:

> Both reviews and the results of primary research are now being used as bases for health care decisions. However, despite this expansion, the quality of literature reviews varies widely, particularly across academic disciplines, and the standard of some published reviews remains poor (Evans & Kowanko, 2000). If reviews are to be considered as evidence and seen as research in their own right, then it follows that the rigor that is expected of primary research must also be applied to literature reviews. (pp. 1284–1285)

Consider the implications of a poorly conducted summary when contrasting the academic and clinical settings. When literature reviews conducted for academic papers lack precision and quality searching, the results often lead to a lower grade. Likewise, when nurses consider decisions about EBP, a poorly conducted literature review may negatively affect patient care.

Reviews can be conducted in a variety of ways. In an article that has become definitive in this field, Whittemore (2005) detailed differences among the major types of reviews. Echoing concerns of Hawker and colleagues (2002), Whittemore also noted that the "literature search stage is a critical element to conducting a quality research review because incomplete and biased searches result in an inadequate database for the review and the potential for faulty conclusions" (p. 58). To make good decisions about best practice, nurses should familiarize themselves with the major types of reviews: narrative, integrative, meta-analysis, and systematic.

Narrative Reviews

Narrative reviews are the most traditional type of review, thus the most familiar. These kinds of reviews are frequently found in trade publications. Because writers judge which works to include and exclude, narrative reviews are subjective. These reviews are often based on only the common or uncommon elements of the various works, and writers are not particularly concerned with widely varying research methods, designs, or settings. For example, the review of literature section in most published articles is a traditional narrative review.

Integrative Reviews

Jackson (1980) defined an *integrative review* as "generalizations about substantive issues from a set of studies directly bearing on those issues" (p. 438). Integrative reviews are scholarly papers that synthesize published studies and articles to answer questions about phenomena of interest. They are typically found in peer-reviewed professional publications. Ganong (1987) is credited with clarifying the steps of conducting integrative reviews in nursing. Ganong's article provided a grid layout that many find useful as a tool to track and compile data from various research papers. Components of the grid include methods, theories, and empirical findings of the reviewed papers. These grids are often included in published integrative reviews. Whittemore (2005) noted that an advantage to integrative reviews "is the ability to combine data from different types of research designs and include theoretical, as well as, empirical literature" (p. 57). In other words, integrative reviews do not need to include works that use the same designs or research methods.

Meta-Analyses

Meta-analyses combine results of studies into a measurable format and statistically estimate the effects of proposed interventions. Often, individual studies about an intervention fail to show statistical significance. But when the results from multiple studies are combined in one large analysis, results may show that the intervention is beneficial (Choi & Lam, 2016). For example, suppose there are 10 studies about the effect of yoga on blood pressure, but none of the studies showed that yoga reduced blood pressure. However, when the results are pooled, data analysis showed statistical significance; then, it could be concluded that yoga can reduce blood pressure. Unlike in an integrative review, meta-analyses include works that are similar or identical so that statistical comparisons can be made. Another difference between these two types of reviews is that meta-analyses include both published and unpublished works. Evans and Kowanko (2000) surmised that meta-analysis reviews grew from narrative reviews when the increasing amounts of numerical data grew too cumbersome. According to Whittemore (2005), meta-analyses are especially useful as sources of evidence when large randomized trials are not feasible.

Systematic Reviews

Systematic reviews combine elements of the three previously discussed methods. These are "scientific tools which are used to summarize and communicate the results and implications of otherwise unmanageable quantities of research" (Evans & Kowanko, 2000, p. 35). Articles included in systematic reviews all address the same clinical problem. "A well-specified clinical question, use of the best available evidence, explicit methods, and an exhaustive search for relevant primary studies are hallmarks of this method" (Whittemore, 2005, p. 58). Systematic reviews adhere to strict eligibility criteria so that bias can be minimized and reliable conclusions can be made (Higgins & Green, 2011). Systematic reviews, combined with other types of guidelines, are sources that can be helpful in situations when evidence is needed quickly. A brief editorial by Cowell (2012) provides a comparative overview of these types of reviews as well as ways in which to assess the quality of such reviews.

KEY TERMS

meta-analyses: A scholarly paper that combines results of studies, both published and unpublished, into a measurable format and statistically estimates the effects of proposed interventions

systematic reviews: Rigorous and systematic syntheses of research findings about a clinical problem

TEST YOUR KNOWLEDGE 4-2

1. Put the following points of the scientific literature publication cycle in order.

   a. Finding cited in textbook
   b. Paper accepted for publication in scholarly journal
   c. Idea for research identified
   d. Article cited in indexes in databases
   e. Findings included in magazine article

2. Which of the following are primary sources? (Select all that apply.)

   a. Biography
   b. Systematic review
   c. Research article
   d. Dissertation

3. Which of the following journals are considered scholarly journals? (Select all that apply.)

   a. *Nursing Research*
   b. *RN Magazine*
   c. *American Journal of Nursing*
   d. *Journal of Nursing Scholarship*

4. What is a review that synthesizes only published articles to answer questions about phenomena of interest?

   a. Narrative review
   b. Integrative review
   c. Meta-analysis
   d. Systematic review

How did you do? 1. c, b, d, e, a; 2. c, d; 3. a, d; 4. b

4.3 How Sources Are Organized

At the end of this section, you will be able to:

‹ Identify and use a variety of sources, both within and outside of the field of nursing, as appropriate
‹ Explain how the sources are structured
‹ Distinguish between the different sources' content, in both topic or subject matter and in format

Consider your first clinical experience with a patient. Before that experience, you were educated about various aspects of patient care and equipment. No one just handed you a stethoscope and a blood pressure cuff and wished you luck.

Most likely, you first read about the various procedures, learned what to expect in typical situations, and then practiced in a laboratory setting. Learning to search for information can be approached in a similar way. Gaining insight about how information resources are structured, what their contents contain, and what search techniques work best increases your skill and efficiency.

> **FYI**
>
> To create an EBP, nurses must be aware of information retrieval options. Librarians are an excellent resource for becoming an effective researcher.

Many factors come into play when conducting a search of the literature. What interests you about the topic should determine the depth and breadth of the search, which sources to search, and the dates of publication to include. Immediate access to sources being sought is not always possible. Sometimes it may take several weeks to acquire sources, while other sources may be unobtainable. Knowing this encourages implementing strategies to ensure that you are able to meet deadlines.

After the research question is developed, the researcher is ready to proceed through the steps of the literature review process. Using selected search words and terms based on the topic, the researcher searches databases, organizes search results, locates full content of the materials, and evaluates the evidence for its usefulness. Being aware of these steps focuses attention on the process and results.

When information applicable to the subject has been gathered, it is important to keep in mind that the process might not be finished. It is not usual for individuals to quit at this point, satisfied that the information they have gathered will somehow work within their needs. Carefully reviewing obtained materials to ensure that they are appropriate can save time and money. Reexamine the original focus and search strategy to ensure that the information obtained is indeed useful. If it is not, determine where the search was flawed and decide whether a new search is necessary.

Finally, make sure that the information gathered is scholarly. Information should be written by knowledgeable authors, published by respected sources, and be appropriately current. The content of information should always be evaluated, appraised on criteria such as intended audience, depth of coverage, objectivity, and related reviews. When you are unsure of the credibility of information, nursing faculty or librarians can provide guidance.

Consult with an Information Resources Expert

Working with a librarian is guaranteed to save you time. Using a systematic review to support their claim, Weightman and Williamson (2005) noted that "there is evidence that library services can lead to time savings for healthcare professionals and, thus, to cost savings and health-care benefits" (p. 5). Few others on a campus or in a healthcare institution know as much about information structure, storage, retrieval, and evaluation as librarians do. Most academic libraries have subject-specialty librarians for specific disciplines, and at health sciences libraries, new roles are emerging that make librarians more specialized (Cooper & Crum, 2013). Whereas reference desk inquiries are appropriate for general questions, an appointment with a subject-specialty librarian is the best way to obtain specific information in a shorter amount of time.

> Impactful use of librarians and library resources isn't limited to academic study. In 1992, hospital librarians in Rochester, New York, initiated what has since become known as "The Rochester Study" in their quest to assess whether or not having a hospital library impacts patient care. "It demonstrated that in the eyes of the information users (in this case, physicians) that library services were valued and that the provided information was seen as making a positive difference in patient care. The Rochester study has been heavily cited, achieving a prominent influence in the field, not only among librarians, but also in the medical literature." (Dunn, Brewer, Marshall, & Sollenberger, 2009, p. 308)

Systematic reviews and other studies, such as "The Health Information Literacy Project," continue to consider and evaluate the value of library use and resources in positively influencing patient care.

To create an EBP, nurses must be aware of information retrieval options. Hospitals often support library resources and a librarian. Academic or health sciences libraries, especially at state-funded institutions, may allow community members access to their holdings. Academic libraries are especially useful because they have strong collections in the scholarly literature, while public libraries have more consumer-oriented materials.

Looking at the Structure of Sources

When information sources are organized using basic principles of consistent record formatting and field labels, searchers can rely on finding similar information each time they perform the same search, even if new information has been added to the system. For example, if the keyword *anxiety* is entered into a database, the searcher would expect the search to yield information such as author, title of article, year of publication, and the abstract each time the keyword is entered. Each time *anxiety* is entered, the same sources should be seen. If any new sources have been added to the database since the previous search, these should also appear.

Considering familiar organizational structures of sources will help in understanding more complex systems. Perhaps the first organizational system you ever learned was the alphabet. Children in kindergarten learn to line up in alphabetical order according to their last names. They do not line up according to height or hair color because those system labels are not as straightforward and consistent as the alphabet is. The phone book is another example of a structure for organizing information. The white pages are arranged in alphabetical order. This is a very effective way to organize information when one knows the name of the business one is seeking. The yellow pages offer another organizational structure for searching. Subject listings in the yellow pages were created so that if one knows the type of business, but not its name, the information can be found. The key to using the yellow pages, though, is to know exactly what terms the creators used for the subject areas. For example, if you need a haircut, would you use "hair," "barber," or "beauty shop" as a keyword? Although this example might seem very elementary right now, understanding how the phone book is organized will be beneficial when considering the most common types of electronic searches.

Structures can also be designed to organize physical objects. For example, in bookstores, books are organized in subject areas around the store, and within each area, they are perhaps grouped into subcategories and shelved by the author's last name. Libraries are arranged in the same manner, but, because there are many more books to organize, a consistent number or letter/number combination system is used. Most public and school libraries use the Dewey decimal system, while most academic libraries in the United States use the Library of Congress system. Many health sciences libraries use the National Library of Medicine system. Here too, when the books are in their general subject areas, they are then categorized into smaller subcategories and shelved according to the author's last name. In the library system, every item has its own unique *call number* according to its subject area and author's last name. No other item will have that same number. Familiarity with the system and knowing which system the library uses make searching for sources more efficient.

Knowing general call numbers of a subject can also expedite searches for items in a library collection. For example, in academic libraries using the Library of Congress method, medical books are located within the R area shelves and nursing books are on the RT shelves. Further knowledge of what subjects the numbers connote can lead to more detailed browsing, such as knowing that the nursing research texts' section is RT 81.5, while writings about nursing history are on the RT 31 shelves. Call numbers for specific books are easily found through searching the library's catalog.

Although the structure used in libraries is quite efficient for locating sources, confusion can occur when sources can be classified in more than one way. Information on a specific topic might be scattered throughout the collection. For example, in a search for sources on the topic of ethical practices and how they relate to health care, it is helpful to browse multiple areas, such as nursing ethics, medical philosophy, medical ethics, law of the United States, and medical legislation.

KEY TERM

call number: Unique identification number assigned to items in a library by subject and author name

Other structures aid in finding information. For example, the table of contents in a book helps readers find information located within the text without having to read every single page. The table of contents narrows the search from hundreds of pages to perhaps 20 or 30 pages. The search can be narrowed even further by using the index, which provides a very detailed listing of subjects contained in the book. The index can narrow the search to a few pages.

The concept of indexes has proved to be a very useful structure to assist researchers with finding scholarly articles and reports. Prior to the electronic age, printed indexes of professional literature covering only the information in one particular discipline provided listings of all information produced in that discipline in a specific time span. For nursing, the most recognized and used *print index* was started in the 1940s and was known as the *Cumulative Index to Nursing and Allied Health Literature*. Today, nurses use the electronic version known as *CINAHL*. *Electronic indexes* are most commonly referred to as databases.

In the print indexes, information is organized three ways: author listings, title listings, and subject listings. In early print indexes, subject listings offered a new organizational structure. Publishers of the indexes began to choose keywords that would always represent the subject regardless of the words used by authors. For example, the term *heart attack* is always listed as "myocardial infarction." The consistent use of keywords provided a solid foundation for the electronic searching conducted today.

With the advent of electronic resources and the Internet, another type of searching became possible. Searching does not need to be limited to keywords because entire bodies of text can be searched. This is known as *keyword* searching. This type of searching in electronic databases allows searching for the author's words, not the subject terms assigned by the database publisher. Keyword searching is not without its challenges. For example, the word *diet* as it is used by the general public usually is defined as a meal plan to lose weight. Healthcare professionals typically use the word *diet* to refer to meal plans that are therapeutic for patients. When conducting a keyword search, entering "diet" will achieve different results depending on the source. Keyword searches also provide results that are exactly what the searcher intends, or not, depending on how the word is used in the text. The source searched does not know the searcher's intent; it only knows what term has been entered.

As electronic search options and resources increase and become integral to today's practice, journal publishers and librarians collaborate to create methods of assisting authors in promoting their articles and researchers in finding them. Grant (2010) detailed the creation of keyword lists, resources that are becoming especially useful when searching for scholarly works on the open Internet. The piece also provides a quick glimpse of the publishing methods of a journal in which submitted articles are reviewed for accuracy and quality while the publisher adds content-rich data that in turn increases findability of articles for keyword searching. Using authoritative keyword lists can save time, whether on the open Internet or when using an institution's databases.

The Internet, while an accessible source of abundant information, has a very unorganized and inconsistent structure. Tools that are comparable to those used in electronic databases are being developed to support Internet searching. Google Scholar and the advanced search options for Google and other Internet search systems give users specific search options, such as searching for phrases, broad subject areas, and document types. As with all organizational structures, knowing how to use the tool results in more productive searches.

Being aware of these simple facts can facilitate searching in indexes and databases. As mentioned earlier, not all electronic resources that were once in print format are comprehensive in their coverage. They may go back in the literature only 20 to 25 years. Foundational or key studies could be missed if they were conducted prior to the date the electronic database began. Keep in mind the frequency with which the database is updated. For example, a database updated monthly will not yield a new search on a daily basis. Searches can be programmed to be performed regularly so that new literature is identified when it is added to the database. Practicing this as a student prepares you to find evidence for implementing best practice.

Databases: The Same but Different

There are variations in databases just as there are variations in the human body. In healthy people there are variations in height, weight, age, and appearance, but overall their organ systems perform in the same manner. Databases also vary in appearance (color, graphics, results display) even though content is the same or very similar. Understanding how a search strategy works in one database can be helpful in understanding how to use another database. If the results of a database search are unsatisfactory, the help feature can offer guidance. Also, it is important to be sure that your topic area fits with the database. For example, when you look for information about anxiety, there may be more citations in a database such as PsycINFO compared to CINAHL (McGrath, Brown, & Samra, 2012).

The fact that not all databases are provided by the same information vendor can be a source of confusion. Consider the many different fast food restaurants that offer variations of the hamburger. Each company touts a special bun, sauce, or grade of hamburger. In the same way, vendors who provide access to the same databases do so in various manners. Companies such as EBSCOhost, Ovid, SilverPlatter, Elsevier, and Thomson Gale purchase database content from the original creator and sell the content with their own design, search options, and date ranges. For example, suppose you are using CINAHL in the EBSCOhost system and a friend at another institution is using it through the Ovid system.

Although the content and search strategies the two of you use will be similar, your resulting searches and appearance of the screens will be very different.

Another cause of confusion for users and librarians alike is that content may change in a database. These changes are caused by interactions among vendors and journal publishers who provide the articles. Sources available in full text one day may be found in a citation-only option the next. When this happens, it may not be the result of errors made while searching. Talking to a librarian may resolve the situation and result in obtaining the information desired.

Topic and Subject Matter

Information about scholarly literature of disciplines is collected and indexed in subject-specific databases, such as CINAHL. Not much, if any, popular-content works are contained in these databases. Additionally, information about works yet to be published, called *grey literature*, includes unpublished reports, conference papers, and grant proposals. Grey literature is often indicative of upcoming hot topics in the field. Databases can also cite professional information, such as organizational guidelines, editorial essays, and letters to the editor. For example, commentaries on author works that have generated controversy can be useful sources.

General content databases offer a mix of scholarly, trade, and popular works. Professional journals, popular magazines, newspapers, and industry bulletins may all be part of the search results (unless you limit the search accordingly). These databases are helpful for gathering information on current news events, government reports, and healthcare topics from the consumer point of view.

Databases also contain citations useful to patient education. In the healthcare literature, distinctions are made between consumer health materials and patient education materials. Consumer health materials are general articles about topics such as maintaining a healthy lifestyle. Patient education materials are items designed to assist patients in making informed decisions regarding their medical care. Nurses are often asked to decipher what patients hear in the news and to refer consumers to additional, reliable information sources.

Format

In print and electronic information sources, the basic building block is called a *record*. Each piece of information contained in the record has been entered into what is referred to as a *search field*, which makes electronic searching possible. Each record minimally consists of a citation of information and a record number. Citations provide author name, title, publication date, and, depending on the type of item, publisher information and page numbers. Citations are the minimal amount of information needed to locate items, and they contain information required for a reference list. Record numbers, similar to call numbers for books, are numbers assigned by the information source and are unique to each record.

Depending on the information source, other fields of information may be available for the citation. Subject terms and *subject headings* are often listed. An abstract may be included and is helpful to quickly determine the item's content. Sometimes references cited in the item are also included in the format. Reference information can be helpful for locating other relevant information. Other fields might be added to the record, such as text language, type of publication, or designation of whether the research is evidence based or peer reviewed. Whereas all databases offer citations, these come in three formats: citation only, citation with full content, or a mix of both. Because print indexes are citation only, an additional step is required to obtain the full content. Most electronic information sources are mixed. Very few databases provide only full-content records, and they are the exception rather than the rule. Because librarians understand the need to have full content available as easily as possible, systems have been created to meet that need. These systems basically tie citations in one database to full content available in other databases or to print resources within the library. If a hyperlink in the record is available to link to full content, no additional step is needed.

When items are not available in full content within any database or within library print holdings, a copy of the item can be retrieved through the *interlibrary loan* system. For your convenience, most records provide a hyperlink to interlibrary loan request forms so that requests can be made immediately when you determine that an item is not available locally. Most of the time, this service is subsidized by the library and is available at no cost. Because it usually takes 7 to 10 days after making a request to receive materials, it is prudent to begin searches well before deadlines. Journal articles are usually copied and sent to the requester to keep. Books, videos, and other such items are sent on loan and must be returned to the lending library. Because each library's procedure is slightly different, it is important to understand how to request materials prior to needing this service. You might not receive everything requested because copyright issues, limited numbers of available copies, and other restrictions can affect requests.

KEY TERMS

subject headings:
A set of controlled vocabulary used to classify materials; organization of databases according to topic

interlibrary loan:
A service whereby libraries provide items in their collections to each other upon request; lending of items through a network of libraries

TEST YOUR KNOWLEDGE 4-3

True/False

1. All libraries use the same system for organizing their collections.
2. Tables of contents and indexes can be useful to narrow searches for evidence.
3. Knowing key terms used in an index can facilitate effective searches.

How did you do? 1. F; 2. T; 3. T

4.4 How to Search for Evidence

At the end of this section, you will be able to:

‹ Perform various types of searches using basic and advanced source tools and search techniques

‹ List four databases where scholarly literature of disciplines is indexed

FYI

Knowing a variety of search techniques—such as use of keywords, Boolean operators, and truncation—is essential to effective research, while accessing the most reliable databases ensures EBP.

Access to Content: Tools and Techniques

There are three types of access to information: free access, access paid by an institution, and access paid by an individual. Most electronic sources provided by the U.S. government are free access. Most libraries grant free access to their holdings to those physically present. If the item is available for borrowing, a library card is needed to check out the item. Although these services are provided to patrons for free, the library is paying the costs. Nurses can often access resources for free at their places of work. Like libraries, the healthcare organization is charged to provide the services. Regardless, access to electronic sources is being paid for by someone. For example, a nurse who is self-employed may have to subscribe as an individual to access CINAHL.

General Search Strategies

Searching for evidence does take time, but knowing the organization of the system and doing a search correctly can improve efficiency (Cleary, Hunt, & Horsfall, 2009; McGrath et al., 2012). Novice searchers often begin by searching for a specific type of document, such as a nursing research article reporting outcomes of an experimental study. Although it is good to have an idea of the evidence that you would like to find, do not discount other evidence uncovered during the search. Sometimes a continuing education article that mentions a particular study or a literature review in an article on a related topic may provide sources not found through other methods of searching.

Another helpful strategy to locate evidence is to build searches both backward and forward in time. This is sometimes called *citation chasing*. For example, a nurse locates a single article about community preparations for bioterrorism. The nurse examines the references listed to determine whether other sources on this topic seem to stand out as foundational or noteworthy. If so, the nurse obtains these sources and proceeds to appraise their reference lists as well. This strategy is an effective way to search previous literature and often identifies the articles

KEY TERM

citation chasing: Using a reference list to identify sources of evidence that were first published about the topic. Forward searching strategies are made possible by electronic databases. For example, the nurse enters information for a single article and uses a hyperlink option "times cited in this database." This link connects to other documents that have cited that article since its publication.

Hints for Searching Print Indexes

Because of the convenience of electronic resources, most individuals are unfamiliar with print indexes. Typically, print indexes are used to search for older literature that has not been indexed in electronic databases. Therefore, perhaps the best strategy when using print indexes is to ask a librarian for help. Librarians are familiar with the sources and know which sources will be most useful. Because older print resources are primarily organized by time, usually in spans of a year or two, knowing the years to search can help immensely. Keeping in mind that search terms change over time is also important when using print indexes. For example, whereas "patient education" is the correct subject term today, if searching records created before 1988, the correct term is "health education, information services."

Hints for Searching Electronic Databases

Parameters of recall and precision provide conceptual baselines for refining search strategies in electronic databases. The successful integration of these parameters results in retrieved records that more closely match the desired focus and number of sources.

Recall describes the broad "catch" of retrieved records. Those records, usually high in number, display a wide range of what has been classified as related records. Recall is a strategy best used when the information being sought is uniquely detailed, a new topic or procedure, or has not been widely written about in the literature. Gathering a large number of records ensures that the information needed is somewhere within them, even though many of the records retrieved will not be relevant.

Precision is a search strategy that narrows the parameters of the search. When a search term displays a precise retrieval, the records are usually smaller in number but more closely matched to the entered search terms. This search strategy is best when the information being sought has been written about in a number of authoritative sources by a number of knowledgeable people. The search can be narrowed without undue concern about the loss of some relevant records because it is likely that the search contained needed information in the retrieved records.

An effective technique, especially for novices whose skills are not yet finely tuned, is to combine these search strategies. Beginning with a recall strategy

KEY TERMS

recall: A strategy used to search for the number of records retrieved with a keyword; the broad "catch" of retrieved records

precision: A search strategy that narrows the parameters of the search

retrieves many records. Following with precision search strategies narrows the field of the originally recalled records.

Basic Searches: Using Keywords

Selecting key terms is critical for achieving successful results when searching for evidence. A good place to begin identifying key terms is the PICOT question (PICOT stands for patient population, intervention of interest, comparison of interest, outcome of interest, and time frame; McGrath et al., 2012). For example, consider the PICOT question, "Does practicing yoga three times a week reduce blood pressure in older adults?" By using the parts of the PICOT question, one can see that concepts such as yoga, blood pressure, and older adults can form the basis for keywords.

There are two basic types of search queries when searching electronic databases: keyword and controlled vocabulary (discussed in the next section). Each has its own benefits and constraints, but the key to successful searching is knowing which type of query to use. Because the Internet is easy to use, bad search habits have resulted. Internet search engines are eager to please and therefore usually produce results for the entered search term. However, the results often include unrelated items, or the definition of terms may not match, the websites identified may be of dubious quality, or perhaps a misspelled search term retrieves matches from others who have misspelled words the same way. Electronic databases hold searchers to a higher level of use. For example, correct spelling really counts. When words are misspelled, databases reply with "zero results retrieved." With the use of good search habits, databases can offer consistency in searching, reliability of information found, and access to information not available on the open Internet.

Keyword searching allows you to enter a search term that best describes a topic as it is used in information source records (Cleary et al., 2009). Although this search strategy retrieves related records, searches also need to include synonyms and variations of the search term to ensure that all relevant records are retrieved. For example, in a search for information about newborns and their mothers, a keyword search using the terms "bonding" and "attachment" would be necessary. Keyword searches are often best for searching full-text or citation records. In most databases, keyword searching also considers words in the title, content notes, and author fields of each item's record.

Search tools are used to refine keyword searches. While the underlying concepts of these tools remain constant across various applications and resources, some electronic databases do not support all of them, or their symbols may be slightly different. To make the best use of powerful search strategies, it is essential to check the database's help files to make sure the tools are available and that the chosen symbols are entered correctly.

Search operators, also known as *Boolean operators*, are words that specify the relationship between two or more search terms. Search terms can be linked in a number of ways using the terms *and*, *or*, and *not*.

Using "and" narrows a search. Both of the search terms entered must be found somewhere in the record, though not necessarily in the same place. For example, terms may be a part of an author's name and part of a title. In most databases, the Boolean operation of "and" is automatically used when two or more keywords are entered. For example, a nurse is searching for information about eating disorders. Entering the keywords "anorexia" and "bulimia" will return only records containing both terms.

Using the Boolean operation of "or" broadens a search. When using this approach, either search term must be found somewhere in the record. This is especially helpful when searching synonyms or words with various forms. Unlike electronic databases, most Internet search engines default to the "or" operation when two or more keywords are entered. This explains why a search can retrieve so many irrelevant records. For example, a search strategy of "anorexia or bulimia" returns records that contain either one or both terms.

Searches can be narrowed by using the Boolean operation of "not." Using this operation, a record can be retrieved only if the first search term is present and the second search term is not present. In the example of eating disorders, entering keywords "anorexia not bulimia" returns results that contain only anorexia.

Search operators can also be used with Internet search engines. It is essential to check the help files of the search engine. Some search engines require that the search operators be typed in all capital letters, some accept two of the three operators and not the other, and some require the combination "and not" for the "not" operator.

Another helpful strategy when conducting basic searches is *truncation*, which is the ability to retrieve records of search terms that share a common root. In each database, a symbol of some sort is placed at the end of the group of letters forming the root search term. The symbol is usually an asterisk, but sometimes a colon, a question mark, a dollar sign, or a pound sign might be used. Check the help files to see which symbol is used in the database. Using the longest root possible increases the accuracy of the search. For example, instead of entering all of the terms "nurse," "nurses," and "nursing" in a search, truncation would replace all three with "nurs*". The challenge with truncation, however, is that it is often surprising to find how many words share common roots. In this example, records that include *nursery* and *nursing home* are also retrieved.

The use of *wildcards* is another strategy that involves substituting symbols for one or more letters in a search term. Many databases use the question mark as a wildcard. The help section provides information about how wildcards are

KEY TERMS

nesting: A strategy best used when a search contains two or more Boolean operators

stopwords: Words, such as *a, the,* and *in,* that are so commonly used that they can hinder accurate record retrieval

controlled vocabularies: Standardized hierarchical lists that represent major subjects within a database

used. For example, instead of entering both "woman" and "women" as search terms, use the wildcard entry "wom?n" instead.

Nesting, or grouping, is a strategy best used when a search contains two or more Boolean operators. Parentheses, and sometimes quotation marks, are used to indicate which search terms are grouped together. Just as in elementary algebra problems, the information within the parentheses is processed first and then applied to the information outside the parentheses. Another way to use nesting is to place the parentheses around a phrase or proper noun to instruct the database to search for the terms exactly as entered. For example, if searching for information about the use of herbal remedies, entering "(herbal remedies)" would generate records about this topic. Nesting is becoming a useful option with many Internet search tools and databases.

In most databases, the first screen allows searchers to apply limits to fields being searched within records, thereby filtering searches from the very start. Limits can be set for fields such as search term, language, publication type, and publication date. Limiting a set after an initial search creates a new, narrower list of records drawn from the original set of records. In some databases, it is possible to apply consecutive limits, which further narrows each subset.

Stopwords are words that are so commonly used in records that they are a hindrance to accurate record retrieval. These words are usually articles of speech, conjunctions, and pronouns. Although database searching has been programmed to ignore stopwords, some databases still show "failed search" when stopwords are used. Although stopwords can vary among databases, the most common ones to avoid are *a, an, and, for, in, of, the, this,* and *to.*

Advanced Searches: Controlled Vocabulary

Controlled vocabularies are standardized, hierarchical lists that have been designated to represent major subject concepts and conditions contained within a database. For a moment, consider the hashtags that you may be familiar with from Twitter, Instagram, or Facebook. People posting comments and photos use hashtags so that searches can retrieve items with matching content. This is basically the same conceptual idea behind controlled vocabularies. Whereas hashtags are chosen by those posting the photo or information, controlled vocabularies are created by those who manage the intellectual content of the index or database.

Vocabularies usually change from database to database. The hierarchical nature of the lists benefits search strategies by allowing broad concepts to be narrowed in a manner that stays consistent within that framework. CINAHL's list is called CINAHL Headings. MEDLINE and the Cochrane Library use Medical Subject Headings (MeSH). Before items are added to a database, subject matter is determined. Specific terms that apply to the determined subjects are chosen from the standardized list, regardless of the terminology used by authors. This approach provides a consistent method for retrieving the records even when different terminology is used in the text. For example, the term *heart attack* is always listed as "myocardial infarction" within a controlled vocabulary structure. Using controlled vocabulary searching is called *subject searching*. Unless otherwise noted, only records that match exactly to the terms as they were entered are displayed. The challenge is to determine which term is being used to represent the subject matter that is being sought.

It is possible to find standardized lists used in databases to determine the best terms to use. In most databases, terms are hyperlinked for ease of use. Do not assume that a keyword in one database is the same one to use in another database. For example, a search conducted in the PsycINFO database may use a different subject term than a search conducted in the MEDLINE database would use, even though both are science-related databases. When this happens, the search "fails" and the searcher is mistakenly led to believe that the second database contains no information on the topic.

Exploding is one of the most powerful techniques for searching subject headings. When a subject term is exploded, the database is instructed to search all the records indexed to that term as well as any terms that are in a related, narrower category. For example, exploding the search term "headache" in a CINAHL search results in a search that includes the terms "rebound headache" and "vascular headache." Exploding can dramatically increase the number of records generated by the search. Most health sciences databases support this technique.

One of the benefits of knowing both keyword and subject searching is that they can be combined to increase the effectiveness and efficiency of the search. Qualification and positional operators are more advanced keyword techniques that can be very powerful when used in combination with subject searching. *Qualification* designates which fields are to be searched in the record. The most common ways to limit searches are by author (au), title (ti), subject (su), publisher, and publication date. Placement of the punctuation can be important when using limiting search terms. These options may be available only using the advanced search methods in databases.

The proximity of search terms to one another can be specified using *positional operators*. The most commonly used are "adj" (adjacent), "near," and "same." Usually, "adj" and "near" can be grouped with a number to specify the number of words that can appear between search terms. "Same" designates that the search terms are found in the same field of the record such as the title or the abstract. Because order is not designated with "same," search terms will

KEY TERMS

subject searching: Searching databases using controlled vocabulary

exploding: Technique for searching subject headings that identifies all records indexed to that term

qualification: Limiting fields of search, commonly using limits such as author, title, or subject

positional operators: Terms that specify the number of words that can appear between search terms

not necessarily be next to one another. When using this technique, it is best to check the help section for instructions.

Best Sources for EBP

Both print and electronic resources contain useful information to answer EBP questions. Many useful encyclopedias, handbooks, guides, and care plan manuals are available in print-only format. Asking a librarian for details on the collection can provide valuable insight. Electronic sources offer a mix of scholarly, trade, and popular works. Professional journals, popular magazines, newspapers, and industry bulletins may all be part of the search results.

The three most commonly found general databases are Academic Search Complete, Expanded Academic ASAP, and LexisNexis Academic. The first two databases contain very similar content and have a higher percentage of scholarly work than does LexisNexis Academic. LexisNexis Academic is all full content and offers a wider range of news, business, and legal sources than do the other two databases. In subject-specific databases, scholarly literature of professions and disciplines is indexed. **Table 4-1** provides categorization and general information about subject-specific databases that are extremely useful when creating EBP. The URL is provided for access to additional information, but if the database is proprietary, it does not provide access to the content. Access may be available through local libraries or places of employment.

After evidence has been gathered, materials must be appraised for their integrity and applicability. Sources chosen by your library, a respected professional organization, or a reputable government agency have already been through an evaluation process. Most individuals struggle with evaluating other Internet sources. A couple of general guidelines can serve you well:

» If you have any doubts at all about the information, do not use it. Or, minimally, verify it elsewhere in a reputable source.
» Ask your nursing faculty or librarian for insight on the situation. Chances are your discussion can clarify your concerns, and as often happens in a discussion of this type, your decision will become apparent.

Librarians create guides to assist users in accessing locally available subscription resources as well as critically evaluated open Internet resources. For example, a categorized listing of recommended sites for other guidelines, systematic reviews, clinical trials, and "free" EBP resources is available through Valparaiso University (http://libguides.valpo.edu/content.php?pid=42078&sid=337662). **Box 4-1** provides recommendations of other EBP sources.

Many guides and resources that help evaluate Internet materials are available in local libraries. Evaluating sources is not as simple as just using a checklist. As noted previously in this chapter, Gilmour and colleagues (2008) stressed

TABLE 4-1	Subject-Specific Databases	
CINAHL	https://www.ebscohost.com/academic/cinahl-plus-with-full-text	CINAHL is the premier database covering the areas of nursing and allied health. Online coverage is usually comprehensive back to 1982 with monthly updates. This proprietary site URL is for information only. Check with your institution's library to determine whether you have subscriber access and through which vendor.
MEDLINE via PubMed Health	http://www.ncbi.nlm.nih.gov/pubmed/	Providing coverage of MEDLINE and other medical sciences and biomedical literature back to the 1950s, PubMed is a service of the U.S. National Library of Medicine, with free access on the Internet to more than 17 million citations. This link is to the free version available on the Internet; your library might provide access to other vendor-created versions that provide a familiar search environment and then also link directly to library resources (and it is called MEDLINE, not PubMed).
PubMed Clinical Queries	http://www.ncbi.nlm.nih.gov/pubmed/clinical	The Clinical Queries search supports specialized PubMed queries for clinicians in areas of clinical studies, systematic reviews, and medical genetics.
Joanna Briggs Institute EBP Database	http://joannabriggs.org/	The institute was established in 1996 to offer collaboration in EBP with healthcare professionals and researchers across the professional continuum in more than 40 countries. JBI is considered one of the foundational providers of EBP information. This proprietary site URL is for information only. Check with your institution's library to determine whether you have subscriber access.
The Cochrane Collaboration and Library	http://www.cochranelibrary.com/	An international not-for-profit organization, the collaboration seeks to provide timely, up-to-date research evidence. Not a physical entity, the Cochrane Library is a database collection, providing access to systematic reviews, controlled trials, methodology registry, technology assessment, and more. DARE (Database of Abstracts of Reviews of Effects) is also part of the library. This proprietary site URL is for information only. Check with your institution's library to determine whether you have subscriber access.
Google Scholar	http://scholar.google.com/	Google Scholar allows you to use the familiarity of Google to search the Internet in an interdisciplinary way. Citation results are scholarly in nature and direct you to full content if it is available on the Internet. Google Scholar also partners with libraries to set up linking with their full-content resources. Your librarian can tell you whether this is possible in your system.

BOX 4-1	Recommended Sources About EBP Clinical Practice Guidelines

Agency for Healthcare Research and Quality (AHRQ) (https://www.ahrq.gov/professionals /clinicians-providers/guidelines-recommendations/index.html)

National Guideline Clearinghouse (http://www.guideline.gov/)

Oncology Nursing Society (ONS) PEP: Putting Evidence into Practice (https://www.ons.org /search?search_api_views_fulltext=Research%20PEP)

Registered Nurses' Association of Ontario (RNAO) (http://rnao.ca/bpg)

Royal College of Nursing (https://www.rcn.org.uk/)

Systematic Reviews and Other Synopses/Syntheses of Evidence

Agency for Healthcare Research and Quality (AHRQ) EPC Evidence-Based Reports (http://www .ahrq.gov/research/findings/evidence-based-reports/index.html)

British Medical Journal (BMJ) Clinical Evidence (http://clinicalevidence.bmj.com/x/index.html)

PubMed Clinical Queries (https://www.ncbi.nlm.nih.gov/pubmed/clinical)

TRIP Database (https://www.tripdatabase.com/)

University of York Centre for Reviews and Dissemination (https://www.york.ac.uk/crd/)

Clinical Trials

ClinicalTrials.gov (https://clinicaltrials.gov/ct2/home)

MedlinePlus: Clinical Trials (https://medlineplus.gov/clinicaltrials.html)

Other EBP Sources

Centre for Evidence Based Medicine (http://www.cebm.net/category/ebm-resources/tools/)

Evidence-Based Nursing (http://ebn.bmj.com/)

National Institute of Nursing Research (https://www.ninr.nih.gov/)

National Quality Measures Clearinghouse (https://www.qualitymeasures.ahrq.gov/)

University of Washington Health Sciences Library EBP guide (http://guides.lib.uw.edu/c .php?g=345956&p=2330155)

Virginia Henderson Global Nursing e-Repository (http://www.nursinglibrary.org/vhl/)

 CRITICAL THINKING EXERCISE 4-1

Which of the following two articles would you recommend to your unit supervisor for changing practice? Explain why you would make this recommendation. One article contains general referrals to the foremost authorities on the topic, and five research studies are cited. The second article contains a summative review of research conducted by authorities in the field, various application scenarios for different institutions, and a comprehensive reference list.

that nurses need to be able to assist patients with their healthcare-information-seeking behaviors. In a qualitative study, Cader (2013) identified six evaluative tasks for nurses when evaluating WWW/Internet resources:

» Assessing user-friendliness of web pages
» Assessing the outlook of web pages
» Assessing authority of web pages
» Assessing relationship to nursing practice
» Appraising the nature of evidence
» Applying cross-checking strategies

In other words, if you discover a piece of evidence that is not confirmed in any other sources and is never mentioned as new, foundational, or ground-breaking, the information may be questionable. The complexity and amount of healthcare-related information available to both professionals and patients are staggering. Nursing professionals will do well to assess such information in a consistent and contextual manner, much as the practice followed in patient assessment.

Formulating a Search Strategy

Creating a plan for searching by combining the suggestions offered in this chapter about where and how to search is wise. Begin by planning the order of databases that will be searched and the key terms that will be used. Keeping notes of the search is recommended, especially because key terms may vary between databases (McGrath et al., 2012). Good notes can be invaluable when there is a need to search in another database.

Searches are rarely completed in one sitting (McGrath et al., 2012); thus referring to notes during subsequent sessions can save time by avoiding duplication. Time can also be used efficiently by saving the search results and having an account for items obtained through interlibrary loan. It is also possible to set up an automatic, periodic search whereby alerts are sent directly to your account.

Mastering the skill of searching databases is important to assure that you have found the best evidence for a PICOT question. It is helpful to use a planned, systematic approach. A worksheet (see **Exhibit 4-1**) assures that a systematic approach is used because each step is documented. It is also helpful because sometimes a search cannot be completed in one sitting. Having a record will be beneficial when you resume the search at a later time. If you encounter difficulties during the search, it will be easier for a librarian to provide assistance. Having a record of the systematic search can save time and effort if you need to retrieve one of the sources at a later time.

Before entering words into a database, it is helpful to reflect on which words are key to the search. Using components of the PICOT question is a good place

EXHIBIT 4-1   Literature Systematic Search Worksheet

STEP 1: Think About the Best Way to Search

A. What is your topic or PICOT question? _____

B. Begin by listing keywords or phrases in the first column. Use words that describe the population, intervention, and outcome. Use words that you think will assist you in finding "the best" evidence on your topic. After you have listed your keywords, use the blanks to the right of your key words to list synonyms (other words) that can be used to say the same thing as the keywords/phrases.

Keywords   Synonyms

P: _____ : _____ OR _____ OR _____

I: _____ : _____ OR _____ OR _____

O: _____ : _____ OR _____ OR_____

C. What are the best information resources/databases/websites for your research?

_____ , _____ , _____

STEP 2: Plan Your First Search

A. List your keywords and synonyms being sure to use symbols (* and "quote marks for more than 1 word") and Boolean operators (OR/AND) to aid your search.

_____ OR _____ OR _____ OR _____

AND _____ OR _____ OR _____ OR _____

AND _____ OR _____ OR _____ OR _____

B. What limiters should you use in the search? (Date range, language, or any other limiting criteria)

_____ , _____ , _____

STEP 3: Begin Your Search

After you've thought about your topic and planned your search, log in and begin your search. Use the keywords and limiters you identified in Step 2. Be sure to avoid typos, as that can ruin your search.

A. What database/resource did you use? _____

B. How many results did you get? _____ Too few results? Too many results?

C. Look at the article citations and identify subject headings (MeSH Terms/CINAHL Headings) that are common across the relevant abstracts/article citations. These should be listed within the citations/records after the Subjects: heading. What is the most common MeSH Term/CINAHL Heading you see? _____

STEP 4: Incorporate a Subject Heading (MeSH Term or CINAHL Heading) within Your Search

Using the same database, incorporate your CINAHL Heading/MeSH Term along with the keywords and phrases you've been using. You may also want to change your limiters depending on the number of results. A simple way to do this is to click on the selected Subjects: term so the database can incorporate the subject into the search box. Then type in the remainder of your keywords, phrases, synonyms, etc.

A. List your MeSH Term/CINAHL Heading with other keywords, synonyms, and phrases used in this refined search.

(MM_____)

AND _____OR _____ OR _____ OR _____

AND_____OR_____ OR _____ OR _____

AND_____OR _____ OR _____ OR _____

B. What limiters did you use in this search?

_____ , _____ , _____

C. Now how many results did you get? _____ Still too few results? Or too many?

STEP 5: Refine Your Search Again

Using the same database, refine your search again. If you've had too many results, try narrowing your population or setting. If you've had too few results, expand your population or setting or add additional subject headings.

A. What keywords, synonyms, phrases and MeSH Terms/CINAHL Headings were used in this even more refined search?

(MM_____)

AND _____OR _____ OR _____ OR _____

AND_____OR_____ OR _____ OR _____

AND_____OR _____ OR _____ OR _____

B. What limiters did you use in this search?

_____ , _____ , _____

C. How many results do you have now? _____

D. Consider the following: Are the results relevant? Current? Of good quality? Appropriate for the assignment? Read the abstracts and then read the full text. If needed, adjust your search more. Consider searching another database/resource to see what other evidence may be available in a different source. Make sure to continue recording your steps.

STEP 6: Search Another Database

Search another database using the keywords, synonyms, phrases, MeSH Terms/CINAHL Headings, and limiters you used in STEP 5.

A. What other database/resource did you search?_____

B. How many results did you get? _____Too few results? Too many results?

C. Think about the following (do not write out answer): How do these results compare to the results you obtained in the other database? Are the results relevant? Current? Of good quality? Appropriate for the assignment? If needed, adjust your search more. Make sure to continue recording your steps.

STEP 7: Reflection

A. Why did you select your specific article?

B. What difficulties did you have locating a single research study that is appropriate for this assignment?

C. The next time you search for evidence, what will you do differently?

Adapted from: Whalen, K. J., & Zentz, S. E. (2014). Five-course meal infused with information skills and resources. In K. Calkins & C. Kvenild (Eds.), *The embedded librarian's cookbook* (pp. 76–79). Chicago, IL: American Libraries Association. Available at http://works.bepress.com/kimberly_whalen/5

to begin. List the population, intervention, and outcome first. Then think of synonyms for those words, and write those words on the worksheet. For the PICOT question, "What are the best strategies for improving handwashing compliance in nursing staff?" a worksheet may begin like this:

P:____nurses____:_____staff_____ OR _registered nurses_ OR _____

I:___strategies___:_interventions_ OR ___education___ OR ___programs___

O: handwashing : hand washing OR _hand hygiene_ OR _hand scrubbing_

Once this step is completed, the next step is to use the words identified and apply advanced search strategies. The worksheet may look like this:

P:_____nurse*___:_____staff_____ OR _"registered nurse*"_ OR _____

I:____strateg*___:_intervention*_ OR _____educat*_____ OR____program*____

O: handwashing : "hand washing" OR "hand hygiene" OR "hand scrubbing"

Once this is step is completed, enter the keywords into a database. As the search progresses, keywords can be added or deleted, MeSH terms or CINAHL headings can be identified, and limiters can be altered to increase or decrease the search results. When a reasonable number of results has been achieved, you are ready to begin skimming abstracts of the articles. If the results are not relevant, try using a different database.

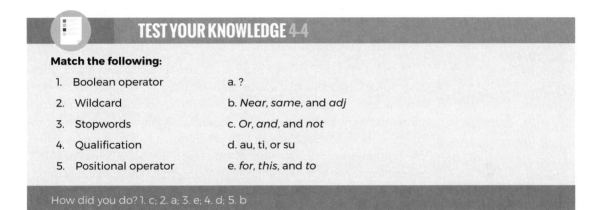

TEST YOUR KNOWLEDGE 4-4

Match the following:

1.	Boolean operator	a.	?
2.	Wildcard	b.	*Near, same,* and *adj*
3.	Stopwords	c.	*Or, and,* and *not*
4.	Qualification	d.	au, ti, or su
5.	Positional operator	e.	*for, this,* and *to*

How did you do? 1. c; 2. a; 3. e; 4. d; 5. b

4.5 Keeping It Ethical

At the end of this section, you will be able to:

‹ Consider the ethical presentation and application of evidence

The phrase "give credit where credit is due" is familiar to most individuals. Few places more stringently apply the concept of attribution than the university setting does. For those new to academic writing, the reference list and citing of sources within papers are confusing and are often considered purposeless tasks imposed by the professor. Often, the citation of references is the last thing done when deadlines are approaching. Consequently, not much thought is given to the importance of attributing information to appropriate sources.

Citations of sources provide acknowledgments of others' ideas and contributions to the subject. Ideas are owned by those individuals who first wrote about them. For example, when you submit a paper to a professor, you have created a piece of original work. No one else has written about the topic in quite the same way, used the same sources in the same way, or drawn conclusions in the same way.

It is considered *plagiarism* to use another's work without giving proper credit. Plagiarism occurs when ideas from others are used without proper

KEY TERM

plagiarism: The use of another's work without giving proper credit

documentation (Horrom, 2012). Intentionally passing off the work of others as your own is unethical. Unintentional plagiarism reflects poor scholarship and laziness. Either way, plagiarism can be illegal because copyright laws may be violated (Horrom, 2012). A simple rule to avoid plagiarism is: If you have read it, heard it, or viewed it and want to include it, cite it. If the thought, wording, or graphic is not your original work, cite the source. Because plagiarism is considered a serious violation of ethical standards, penalties can be severe. Plagiarism is easy to avoid by providing proper citations.

Things get a little less clear when it comes to paraphrasing the work of others. This is when unintentional plagiarism can occur, even by the most conscientious students. There are examples of both direct quotes and paraphrasing in this chapter. Paraphrasing can be identified by noting the citation for the author names and publication dates. Depending on the sentence construction, paraphrasing either precedes or follows those indicators. Paraphrasing can be very challenging. If you have difficulty with this technique, use direct quotes or seek assistance from your school's writing center.

Using the common knowledge test can help determine whether a citation is required. Like paraphrasing, over time you will become more comfortable with this. As you become more knowledgeable about accepted facts in nursing, you will be able to recognize common knowledge situations. Another simple rule is: If you have to look it up, cite it. For example, it is common knowledge that antibiotics are used to treat infections. But if information is presented about a new antibiotic that is not well known, a citation would be required. It is better to err on the side of caution and write a paper with too many citations than to accidentally plagiarize.

There are several strategies one can use to avoid plagiarism. One major way is not to cut and paste content from the original source (Horrom, 2012). By avoiding cut and paste, writers are more likely to put ideas into their own words. Another way to avoid plagiarism is to ensure that all sources are cited appropriately. Following style guidelines, such as APA (from the American Psychological Association) or MLA (from the Modern Language Association), helps to eliminate plagiarism. Checking your paper with plagiarism detection software is another way to ensure that ideas are expressed in your own words.

Your authority as a writer in the discipline is increased when you give proper credit to the work of others. Practiced professionals often skim a reference list to see if foundational studies are included, and if not, they may disregard the paper. By placing your original thoughts within the context of others who are already known and respected, you are continuing the scholarly conversation from your perspective. Given the increase in undergraduate research, your contributions could provide a new insight that results in being cited by others.

FYI

Keeping the review of the literature ethical requires giving full credit to sources, which entails keeping accurate citations.

Citation formatting is not just busywork to add stress to the task of completing a paper. Just as providing the proper information in search fields increases consistency and reliability in searching, providing citation information that is correct and in the right format increases the reliability and ease of locating those sources if desired. Providing the correct citation information allows your work to serve as a conduit for those who are citation chasing.

TEST YOUR KNOWLEDGE 4-5

1. How can plagiarism be avoided? (Select all that apply.)
   a. By using quotations with proper citations
   b. By paraphrasing the work of others
   c. By erring on the side of caution
   d. By cutting and pasting from websites

How did you do? 1. a, b, c

Apply What You Have Learned

Members of the EBP committee have searched the literature and compiled a list of articles. As a committee member, you have agreed to retrieve these articles and distribute copies to all committee members. The first column of the table provided here has a list of the citations. The second column of the table has search terms and limiters to help you search.

Citation	Search Term (Limiter)
Al-Hussami, M., Darawad, M., & Almhairat, I. I. (2011). Predictors of compliance handwashing practice among healthcare professionals. *Healthcare Infection, 16,* 79–84.	Al-Hussami (author) "handwashing practice" (all fields)
Chun, H., Kim, K., & Park, H. (2015). Effects of hand hygiene education and individual feedback on hand hygiene behavior, MRSA, acquisition rate, and MRSA colonization pressure among intensive care unit nurses. *International Journal of Nursing Practice, 21,* 709–715.	Chun (author) "individual feedback" (all fields)
Dyson, J., Lawton, R., Jackson, C., & Cheater, F. (2013). Development of a theory-based instrument to identify barriers and louvers to best hand hygiene practice among healthcare practitioners. *Implementation Science, 8*(111), 1–9.	Dyson (author) Lawton (author) "barriers" (all fields)

(continued)

Apply What You Have Learned *(continued)*

Citation	Search Term (Limiter)
Fakhry, M., Hannah, G. B., Anderson, O., Holmes, A., & Nathwain, D. (2012). Effectiveness of an audible reminder on hand hygiene adherence. *American Journal of Infection Control, 40,* 320–323.	"audible reminder" (title) "hand hygiene" (title)
Huis, A., Schoonhoven, L., Grol, R., Donders, R., Hulscher, M., & van Achterber, T. (2014). Impact of a team and leaders-directed strategy to improve nurses' adherence to hand hygiene guidelines: A cluster randomized trial. *International Journal of Nursing Studies, 50,* 464–474.	Huis (author) Donders (author)
Jackson, C., Lowton, K., & Griffiths, P. (2014). Infection prevention as "a show": A qualitative study of nurses' infection prevention behaviours. *International Journal of Nursing Studies, 51,* 400–408.	Jackson (author) Lowton (author) "International Journal of Nursing Studies" (publication name)
Johnson, L., Jrueber, S., Schlotzhauer, C., Phillips, E., Bullock, P., Basnett, J., & Hahn-Cover, K. (2014). A multifactorial action plan improves hand hygiene adherence and significantly reduces central line-associated bloodstream infections. *American Journal of Infection Control, 42,* 1146–1151.	Johnson (author) "multifactorial action plan" (all fields)
Kingston, L., O'Connell, N. H., & Dunne, C. P. (2016). Hand hygiene-related clinical trials reported since 2010: A systematic review. *Journal of Hospital Infection, 92,* 309–320.	Kingston (author) "systematic review" 2016 (publication date)
Whitby, M., & McLaws, M. (2007). Methodological difficulties in hand hygiene research. *Journal of Hospital Infection, 67,* 194–195.	Whitby (author) "methodological difficulties" (title)

To retrieve these articles, you will need to sign into a database for nursing literature (i.e., CINAHL, Proquest, PubMed). Once you have signed in, enter a search term in a blank box that appears. Then, using the drop down menu, enter the limiter that is suggested for that search term. Here is an example from CINAHL to show you how to enter the search terms and limiters for the first article by Al-Hussami, Darawad, & Almhairat (2011).

When you obtain the article, it is helpful to save it as a PDF file. As you save each article, it is wise to identify the file using the name of the first author followed by the year of publication. For example, the first article could be saved as "Al-Hussami (2011).pdf." Naming files in this manner will save you time and frustration later when you want to find a particular article referenced in Apply What You Have Learned. Continue this process for the remaining articles shown in the table.

The next task for the EBP committee members is to read and analyze each piece of evidence. The EBP committee has decided to use a grid to organize and summarize the evidence so that

Apply What You Have Learned *(continued)*

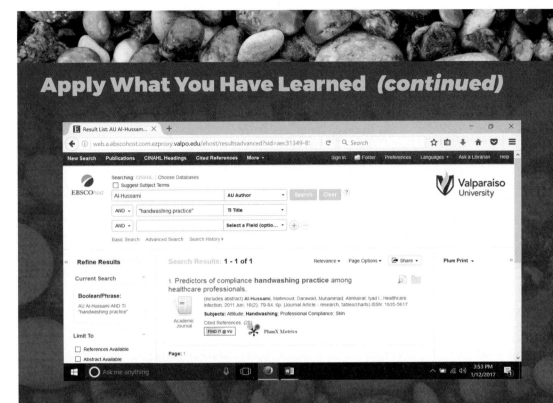

the information is presented in a consistent and succinct format. This is helpful because trends can be easily identified, and gaps in the knowledge base are made apparent. Organizing the review with a grid is a positive strategy to overcome the barrier of lack of time because it reduces the need to repeatedly sort through articles during future discussions. On the text's digital resources, you will also find a grid to use for this exercise. Two articles (Chhapola & Brar, 2015; Salmon & McLaws, 2015) are summarized as an example.

Read Chun, Kim, and Park (2015). Enter information about this article into the first column. In this column, one uses APA format because this is the most commonly used style for nursing publications.

⚡ *RAPID REVIEW*

» Today's work environment requires that nurses be adept at gathering and appraising evidence for clinical practice and assisting patients with healthcare information needs.

» Literature reviews provide syntheses of current research and scholarly literature. A well-done literature review can provide support for EBP.

» An understanding of the scientific literature publication cycle provides a basis for making decisions about the most current information on a topic.

» Primary sources are original sources of information presented by the people who created them. Secondary sources are resulting commentaries, summaries, reviews, or interpretations of primary sources.

» Many research journals involve peer review.

» There are many ways to categorize sources. Scholarly, trade, and popular literature is one way. Another categorizing system involves periodicals, journals, and magazines.

» There are four types of review: narrative, integrative, meta-analysis, and systematic.

» Understanding how sources are structured can simplify a search of the literature.

» Sources can be identified through both print indexes and electronic databases. Topics, subject matter, and format may vary but all include citation information.

» Helpful strategies to use when conducting a search include citation chasing, measurements of recall and precision, keyword and controlled vocabulary searches, Boolean operators, truncation, wildcards, nesting, limits, stopwords, exploding, qualification, and positional operators.

» Databases can be either general content sources or subject-specific content sources. CINAHL is nursing's premier subject-specific database.

» By interacting with professional literature through writing, creating literature reviews, and conducting research, nurses are part of the scholarly conversation taking place within their discipline. Correct attribution of others' original work, as well as proper construction of citations, demonstrates the ethical sense of responsibility and professionalism.

REFERENCES

Burt, H. A. (2013). *The patient safety perspective: Health information and resources online and in print*. Chicago, IL: Medical Library Association.

Cader, R. (2013). Judging nursing information on the World Wide Web. *Computers, Informatics, Nursing, 31*(2), 66–73.

Choi, S. W., & Lam, D. M. H. (2016). Statistically speaking. *Anaesthesia, 71*, 228–231.

Christie, J., Hamill, C., & Power, J. (2012). How can we maximize nursing students' learning about research evidence and utilization in undergraduate, preregistration programmes? A discussion paper. *Journal of Advanced Nursing, 68*, 2789–2801.

Cleary, M., Hunt, G. E., & Horsfall, J. (2009). Conducting efficient literature searches: Strategies for mental health nurses. *Journal of Psychosocial Nursing and Mental Health Services, 47*(11), 34–41.

Cohen, H., & Shastay, D. (2008). Getting to the root of medication errors. *Nursing, 38*(12), 39–49.

Cooper, D., & Crum, J. A. (2013). New activities and changing roles of health science libraries: A systematic review, 1990–2012. *Journal of the Medical Library Association, 10*, 268–277.

Cowell, J. (2012). Literature reviews as a research strategy. *Journal of School Nursing, 28*(5), 326–327.

Dunn, K., Brewer, K., Marshall, J., & Sollenberger, J. (2009). Measuring the value and impact of health sciences libraries: Planning an update and replication of the Rochester study. *Journal of the Medical Library Association, 97*(4), 308–312.

Evans, D., & Kowanko, I. (2000). Literature reviews: Evolution of a research methodology. *Australian Journal of Advanced Nursing, 18*(2), 33–38.

Ganong, L. H. (1987). Integrative reviews of nursing research. *Research in Nursing and Health, 10*(1), 1–11.

Gilmour, J. A., Scott, S. D., & Huntington, N. (2008). Nurses and Internet health information: A questionnaire survey. *Journal of Advanced Nursing, 61*(1), 19–28.

Grant, M. (2010). Key words and their role in information retrieval. *Health Information and Libraries Journal, 27*(3), 173–175.

Hawker, S., Payne, S., Kerr, C., Hardey, M., & Powell, J. (2002). Appraising the evidence: Reviewing disparate data systematically. *Qualitative Health Research, 12*(9), 1284–1299.

Higgins, J. P. T., & Green, S. (2011). *Cochrane handbook for systematic reviews of interventions* (Version 5.1.0). Retrieved from http://handbook.cochrane.org/

Hill, S., & Cochrane Collaboration. (2011). *The knowledgeable patient: Communication and participation in health.* Chichester, West Sussex, United Kingdom: Wiley.

Horrom, T. A. (2012). The perils of copy and paste: Plagiarism in scientific publishing. *Journal of Rehabilitation Development, 49*(8), vii–xii.

Jackson, G. B. (1980). Methods for integrative reviews. *Review of Educational Research, 50*, 438–460.

Jordan-Marsh, M. (2011). *Health technology literacy: A transdisciplinary framework for consumer-oriented practice.* Sudbury, MA: Jones & Bartlett Learning.

Kimbrough Kushner, T. (2010). *Surviving health care: A manual for patients and their families.* New York, NY: Cambridge University Press.

Kliger, J., Blegen, M. A., Gootee, D., & O'Neil, E. (2009). Empowering frontline nurses: A structured intervention enables nurses to improve medication administration accuracy. *Joint Commission Journal on Quality and Patient Safety, 35*, 604–612.

Lander, J. (2005). Finding, evaluating, and using research for best practice. *Clinical Nursing Research, 14*, 299–302.

McGrath, J. M., Brown, R. E., & Samra, H. A. (2012). Before you search the literature: How to prepare and get the most out of citation databases. *Newborn and Infant Nursing Reviews, 12*(3), 162–170.

Tomietto, M., Sartor, A., Mazzocoli, E., & Palese, A. (2012). Paradoxical effects of a hospital-based, multi-intervention programme aimed at reducing medication round interruptions. *Journal of Nursing Management, 20*(3), 335–343.

University of Washington Libraries. (1999). *Scientific publication cycle.* Retrieved 6/23/17 from http://guides.lib.uw.edu/c.php?g=345956&p=2330155

Weightman, A. L., & Williamson, J. (2005). The value and impact of information provided through library services for patient care: A systematic review. *Health Information and Libraries Journal, 22*(1), 4–25.

Whalen, K. J., & Zentz, S. E. (2014). Five-course meal infused with information skills and resources. In K. Calkins & C. Kvenild (Eds.), *The embedded librarian's cookbook* (pp. 76–79). Chicago, IL: American Libraries Association. Available at http://works.bepress.com/kimberly_whalen/5

Whittemore, R. (2005). Combining evidence in nursing research. *Nursing Research, 54*, 56–62.

At the end of this chapter, you will be able to:

< Define the terms *theory* and *research* as they relate to the practice of nursing

< Distinguish between conceptual and empirical definitions

< Describe how theory and research influence each other in a professional discipline

< Apply the language of the discipline in describing the relevance of linking theory, research, and practice in nursing

< Discuss how honoring prior work ethically builds nursing knowledge

KEY TERMS

concepts
conceptual definitions
construct
empirical indicators

metaparadigm
model
operational definitions
proposition

theoretical framework
theory

CHAPTER 5

Linking Theory, Research, and Practice

Elsabeth Jensen

5.1 How Are Theory, Research, and Practice Related?

At the end of this section, you will be able to:

< Define the terms *theory* and *research* as they relate to the practice of nursing
< Distinguish between conceptual and empirical definitions
< Describe how theory and research influence each other in a professional discipline
< Apply the language of the discipline in describing the relevance of linking theory, research, and practice in nursing

"The bringing together or nexus of nursing theory, practice and research creates a true integration of knowledge designed to support the service to clients and the health of society" (Butcher, 2006, p. 112). In the profession of nursing, theories and research provide an essential foundation for practice and exist to serve the goals of practice. At the same time, practice is the source of the questions to be addressed by research. The relationships between theory, research, and practice are reciprocal in that each informs the other in the development of disciplinary knowledge. Practice is also the testing ground for theory, where only those theories found helpful to practice survive and evolve. Practice is also a source for new theories.

FYI

Knowledge is not static, but rather it develops out of asking questions and seeking answers. Learning to ask good questions is as essential as learning how to find good answers.

In the same way, the disciplinary knowledge that is nursing knowledge is also dynamic and evolving. As students prepare for practice as nurses, it is easy for them to believe that what is being learned is sound and should never be questioned. Learning to ask good questions and developing a critical mind are essential. A curious mind is invaluable in the pursuit of providing the best nursing service possible.

Knowledge is not static, but rather it develops out of asking questions and seeking answers. Learning to ask good questions is as essential as learning how to find good answers.

Understanding Theory, Research, and Practice from a Practice Perspective

There are terms applicable when discussing theory, research, and practice. Understanding these terms allows nurses to communicate ideas effectively with other members of the healthcare team to develop an evidence-based practice.

The Special Language of Theory

A *theory* is a set of concepts linked through propositions to provide an explanation of a phenomenon. Nursing theories are belief systems that guide practice (Parse, 2014). Theory provides the lens through which nurses view clients. In any discipline there is usually one model that defines it at any point in time (Butcher, 2006). Currently in nursing, the concepts of person, environment, health, and nursing are the focus of the development of disciplinary knowledge (Fawcett, 1984; Graham, 2003). These four concepts have been present from the time of Nightingale (1859/1969). Nurses have many formal nursing theories available from which to choose. Although it is beyond the scope of this chapter to describe them, it is important for students and nurses to study them because they represent the many ways that nursing practice can be approached.

Using theory in practice provides a framework to nurses as they assess and provide care. The study of theory introduces a new language that is specific to nursing. Fawcett and Downs (1992) are considered to be authorities on the study of theory and research. As mentioned earlier, the concepts that are core to nursing are person, environment, health, and nursing. These are known as the *metaparadigm* of nursing. The concepts are very broad, and each nursing theory provides definitions for how they are used in that model. *Concepts* are the words or phrases that convey a unique idea or mental image that is relevant to the theory. For example, Hildegard Peplau (1952) defined health as the forward movement of personality, whereas Martha Rogers (1970) defined health as being what the person says it is; that is to say, individuals define health for

CRITICAL THINKING EXERCISE 5-1

In your nursing program, how are the concepts of the metaparadigm defined? Is there a model or theory that is used?

themselves, and nurses need to know what that definition is for each person. As another example, Nightingale defined environment as everything outside the person, whereas Rogers defined environment as being integral with the person. These are different views and lead to some differences in the focus of practice of nurses guided by each of these theories.

Concepts are individual building blocks joined together in statements to create propositions. A *proposition* is a statement about the relationship between two or more concepts. For example, Nightingale (1859/1969) linked a concept from the environment, sunlight, to the concept of health when she wrote:

> It is the unqualified result of all my experience with the sick, that second only to their need of fresh air is their need of light . . . not only light, but direct sunlight they want. . . . People think the effect is upon the spirits only. . . . we must admit that light has quite as real and tangible effects upon the human body. (p. 84)

Nightingale's proposition is that exposure to sunlight promotes healing and recovery in the person. Knowing this, nurses will expose people to sunlight to promote health.

Another important word in the language of theory is *construct*. A construct is a property that is neither directly nor indirectly observed. It is a word or phrase to communicate a specific, key idea to others. One example of a construct is social support. Social support cannot actually be seen, but it can be inferred through assessment of other observable attributes. To assess social support, nurses could count the number of people in a patient's circle of family and friends or could ask patients about their perceptions of the support they receive.

The Importance of Testing Theory

Nurses look to research to develop and test ideas that may be useful and also look to researchers to address practice questions for which there are no answers. Nursing researchers are responsible for developing and testing knowledge to guide nursing practice (Butcher, 2006). There are important distinctions to note in order to understand what is and what is not nursing research. Nursing research is research that provides results that are relevant for practice, either at the level of basic research or at the level of applied research. Some researchers claim their work is nursing research because the researcher is a nurse or because the researcher studied nurses. But it is the focus on nursing practice that defines nursing research. The mere fact that the research was conducted by a nurse or

KEY TERMS

proposition: A statement about the relationship between two or more concepts

construct: A word or phrase used to communicate a specific key idea to others

that nurses were studied does not necessarily qualify the research as nursing research. Historically, and even today, approaches to practice are often based on "professional opinion" when research is absent. **Case Example 5-1** provides such a historical illustration. It also demonstrates the value of systematically studying the effects of interventions.

This case example clearly illustrates how knowledge changes over time and how ineffective practices are replaced with innovations. What is considered to be state-of-the-art practice at one time is replaced when new knowledge based on evidence emerges. Understanding the cycle of science compels nurses to continue learning throughout their careers to avoid becoming laggards. This case also underscores the importance of ordinary observations in the field of practice. In this case example, postmortem observations pointed to the need for another, sounder approach to resuscitation. This case also illustrates how

CASE EXAMPLE 5-1

Early Methods of Resuscitation: An Example of Practice Based on Untested Theory

Throughout the past century, nursing students have been taught how to resuscitate patients who stop breathing. As early as 1912, students were taught a variety of methods for providing artificial respiration. It was theorized that moving air in and out of the lungs would be effective. One of these techniques was designed for resuscitating infants. Byrd's Method of Infant Resuscitation (Goodnow, 1919) directed the nurse to hold the infant's legs in one hand, and the head and back in the other. The nurse would then double the child over by pressing the head and the knees against the chest. Then the nurse would extend the knees to undouble the child. This would be repeated, but "not too rapidly" (Goodnow, 1919, p. 305). At intervals, the nurse would dip the child into a mustard bath in the hope that this would also stimulate respiration. The nurse would continue this until help arrived.

Other methods of artificial respiration taught included Sylvester's method for adults (Goodnow, 1919). The patient was placed flat on his back. The nurse would grasp the patient's elbows and press them close to his sides, pushing in the ribs to expel air from the chest. The arms would then be slowly pulled over the head, allowing the chest to expand. The arms would be lowered to put pressure on the chest, and the cycle was then repeated. This was to be done at the rate of 18 to 20 cycles per minute.

By 1939, postmortem examinations after unsuccessful resuscitations showed veins to be engorged while the arteries were empty (Harmer & Henderson, 1942). Although this evidence indicated other factors needed to be considered, resuscitation techniques continued to focus only on the respiratory system. The same methods of resuscitation that were in use in 1919 were still being taught in 1942. Although students were still being taught the Sylvester method, they were also learning the new "Schäfer method" (Harmer & Henderson, 1942, p. 9401). This method involved placing the patient in a prone position. The nurse would straddle the thighs, facing the patient's head, and alternatively apply and remove pressure to the thorax.

Eventually, it was noted that what was believed to be best practice was not effective. Results of postmortem examinations indicated that something was missing in the techniques, and therefore research was begun to determine best practice. Today, nursing students are taught cardiopulmonary resuscitation techniques based on updated research and theories.

slowly innovations are adopted, even with evidence that a current practice is unsound.

Another area of nursing that has seen many changes over time is wound care. Daunton, Kothari, Smith, and Steele (2012) reviewed the approaches to wound care from 2500 BC to the present. One can see that some old approaches may have been on the right track, such as ancient Egyptians putting moldy bread into a wound (we now know bread mold can be a source of penicillin). Other approaches, such as the use of dry gauze, also have long roots but are now falling out of favor. For example, removal of dry gauze from the wound damages the tissue, slowing healing; the move is now toward use of newer products and less frequent dressing changes. Kohr (2001) demonstrated both effectiveness in practice and efficiency in cost reductions in the use of these new approaches in a practice setting.

> ### FYI
>
> Nursing research provides results that are relevant to and expand or enhance practice. For research to be considered *nursing research*, the focus is on nursing practice rather than that the research happens to be conducted by a nurse.

The Special Language of Research

It is important to understand the special language associated with research (Fawcett & Downs, 1992). Research can be either deductive or inductive. It can be quantitative, qualitative, or a combination of both approaches. Regardless of the approach used, theory provides a framework for the design.

Deductive research typically involves quantitative designs and begins by deriving testable ideas from theories (**Case Example 5-2**). Reports of deductive research describe the theoretical assumptions used to guide the study in the introduction section. Reports also include a critical review of previous research that both supports and refutes aspects of the theory. Because theories are abstract in nature, there is a language of research that corresponds to the language of theory. Unlike terms associated with theory, the language of research refers to the empirical, or that which can be observed.

CASE EXAMPLE 5-2

Nightingale's Work to Reduce Death Rates During War: An Example of Theory and Deductive Research

Nightingale theorized that five factors were essential for promoting health: pure or fresh air, pure water, efficient drainage, cleanliness, and light—especially direct sunlight (Nightingale, 1859/1969). Through the application of her theory about what was required for the sick to recover, the death rate at Barrack Hospital during the Crimean War dropped from 42% to 2.2% in the first 6 months after her arrival. Nightingale was able to document this through the use of statistics (Strachey, 1918). Through careful collection and tracking of data, she was able to confirm that nursing interventions based on her theory were effective. Nightingale remains the first known quantitative researcher in nursing. Her work is an excellent example of developing theory, applying theory to practice, and finding support and validation through systematic research.

Researchers cannot measure concepts; however, they can measure variables. A variable is an observation that can be measured by assigning a number to each dimension. For example, a researcher may choose to study the abstract concept of health by measuring the empirical variable of number of acquired upper respiratory infections per year. A hypothesis is a special type of proposition that can be tested empirically. There should be a theoretical basis for hypotheses. For example, to test Nightingale's (1859/1969) observations, a nurse may wish to test the relationship between exposure to sunlight and number of acquired upper respiratory infections per year in people receiving nursing care. The stated hypothesis could be that there is a relationship between exposure to sunlight and the number of acquired upper respiratory infections per year. The researcher would statistically test the null hypothesis that exposure to sunlight does not affect the acquisition of upper respiratory infections.

Statistical methods are such that a hypothesis, and by extension, a theory, is never proved. Hypotheses can only be supported. A theory holds only until evidence comes forward to refute it (Johnson, 1983). This is a hard concept for students to grasp because the logic of building knowledge by rejecting opposite ideas seems backward. This is one reason why research can be slow and painstaking.

Using deduction, researchers formulate hypotheses based on clear definitions of concepts and variables. Often, formulating hypotheses coincides with stating definitions. There are two kinds of definitions: conceptual and operational. *Conceptual definitions* are the definitions of concepts contained in the theory that is being used. These definitions sound like those found in dictionaries. *Operational definitions* are definitions that explicitly state how the variable will be measured or operationalized. For example, using Nightingale's theory (1859/1969), the conceptual definition of health would be the absence of disease. A researcher could operationalize health as the number of self-reported upper respiratory infections per year. Environment was defined as everything outside the person (Nightingale, 1859/1969); this is the conceptual definition. The number of hours a person is in the light of the sun is an operational definition of environment. Defining concepts and variables allows researchers to collect quantitative data and apply statistics to learn about the phenomenon of interest.

Operational definitions can vary across studies because there are many different ways to measure any given concept. In the example, exposure to sunlight could also be measured using an instrument that would provide a value for the intensity of sunlight over a period of time. The researcher would need to decide whether exposure to sunlight through a glass window is appropriate or whether exposure needs to be unobstructed by glass. The instruments used to measure the amount of time exposed to sunlight and the method of recording the number of self-reported acquired upper respiratory infections would be considered the *empirical indicators* of the variables being studied.

KEY TERMS

conceptual definitions: Definitions of concepts contained in a theory that sound like dictionary definitions

operational definitions: Definitions that explicitly state how the variable will be measured or operationalized; empirical definitions

empirical indicators: Measures of the variables being studied

When researchers formulate their plans of research, they use theories to create *theoretical frameworks*. A theoretical framework provides the structure for the study by linking the abstract to the empirical. Sometimes researchers depict their frameworks using a *model*, which is essentially a pictorial representation of the concepts and their interrelationships.

Inductive research is used to develop theory and is usually qualitative. Researchers typically begin data collection before reading the literature to avoid biasing the data collection process. When reporting inductive research, authors use quotations to highlight key points of the theory that has emerged. An example of how a theory can be developed inductively using one particular qualitative method follows (**Case Example 5-3**).

There are also researchers who use both qualitative and quantitative methods in the same study. Studies can also have both deductive and inductive elements. The development of the transitional discharge model in mental health is an example of this mixing of methods and approaches (Forchuk & Brown, 1989; Forchuk, Chan, et al., 1998; Forchuk, Jewell, Schofield, Sircelj, & Valledor, 1998; Forchuk, Martin, Chan, & Jensen, 2005).

Case Example 5-4 illustrates how researchers might use multiple approaches when addressing clinical questions. It also demonstrates that it takes more than one study to build knowledge. Work replicated in Scotland with similar positive results (Reynolds et al., 2004) lends further support to the transitional discharge model for mental health.

Theory in Practice

The American Nurses Association (ANA) has defined the practice of nursing as the "protection, promotion, and optimization of health and abilities, prevention of illness and injury, facilitation of healing, alleviation of suffering through the diagnosis and treatment of human response, and advocacy in the

KEY TERMS

theoretical framework: The structure of a study that links the theory concepts to the study variables; a section of a research article that describes the theory used

model: Pictorial representation of concepts and their interrelationships

---

CASE EXAMPLE 5-3

Understanding and Helping Depressed Women: An Example of Theory and Inductive Research

Schreiber, a clinical nurse specialist, noticed that twice as many women as men suffered from depression. She found little in the way of nursing research that could help her care for these women. In order to better understand the recovery process for these women, she used a grounded theory approach (Glaser & Strauss, 1969) to guide her work (Schreiber, 1996). A sample of 21 women who had recovered from depression was interviewed for the study. Schreiber identified that women need to tell their story, and "seek understanding," in order to proceed to the stage of "cluing in," which is a stage of recovery. By identifying stages of recovery and formulating a theory about the process of recovery, specific nursing interventions were able to be identified. For example, implications for nursing practice include recognizing the importance of facilitating women telling their stories.

CASE EXAMPLE 5-4

A Transitional Discharge Model for Mental Health: An Example of Theory and Research Using Mixed Methods

As an advanced practice nurse in a tertiary care mental health setting, Forchuk noted that more clients left the unit because of death than by discharge. Those who had been discharged were often readmitted within a month of leaving the hospital. Her challenge was to find a way to help discharged clients return to the community and successfully remain there. She worked systematically with staff, clients, family members, and former clients in the community to discover what interventions might be helpful. From these efforts, it became clear that patients were discharged to an environment where all of their relationships were within a community in which they felt alone and isolated. This conclusion was reached inductively.

Because no nursing theory could be found to effectively explain the observations, Forchuk began developing a model to explain successful discharge of mental health clients. The model combined continuing staff support from professionals who had established therapeutic relationships with the clients with peer support from former users of mental health services who had successfully transitioned to the community. Professionals continued interactions with clients until the clients established a working relationship with the community. The model was piloted and the results were impressive (Forchuk & Brown, 1989). All nine clients discharged during the study year were successful in their return to the community, reducing the cost of their care (Forchuk, Chan, et al., 1998; Forchuk, Jewell, et al., 1998; Schofield et al., 1997). Both quantitative and qualitative measures were used to collect data. As a result of the pilot, funding for a large clinical trial to test the model in an experimental study was obtained (Forchuk et al., 2005).

care of individuals, families, groups, communities, and populations" (ANA, 2017). From the early days of the profession, students have been taught that a scientific attitude and method of work combined with "experience, trained senses, a mind trained to think, and the necessary characteristics of patience, accuracy, open-mindedness, truthfulness, persistence, and industry" (Harmer, 1933, p. 47) are essential components of good practice. Harmer goes on to say, "Each time this habit of looking, listening, feeling, or thinking is repeated it is strengthened until the habit of observation is firmly established" (p. 47). This still holds true today. Benner (1984) studied nurses in practice and concluded that to become an expert nurse one has to practice nursing a minimum of 5 years. There are no shortcuts to becoming an expert in one's field. The development of knowledge and skill takes time and work. As nurses encounter new situations, learning takes place. Nursing knowledge develops and is refined as nurses practice (Waterman, Webb, & Williams, 1995). In this way, nurses adapt theories to fit their practices. Unfortunately, much that is learned about theory during practice remains with the nurse because nurses rarely share their practice expertise through conference presentations and publications. The discipline will be enriched when nurses engage more formally in disseminating their knowledge about theory in practice.

CRITICAL THINKING EXERCISE 5-2

A nurse on a surgical floor observes that several new approaches are being used to dress wounds. She observes that some methods appear to promote healing faster than others do. While reviewing the research literature, she is unable to locate any research about the dressings she is using. How might she go about testing her theory that some methods are better than others? Can this be done deductively, inductively, or using mixed methods? Are any theories presently available related to wound healing, and if so, where might she locate these? What concepts might be important in forming the question?

The Relationships Among Theory, Research, and Practice

Practice relies on research and theory and also provides the questions that require more work by theorists and researchers. Each informs and supports the other in the application and development of nursing knowledge. When the relationships among theory, research, and practice are in harmony, the discipline is best served, ultimately resulting in better patient outcomes (Maas, 2006). The relationships are dynamic and flow in all directions. Practice informs and is informed by theory development as well as research. Research and theory development inform and are informed by each other (see **Figure 5-1**). Inclusion of practitioner perspectives, experiences, and insights in education helps students to understand how theory and research are applied to practice and informed by it (Chan, Chan, & Liu, 2012).

FIGURE 5-1   The Relationships of Theory, Research, and Practice

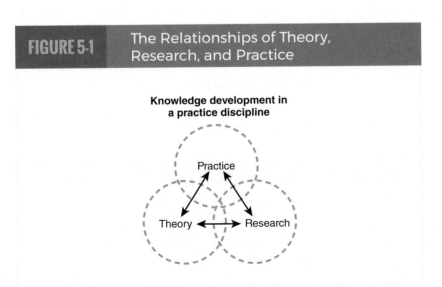

The literature continues to reflect that in the nursing profession there is tension about the relationships among theory, research, and practice (McCrae, 2012). Too often theorists, researchers, and nurses work in isolation from each other. Some see research as serving to develop theory that should then drive practice (Mitchell, 1997), while others see theory as driving research that should then drive practice (Billings & Kowalski, 2006). Still others see practice as informing and being informed by research and theory (Schmelzer, 2006). As Butcher (2006) pointed out, practicing nurses focus on unique individuals, researchers focus on systematically collecting knowledge about samples and populations, and theorists focus on abstract and general concepts and their interrelationships. Understanding the different perspectives of each of these groups in knowledge building shows their activities to be complementary.

At a micro level, each nurse engages in research and theory development. For example, each patient encounter can be considered a study with one subject. Assessment can serve as data collection involving both quantitative and qualitative data, and the plan of care emerges from the analysis. The result is a theory of what will work for this person. The theory is tested as care is delivered, and if positive outcomes are achieved, the theory is validated. If outcomes are not positive, the theory is refuted and a new theory is created, resulting in a revised plan of care. Learning from each patient encounter is applied to new encounters. Case by case, the nurse learns about both the unique and universal characteristics of individuals.

Researchers engage in a similar process, but from a different perspective. Nursing researchers systematically study individuals in groups, or in samples representing larger populations, to uncover knowledge about universal characteristics of individuals as these apply to people's health. Knowledge from research assists nurses to choose interventions that have a known probability of success. Although research findings help nurses predict what will be successful for the majority of individuals, outcomes cannot be predicted for an individual. When an individual does not respond like the majority of people do, a nurse will rely more on clinical judgment and patient preferences.

Like researchers, theorists also work at a macro level building knowledge that can be universally applied. Theory provides understanding and

 CRITICAL THINKING EXERCISE 5-3

Reflect on your most recent patient encounter. When you assessed your patient, what theoretical assumptions guided your data collection? Were there questions you had about nursing needs or health circumstance that puzzled you? How did you go about addressing these questions? How might you go about that in the future? Who might you involve in addressing questions? What did you do that worked when providing care for this patient? Would you use the approach with another patient? Why or why not?

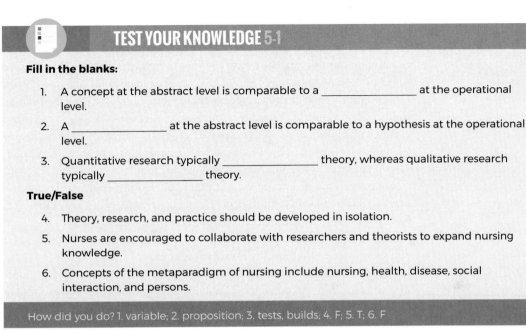

TEST YOUR KNOWLEDGE 5-1

Fill in the blanks:

1. A concept at the abstract level is comparable to a _____ at the operational level.

2. A _____ at the abstract level is comparable to a hypothesis at the operational level.

3. Quantitative research typically _____ theory, whereas qualitative research typically _____ theory.

True/False

4. Theory, research, and practice should be developed in isolation.

5. Nurses are encouraged to collaborate with researchers and theorists to expand nursing knowledge.

6. Concepts of the metaparadigm of nursing include nursing, health, disease, social interaction, and persons.

How did you do? 1. variable; 2. proposition; 3. tests, builds; 4. F; 5. T; 6. F

guidance to the practice of nursing. It also provides language for describing nursing's work.

It is clear from the debate in the literature that nurses, researchers, and theorists can work more closely together and that such partnerships will be very fruitful for the development of nursing knowledge. Schmelzer (2006) encouraged nurses to collaborate with researchers to find answers for practice problems. Waterman and associates (1995) also supported closer working relationships among nurses, researchers, and theorists. It is quite reasonable for nurses to be members of formal research teams as content experts. Another way to increase collaboration is for more researchers and theorists to engage in practice.

5.2 Keeping It Ethical

At the end of this section, you will be able to:

‹ Discuss how honoring prior work ethically builds nursing knowledge

Students of any discipline are taught the body of knowledge that has been built over time, including the origins of the ideas that comprise that body of knowledge. As individuals contribute to the body of knowledge, credit should be given to those on whose work they are building.

FYI

Credit must be given for ideas built on earlier work as well as for new ideas generated by challenging old ideas.

Knowledge in a discipline is built in small steps that in time mark a long and fruitful journey of discovery. When reading the works of nurses, researchers, and theorists, students of the discipline should be able to trace the evolution of ideas. Credit must be given for ideas built on earlier work as well as for new ideas generated by challenging old ideas. This trail can be followed by examining references and reading the work of those who made earlier contributions. Sadly, nurses have been poor at leaving such a trail. Few theorists cite the nurses who influenced their thinking. For example, Peplau (1952) gives credit to Adler, a psychologist, for influencing her thinking, but she makes no mention of nurses who may have influenced her despite the fact that she published for nurses practicing in mental health areas. Likewise, Rogers (1970) does not credit the sources of her nursing knowledge even though she published a model for nurses in all settings. In other cases, an author may state that an idea came from another individual but does not provide a reference, or an author may use a secondary source for a quotation when a primary source is available. Failure to honor the work of others creates problems for nurses trying to understand the evolution of nursing knowledge and practice.

Here is a very good example of how the knowledge train can get derailed. McCrae (2012) credited Virginia Henderson as publishing the first definition of nursing as "to attend to the functional needs of patients." McCrae cited the 1955 version of the text Henderson coauthored with Bertha Harmer. However, the credit for this definition really should go to Harmer. Harmer had first published this definition as a sole author in 1925 and had clearly linked her work to Nightingale's work.

> Nursing is rooted in the needs of humanity and is founded on the ideal of service. Its object is not only to cure the sick and heal the wounded but to bring health and ease, rest and comfort to mind and body, to shelter, nourish, and protect and to minister to all those who are helpless or handicapped, young, aged or immature. Its object is to prevent disease and to preserve health. (Harmer, 1925, p. 3)

Not until 1942 when Harmer brought in Henderson to take over her work was Henderson associated with this definition (Harmer & Henderson, 1942). A much later edition by these two authors from 1955 is where McCrae in 2012 obtained her citation. This example shows the importance of following the knowledge trail with curiosity and diligence in order to truly understand the foundations of current nursing knowledge. Honoring the work of earlier nurses honors the profession itself, and all who are part of it.

When studying the writings of nurses who are contributors to disciplinary knowledge, it is important to look for the foundation of their ideas. Where information about these ideas is lacking, nurses should critically appraise claims that the work is a legitimate part of the disciplinary knowledge of nursing. To write as a contributor to the disciplinary body of knowledge without giving proper credit to those who provided the basis for the ideas is not just poor or dishonest practice but is unethical and, in fact, plagiarism.

FYI

To write as a contributor to the disciplinary body of knowledge without giving credit to those who provided the basis for the ideas is not just poor practice but is unethical and, in fact, plagiarism.

TEST YOUR KNOWLEDGE 5-2

True/False

1. In the discipline of nursing, it is easy to follow how knowledge has developed because theorists have carefully provided citations for their ideas.

2. Giving credit to those who provide the basis for ideas is ethical practice.

How did you do? 1. F; 2. T

RAPID REVIEW

» Theories are sets of concepts linked by propositions that explain phenomena. They provide a belief system to guide practice.

» Concepts are words or phrases conveying unique ideas or mental images. They are the building blocks of theories.

» The metaparadigm of nursing has four concepts: person, health, environment, and nursing.

» Propositions are statements describing relationships between two or more concepts.

» Constructs are properties that are inferred because they cannot be directly observed.

» Variables describe how concepts will be measured at the empirical level, and hypotheses are propositions that can be tested empirically.

» Concepts, propositions, variables, and hypotheses form theoretical frameworks that provide structure for research studies. Models are pictorial representations of theoretical frameworks.

» Conceptual definitions are like definitions found in dictionaries and are abstract in nature. Operational definitions specify how variables will be measured. Empirical indicators are the instruments used to measure variables.

» Deductive quantitative research is typically used to test theory, whereas inductive qualitative research can be used to build theory. Mixed methods can also contribute to the development of theory.

» In practice, nursing knowledge is developed and refined through patient encounters.

» The relationships of theory, research, and practice are dynamic and complementary.

» In practice, nurses learn about unique and universal characteristics of individuals. Researchers use systematic study to discover knowledge about universal characteristics of people. Theorists build knowledge that can be universally applied.

» The ethical practice of honoring the work of others creates a trail whereby nurses can follow the building of nursing knowledge.

Apply What You Have Learned

An EBP committee member tells you she has found an article (Al-Tawfiq & Pittet, 2013) that describes how behavioral theories are applied to improve hand hygiene compliance. She is excited about this, and she would like the committee to consider how these models might be useful to its work. To prepare for the next meeting, read the article and consider how these models could be used as frameworks for designing interventions.

REFERENCES

Al-Tawfiq, J. A., & Pittet, D. (2013). Improving hand hygiene compliance in healthcare settings using behavior change theories: Reflections. *Teaching and Learning in Medicine, 25*, 374–382.

American Nurses Association. (2017). What is nursing? Retrieved 6/22/17 from http://www.nursingworld.org/EspeciallyForYou/What-is-Nursing

Benner, P. (1984). *From novice to expert: Excellence and power in clinical nursing practice.* Menlo Park, CA: Addison-Wesley.

Billings, D. M., & Kowalski, K. (2006). Bridging the theory–practice gap with evidence-based practice. *Journal of Continuing Education in Nursing, 37*, 248–249.

Butcher, H. (2006). Integrating nursing theory, nursing research, and nursing practice. In P. S. Cowen & S. Moorhead (Eds.), *Current issues in nursing* (pp. 112–122). St. Louis, MO: Mosby.

Chan, E. A., Chan, K., & Liu, Y. W. J. (2012). A triadic interplay between academics, practitioners and students in the nursing theory and practice dialectic. *Journal of Advanced Nursing, 68*(5), 1038–1049.

Daunton, C., Kothari, S., Smith, L., & Steele, D. (2012). A history of materials and practices for wound management. *Wound Practice and Research, 20*(4), 174–186.

Fawcett, J. (1984). The metaparadigm of nursing: Current status and future refinements. *Image: Journal of Nursing Scholarship, 16,* 84–87.

Fawcett, J., & Downs, F. S. (1992). *The relationship of theory and research* (2nd ed.). Philadelphia, PA: Davis.

Forchuk, C., & Brown, B. (1989). Establishing a nurse–client relationship. *Journal of Psychosocial Nursing, 27*(2), 30–34.

Forchuk, C., Chan, L., Schofield, R., Sircelj, M., Woodcox, V., Jewell, J., . . . Overby, B. (1998). Bridging the discharge process. *Canadian Nurse, 94*(3), 22–26.

Forchuk, C., Jewell, J., Schofield, R., Sircelj, M., & Valledor, T. (1998). From hospital to community: Bridging therapeutic relationships. *Journal of Psychiatric and Mental Health Nursing, 5,* 197–202.

Forchuk, C., Martin, M. L., Chan, Y. L., & Jensen, E. (2005). Therapeutic relationships: From psychiatric hospital to community. *Journal of Psychiatric and Mental Health Nursing, 12,* 556–564.

Glaser, B., & Strauss, A. (1969). *The discovery of grounded theory.* Chicago, IL: Aldine.

Goodnow, M. (1919). *First-year nursing* (2nd ed.). Philadelphia, PA: Saunders.

Graham, I. W. (2003). The relationship of nursing theory to practice and research within the British context: Identifying a way forward. *Nursing Science Quarterly, 16,* 346–350.

Harmer, B. (1925). *Text-book of the principles and practice of nursing.* New York, NY: Macmillan.

Harmer, B. (1933). *Textbook of the principles and practice of nursing* (2nd ed.). New York, NY: Macmillan.

Harmer, B., & Henderson, V. (1942). *Textbook of the principles and practice of nursing* (4th ed.). New York, NY: Macmillan.

Johnson, M. (1983). Some aspects of the relation between theory and research in nursing. *Journal of Advanced Nursing, 8*(1), 21–28.

Kohr, R. (2001). Moist healing versus wet-to-dry [Standard protocol for chronic wounds]. *Canadian Nurse, 97*(1), 17–19.

Maas, M. L. (2006). What is nursing, and why do we ask? In P. S. Cowen & S. Moorhead (Eds.), *Current issues in nursing* (pp. 5–10). St. Louis, MO: Mosby.

McCrae, N. (2012). Whither nursing models? The value of nursing theory in the context of evidence-based practice and multidisciplinary health care. *Journal of Advanced Nursing, 68*(1), 222–229.

Mitchell, G. J. (1997). Questioning evidence-based practice for nursing. *Nursing Science Quarterly, 10,* 154–155.

Nightingale, F. (1969). *Notes on nursing: What it is, and what it is not.* New York, NY: Dover. (Original work published 1859)

Parse, R. R. (2014). *The humanbecoming paradigm: A transformational worldview.* Pittsburgh, PA: Discovery International Publications.

Peplau, H. E. (1952). *Interpersonal relations in nursing: A conceptual frame of reference for psychodynamic nursing.* New York, NY: Putnam.

Reynolds, W., Lauder, W., Sharkey, S., MacIver, S., Veitch, T., & Cameron, D. (2004). The effect of transitional discharge model for psychiatric patients. *Journal of Psychiatric and Mental Health Nursing, 11,* 82–88.

Rogers, M. E. (1970). *An introduction to the theoretical basis of nursing.* Philadelphia, PA: Davis.

Schmelzer, M. (2006). Personal reflections about the theory–research–practice connection. *Gastroenterology Nursing, 29*, 489–491.

Schofield, R., Valledor, T., Sircelj, M., Forchuk, C., Jewell, J., & Woodcox, V. (1997). Evaluation of bridging institution and housing—a joint consumer care provider initiative. *Journal of Psychosocial Nursing, 35*, 9–14.

Schreiber, R. (1996). Understanding and helping depressed women. *Archives of Psychiatric Nursing, 10*, 165–175.

Strachey, L. (1918). *Eminent Victorians.* New York, NY: Garden City.

Waterman, H., Webb, C., & Williams, A. (1995). Parallels and contradictions in the theory and practice of action research and nursing. *Journal of Advanced Nursing, 22*, 779–784.

Persuasion

Persuasion is the art of using facts to promote change.

CHAPTER 6

Key Principles of Quantitative Designs

Rosalind M. Peters

6.1 Chart the Course: Selecting the Best Design

At the end of this section, you will be able to:

< Explain the relationships among the study purpose, literature review, research questions or hypotheses, study framework, and the study design
< Define key concepts relevant to quantitative research designs including experimental, nonexperimental, causality, probability, control, manipulation, bias, randomization, between-subjects, within-subjects, and study validity
< List elements to be considered when appraising quantitative designs

You will see the term *research design* used two different ways. Many people use the term broadly to encompass multiple aspects of the research process including the sampling plan, data collection procedures, implementation strategies, and data analysis. In this context, the broad use of the term implies the overall method of the research study. Another way the term can be used is to refer to the specific plan or blueprint that will be used to meet the stated purpose of the study. When you evaluate the appropriateness of the research design, it is important to realize that the design is not developed in a vacuum. Instead, it should reflect an integration of the theoretical and empirical literature that was presented in the review of the literature section of the study. This section usually ends by identifying a gap in current knowledge about the phenomenon of interest. The purpose of the proposed study should be to fill some portion of that gap in knowledge with the research questions or hypotheses determining what specific new knowledge will be generated. The research design should flow from the stated purpose and provide a plan that can answer the research questions and test the stated hypotheses.

Quantitative designs used to examine relationships among variables are categorized as experimental or nonexperimental. These designs can be used to meet four key purposes. Experimental designs are used for the purpose of examining causality. Nonexperimental designs can be used for the purposes of describing a phenomenon in detail, explaining relationships and differences among variables, and predicting relationships and differences among variables. The major difference between nonexperimental and experimental designs is the role of the researcher. In experimental designs, researchers actively manipulate the independent variable (IV), sometimes known as the causal variable, to determine its effect on the dependent variable (DV), or outcome variable. Experimental designs also involve randomization and the use of a control group whose results can be compared to the group receiving the experimental intervention. Quasi-experimental designs also involve the manipulation of the IV but lack either randomization or a control group. In nonexperimental designs, researchers are observers noting the occurrence of the variables of interest and trying to determine relationships and differences. Other quantitative designs are used to address methodological issues such as instrument development or in the case of meta-analyses to examine outcomes across a number of studies.

As you appraise an article for the quality of the study presented, you should find that there is a logical flow of information presented. Information from the literature reviewed and discussion of the study framework should lead you to agree that the study is needed, that the purpose is appropriate given the literature presented, and that the planned design will be able to generate quantitative information to address the stated research questions and hypotheses.

Understanding Key Concepts in Quantitative Designs

Best practice means that nurses must have confidence in the evidence that they are applying to patient care. Having confidence in findings requires that nurses be able to critically appraise quantitative studies before applying findings to practice. Therefore, understanding key concepts and principles related to the design of quantitative studies is necessary.

Causality and Probability

Causality refers to the relationship that exists between a cause and its effect. The cause has the ability or power to produce a specific effect. The assumption is made that the cause precedes the effect. Being able to determine causality requires that the variables of interest are studied in chronological order: the causal variable, or IV, has to occur prior to the occurrence of the DV, or the effect. From a research perspective, causality is the belief that researchers, using stringent controls, can manipulate a cause to produce the effect or result that can be repeated. Experimental designs are used to examine causality, with researchers manipulating the IV while observing its effect on the DV. When working with people, nurse researchers recognize that there are multiple factors that can contribute to an outcome. Rarely do nurses deal with problems that have only one cause and one effect. When outcomes have many causes, it is known as multicausality. Therefore, it is important to consider multicausality when evaluating research designs. Because it is possible that there are multiple, interrelated factors causing an outcome, it is important for researchers to try to identify and control for as many of those factors as possible. When appraising research studies, nurses need to familiarize themselves with the variables included in the study and evaluate the discussion section of the study report to determine whether researchers identified other possible causes for the results. **Box 6-1** outlines points that should be considered when appraising quantitative designs.

Closely related to the idea of multicausality is the idea of *probability*. Again, because nursing is a human science rather than a basic science, such as biology or chemistry, nurse researchers are unlikely to be able to assert with absolute certainty that the IV caused the effect in the DV. Instead, research related to human health and functioning results in assertions of probability or how likely it is that the change in the DV was caused by the IV. Probability assertions

KEY TERMS

causality: The relationship between a cause and its effect

probability: Likelihood or chance that an event will occur in a situation

BOX 6-1	Elements to Consider When Appraising Quantitative Designs

What type of quantitative design is being used?

Can causality be inferred?

Did researchers use the highest level of design possible to answer the research questions?

What strategies did the researcher use to control for the effects of extraneous variables?

What threats to internal and external validity might be present, and were any strategies used to reduce them?

Were there any ethical concerns about the design?

leave open the possibility that there are other causes and factors affecting the result seen in the DV.

Control, Manipulation, and Bias

Control refers to the ability to manipulate, regulate, or statistically adjust for the multitude of factors that can influence the DV. Control is necessary to make assertions about cause and effect. *Manipulation* is an important aspect of control in experimental designs and refers to the ability of researchers to control the IV. The IV is considered to be the intervention, or treatment, that is being tested in an experimental study. The intervention may be physiological, psychological, behavioral, educational, or a combination of these.

For example, a researcher hypothesizes that educational interventions will result in increased condom use among sexually active teens and wants to test a newly developed computer-based intervention. The researcher manipulates the IV, the educational intervention, by determining what content will be included, how it will be delivered, in what environment it will be delivered, and who will receive it. The researcher in this example would then compare preintervention condom usage with postintervention usage. The researcher also could compare the difference in condom usage between the intervention group and a control group. In health-related experimental designs, the control group of subjects usually receives the standard of care but does not get the intervention. The control group of teens, in this example, would participate in the traditional sex education classes offered in their school but would not be able to access the computer-based program. However, because factors other than education can affect condom use, the researcher also needs to control for these extraneous or confounding factors.

Extraneous variables are those that confound, or confuse, the effect of the IV on the DV. Researchers can control for extraneous variables through careful selection of participants, use of consistent data collection procedures, randomization, or use of certain statistical tests. Examples of confounding variables in the example might be the age of the teen, religious beliefs, self-efficacy for resisting peer pressure, cost of condoms, ease of purchasing them, and whether or not the teen has a current sexual partner. Without careful control of extraneous variables, bias can be introduced into the study.

Bias results when extraneous variables influence and distort the relationship between the IV and the DV so that the findings are not really reflecting the true relationship. For example, if the study included students without a current sexual partner, it would be highly likely that the intervention would result in no significant difference in condom use. This lack of difference might be attributed to the intervention being ineffective when it is actually caused by the fact

KEY TERMS

control: Ability to manipulate, regulate, or statistically adjust for factors that can affect the dependent variable

manipulation: The ability of researchers to control the independent variable

extraneous variables: Factors that interfere with the relationship between the independent and dependent variables; confounding variable; Z variable

bias: When extraneous variables influence the relationship between the independent and dependent variables

that the teen is not currently engaging in sexual activity requiring a condom. Researchers control for this type of bias by clearly specifying criteria required for subjects to be included in a study. After subjects are enrolled in a study, it is important for researchers to control how the study is actually conducted. This includes controlling the environment in which the study is conducted, providing consistency in how interventions are delivered, and collecting data in a careful and consistent manner. For example, asking students to report their condom use during an interview where others might hear their responses could bias the results because students may not feel comfortable responding truthfully. A better way to obtain this information may be to have students complete a self-report of their condom use on an anonymous questionnaire.

Randomization

Randomization is an effective way to control extraneous variables. Randomization can occur either with random sampling of the subjects to be studied or by random assignment of subjects to the intervention or control group. *Random sampling* means that all people in the population of interest have the same probability of being selected to be included in the study. This occurs infrequently in health-related research because researchers usually do not have the time or money to randomly sample all people who could potentially participate. For example, it would be very difficult to randomly sample sexually active teens from around the country. Instead, in this example the researcher would most likely use a convenience sample of students from high schools within the area. The researcher would then randomly assign the students into the intervention and the control groups. *Random assignment* means that all subjects in the sample (not the population) have an equal chance of being assigned to either the treatment or the control group. Random assignment increases the likelihood that extraneous variables that may affect the DV will be equally distributed between the two groups. Using random assignment allows researchers to be more confident that the IV rather than the extraneous variables caused the effect on the DV. Although researchers may be very careful about selecting representative samples and using random assignment to groups to control for extraneous variables, these techniques do not guarantee that extraneous variables will be equally distributed between the two groups. When groups are different, researchers need to apply certain statistical tests to control for the effect of extraneous variables on the DV.

Between-Groups and Within-Groups

Quantitative studies often are designed for the purpose of making comparisons either by comparing different groups of subjects or by comparing the same subject at different points in time. Studies developed to compare two different

KEY TERMS

randomization:
The selection, assignment, or arrangement of elements by chance

random sampling:
Technique for selecting elements whereby each has the same chance of being selected

random assignment:
Assignment technique in which subjects have an equal chance of being in either the treatment or the control group

groups of subjects use a *between-groups design*. For example, a researcher who is studying condom use among adolescents may wish to know the practices of high school juniors and seniors as well as college freshmen and sophomores. The researcher could make comparisons among these four groups about the frequency of condom use.

Although comparisons among diverse subjects are important, there may be other situations when researchers are more interested in making comparisons within the same subject. For example, a researcher is interested in the effect of music therapy on patients' levels of pain. Using a *within-groups design*, the researcher would measure the subjects' levels of pain before the intervention, conduct the intervention, and then measure pain levels after the intervention. By comparing the subjects' pain scores before and after the intervention, the researcher is able to determine the effectiveness of music therapy as a pain relief measure.

TEST YOUR KNOWLEDGE 6-1

1. When designing a study, which of the following should the researcher consider? (Select all that apply.)
   a. Research question
   b. Review of the literature
   c. Theoretical framework
   d. Study purpose

2. Which of the following is *not* a purpose of nonexperimental designs?
   a. Describe phenomenon
   b. Explain relationships
   c. Predict relationships
   d. Examine causality

3. What is the researcher's ability to manipulate or regulate extraneous variables known as?
   a. Control
   b. Manipulation
   c. Bias
   d. Probability

4. When a researcher assigns subjects to groups by tossing a coin, the researcher is using which technique?
   a. Random selection
   b. Random assignment
   c. Bias
   d. Within-groups design

How did you do? 1. a, b, c, d; 2. d; 3. a; 4. b

Researchers can combine between-groups and within-groups designs within the same study to compare the effectiveness of more than one intervention. In the pain example, the researcher might offer music therapy as an intervention to one group of subjects and relaxation therapy as another intervention to a different group of subjects. The researcher could analyze the within-groups results to determine the level to which each intervention reduced pain, and the researcher could compare between-groups results to determine whether there was a difference in the amount of pain relief provided by the music and relaxation.

6.2 What Is Validity?

At the end of this section, you will be able to:

< Define the two types of validity
< Describe seven threats to internal validity
< Describe five threats to external validity
< Identify strategies used to reduce threats to internal and external validity

Exerting control over extraneous variables affecting the DV is one important factor to ensure valid results. *Study validity* refers to the ability to accept results as logical, reasonable, and justifiable based on the evidence presented. Validity is sometimes described as the truth or accuracy of the results. Evaluating the quality of quantitative evidence requires nurses to identify potential threats to validity, evaluate the seriousness of those threats, and determine whether results are valid for application to patient care. Threats are forces that can change the results of studies. Campbell and Stanley (1966) identified two major types of validity: internal and external (see **Table 6-1**). Internal and external validity were originally developed to evaluate cause-and-effect relationships, making them most relevant for experimental designs. However, validity should be considered with all quantitative designs. It is important when appraising research articles to identify threats and consider how these threats may have influenced the relationship between the IV and DV or the interpretation of results.

Internal Validity

Internal validity is the degree to which one can conclude that it was the IV, not extraneous variables, that produced the change in the DV (Cook & Campbell, 1979). To establish internal validity, researchers must demonstrate that results obtained were caused by the IV. Seven common threats to internal validity include selection bias, history, maturation, testing, instrumentation, mortality, and statistical conclusion validity.

KEY TERMS

study validity:
Ability to accept results as logical, reasonable, and justifiable based on the evidence presented

internal validity:
The degree to which one can conclude that the independent variable produced changes in the dependent variable

TABLE 6-1	Summary of Design Threats

Threats to Internal Validity	**Threats to External Validity**
‹ Selection bias	‹ Construct validity
‹ History	— Bias
‹ Maturation	— Confounding
‹ Testing	— Reactivity
‹ Instrumentation	‹ Effects of selection
‹ Mortality	‹ Interaction of treatment and selection of subjects
‹ Statistical conclusion validity	‹ Interaction of treatment and setting
	‹ Interaction of treatment and history

KEY TERMS

selection bias: A threat to internal validity when the change in the dependent variable is a result of the characteristics of the subjects before they entered a study

history: A threat to internal validity when the dependent variable is influenced by an event that occurred during the study

Selection Bias

Selection bias occurs when the change in the DV is a result of differences in the characteristics of subjects before they entered a study rather than a result of the IV. Suppose a researcher wants to compare the effectiveness of group teaching to one-on-one teaching. At the hospital where the study is being conducted, patients are allowed to choose the kind of teaching they want. It is possible that people who select group teaching are different on some characteristics from those who select one-on-one teaching. Selection bias can be minimized somewhat by the use of random assignment to groups.

History

The threat of *history* occurs when the DV may have been influenced by some event other than the IV that occurred during the course of the study. In the example of condom use, it might be difficult to attribute increased use of condoms to the computer intervention if during the same time as the study was being conducted MTV or VH1 aired public service announcements encouraging safe sex practices. In such a situation, it is difficult for the researcher to know whether the IV or the increased awareness from television produced the change in the DV. The threat of history could have been decreased by including a control group that was exposed to the television ads but that did not receive the computer intervention.

FYI

Evaluating the quality of quantitative evidence requires nurses to identify potential threats to validity, evaluate the seriousness of those threats, and determine whether results are valid for application to patient care. The two primary types of validity are internal validity and external validity.

Maturation

Over the course of a study, subjects may change either by growing or becoming more mature. This is known as the threat of *maturation*. Changes such as these are more likely to influence the DV when a study continues over time. For example, if subjects during the study on condom use came of age to obtain a driver's license and get a job, it would be difficult to determine whether an increase in condom use was a result of the IV or of the subjects' increased ease of purchasing condoms for use. A control group may help limit this threat to internal validity.

Testing

The threat of *testing* occurs when a pretest influences the way subjects respond on a posttest. Repeated testing can cause familiarity with the test itself, and answers may reflect subjects' abilities to remember how questions were answered previously rather than reflecting current knowledge and beliefs.

Instrumentation

When there are changes made in the way variables are measured, the threat of *instrumentation* can occur. For example, in a study measuring blood pressure, if the original measurement is taken using an aneroid sphygmomanometer but later measurements are taken using an automated device, it makes it difficult to determine whether any change in blood pressure readings is a result of the IV or the change in devices. Another potential instrumentation threat arises when data are collected by observation or interview using different data collectors. To control for this threat, researchers need to ensure all data collectors are comprehensively trained. Researchers also evaluate interrater reliability to determine the degree of consistency among individuals collecting data.

Mortality

Mortality refers to the loss of subjects before the study is completed. Loss of subjects may be a threat to internal validity if there is a difference in the characteristics of the subjects who dropped out compared to those who completed the study. Internal validity is also threatened when there is a difference in the loss of subjects between the experimental and control groups. Mortality tends to increase the longer a study lasts. In health-related research, emotional states such as depression and anxiety, as well as physical states such as fatigue, may influence dropout rates. When appraising a study for the threat of mortality, it is important to compare the number of subjects who entered the study with the number of subjects in the final sample. In a research article, the term *attrition rate* refers to the dropout rate. If the attrition rate is high, the author of the article should provide an analysis and explanation for the dropout rate.

KEY TERMS

maturation: A threat to internal validity when subjects change by growing or maturing

testing: A threat to internal validity when a pretest influences the way subjects respond on a posttest

instrumentation: A threat to internal validity when there are inconsistencies in data collection

mortality: A threat to internal validity when there is a loss of subjects before the study is completed; attrition rate

attrition rate: Dropout rate; loss of subjects before the study is completed; threat of mortality

Statistical Conclusion Validity

Statistical conclusion validity refers to the confidence one has that the results of the statistical analysis accurately reflect the true relationship between the IV and DV. This does not happen when researchers make a *type II error*. Type II errors occur when researchers inaccurately conclude that there is no relationship between the IV and DV when an actual relationship does exist. A type II error is more likely to occur when the sample size is small. Often large samples are needed in order to detect the effect of the IV on the DV. Low reliability of the measures is another factor that can interfere with researchers' abilities to draw accurate conclusions about relationships between the IV and DV. When appraising research articles for threats to statistical conclusion validity, it is important for readers to consider the information presented in the methods section that details the reliability of instruments. Researchers can control for low reliability of the measures by using well-established and well-designed instruments.

External Validity

External validity refers to the degree to which the results of the study can be generalized to other subjects, settings, and times (Cook & Campbell, 1979). There are five major threats to external validity. Construct validity is concerned with whether the instruments are really measuring the theoretical concepts under investigation. Other threats to external validity include threats related to selection of subjects for the study and ones that occur because of interactions between the IV and the subjects, the setting, or history.

Construct Validity

Construct validity is an important consideration when evaluating external validity. Assessing construct validity allows researchers to determine whether instruments are actually measuring the theoretical cause or effect concepts that are intended to be measured. A threat of construct validity can lead to bias or unintentional confounding of the results.

Bias refers to a systematic error in subject selection, measurement of variables, or analysis. For example, a researcher is studying the effect of anger on blood pressure; however, the instrument used to measure anger contains some items that might also reflect depression. The relationship between anger

CRITICAL THINKING EXERCISE 6-1

A researcher is interested in studying the effect of hearing loss on self-esteem in adolescents attending grades 6–12. What threats to internal validity should the researcher address? What controls could the researcher use to minimize these threats?

and blood pressure is biased because the instrument measures two different theoretical concepts. Therefore, the researcher would be unable to determine whether changes in blood pressure were a result of anger or depression. When appraising an article for threats to construct validity, it is important for readers to consider information presented in the methods section of the article. This section should contain information on the reliability of the instrument used and details on how the validity of the instrument was established.

Confounding means there is a possible error in interpretation of the results (Cook & Campbell, 1979). This can occur when experimental controls do not allow the researcher to eliminate possible alternative explanations for the relationship between the IV (cause variable) and the DV (effect variable). Subject reactivity and experimenter reactivity are two examples of unintentional confounding.

Subject reactivity means that sometimes subjects are influenced by participating in a study. Changes noted in the DV can be a result of subject *reactivity* and not a result of the IV. This is known as the *Hawthorne effect*. The Hawthorne effect was first recognized in studies done at the Western Electric Corporation's Hawthorne plant (Mayo, 1933). One of the studies attempted to determine whether changing the amount of lighting (IV) in the work environment changed worker productivity (DV). In this study, productivity increased regardless of changes made to lighting. Thus, one explanation was that increased lighting caused increased productivity as was hypothesized, but that interpretation did not explain why productivity increased in the control group. An alternative explanation for this result was that the increased productivity occurred not because of changes in illumination but because the employees in both groups knew they were being studied. Therefore, the effect of the IV on the DV was confounded by the subjects' behavior. The behavior of subjects in a study may be affected by their personal values, their desires to please the experimenter or provide the results the experimenter wants, and congruence of the study with subjects' personal interests and goals.

Experimenter reactivity is another type of reactivity that threatens external validity. When researchers have expected or desired outcomes in mind, they may inadvertently affect how interventions are conducted and how they interact with subjects. For example, a researcher may be friendlier to subjects in the experimental group than to subjects in the control group. As a result, subjects in the experimental group may perceive involvement in the study more positively than do subjects in the control group.

> **KEY TERMS**
>
> **reactivity:** The influence of participating in a study on the responses of subjects; Hawthorne effect
>
> **Hawthorne effect:** Subjects' behaviors may be affected by personal values or desires to please the experimenter; reactivity

CRITICAL THINKING EXERCISE 6-2

Have you ever participated in a research study? Do you think your behaviors were different because you knew you were being studied?

KEY TERMS

double-blind experimental designs: Studies in which subjects and researchers are unaware whether subjects are receiving experimental interventions or standard of care

effects of selection: Threats to external validity when the sample does not represent the population

interaction of treatment with selection of subjects: A threat to external validity where the independent variable might not affect individuals the same way

interaction of treatment and setting: A threat to external validity when an intervention conducted in one setting cannot be generalized to a different setting

Double-blind experimental designs have been used in health research to control for threats of reactivity. In double-blind studies, neither subjects nor individuals administering the treatments know whether subjects are receiving experimental interventions or standard of care. This design is fairly common in drug studies where a placebo pill can be manufactured to appear exactly like the drug being studied.

Effects of Selection

Because researchers most often study samples rather than an entire population, representativeness of the sample is essential. If the sample does not represent the population, *effects of selection* limit whether the study can be generalized to the population. For example, a researcher is interviewing mothers. Because interviews are being conducted only during the day and no child care is provided, individuals who work during the day or who have small children are less likely to participate in this study. Consequently, researchers would not be able to generalize to all mothers but only to mothers who do not work during the day and mothers without young children.

Interaction of Treatment with Selection of Subjects

Because external validity is concerned with generalizing to other individuals, it is only natural to ask, "Will this IV affect other people in the same way?" The *interaction of treatment with selection of subjects* must be considered (Cook & Campbell, 1979). This requires consideration of the difference between the accessible population and the target population of interest (Kempthorne, 1961). In the condom use example, the target population is all sexually active teens. The accessible population is the group of teens from which the researcher is actually able to obtain a sample of subjects. So, if the computer-based intervention is found to be effective in increasing condom use in a sample of students from a Midwestern suburban high school, how generalizable are those findings to teens living in urban centers in the West or rural areas of the South?

Interaction of Treatment and Setting

Sometimes an *interaction of treatment and setting* can affect external validity. This interaction is concerned with whether results from an intervention conducted in one setting can be generalized to another setting where the same intervention is used. If the study on condom use was conducted with teens waiting to be seen in a family planning clinic, can the findings from that study be generalized to teens in a high school setting?

Interaction of Treatment and History

Interactions of treatment and history can also occur. This threat is concerned with how the effects from the intervention might be changed by events occurring in the past or in the future. For example, if the researcher found that the computer-based intervention increased condom use, would those results be generalizable to the future if a cure for HIV were to be discovered?

> **KEY TERM**
>
> **interaction of treatment and history:** A threat to external validity when historical events affect the intervention

TEST YOUR KNOWLEDGE 6-2

1. What is the degree to which the results of studies can be generalized to other individuals, settings, or time called?
   a. External validity
   b. Construct validity
   c. Internal validity
   d. Statistical conclusion validity

2. During a study examining nurses' job satisfaction, the union decides to hold a strike. This is which type of threat to internal validity?
   a. Selection bias
   b. Mortality
   c. History
   d. Testing

3. A researcher plans to observe children in a kindergarten class. Students have always been told to be on their best behavior when guests are present in the classroom. What is the greatest threat to external validity?
   a. Construct validity
   b. Hawthorne effect
   c. Selection
   d. Interaction of treatment setting

How did you do? 1. a; 2. c; 3. b

6.3 Categorizing Designs According to Time

At the end of this section, you will be able to:

< Differentiate the time dimension of data collection across retrospective, cross-sectional, and longitudinal and prospective designs

Evaluating the strength of the evidence obtained with quantitative designs includes evaluating the timing of data collection. The time dimension of a study may be classified as retrospective, cross-sectional, and longitudinal or prospective.

Retrospective Designs

Retrospective designs may also be referred to as *ex post facto*, which means after the fact. When designing retrospective studies, researchers start with the DV and look back in time to determine possible causative factors. Retrospective designs are considered to be after the fact because the DV has already occurred, which means that the IV cannot be manipulated and subjects cannot be randomly assigned. Thus, retrospective designs are never experimental in nature.

Retrospective designs are often used in epidemiological studies. For example, causes of AIDS were discovered by researchers who started noticing an unusual increase in the number of cases of Kaposi's sarcoma occurring in young men (Gallo & Montagnier, 2003). By taking careful histories, researchers were able to look back in time to determine behaviors and risk factors common to men who developed AIDS. Behaviors were compared with behaviors of men who did not have the disease. This type of retrospective study is called a *case-control* study because researchers started with a group of people who already had the disease. Identifying smoking as a cause of lung cancer also resulted from examining retrospective data. In both of these examples, retrospective designs were appropriate because it would have been unethical for researchers to deliberately expose subjects to either the HIV virus or tobacco smoke.

When conducting quality control studies, researchers often use retrospective designs. In these types of studies, researchers may want to gather information about an organization's status related to a patient problem such as falls. Chart audits can be done to determine the number of falls that occurred in the past 6 months. Information can be gathered on patients who have fallen to identify potential causative factors such as age, diagnoses, units where falls occurred, and staffing levels at the time of falls. Thus, retrospective studies can provide important data using nonexperimental designs. However, because retrospective designs are not experimental, a disadvantage is that researchers cannot say definitively that the IV caused the DV. Instead, researchers can conclude that there is an increased likelihood or probability that the IV caused the outcome in the DV.

Cross-Sectional Designs

Cross-sectional studies are nonexperimental designs that researchers use to gather data from a group of subjects at only one point in time. Cross-sectional designs provide a snapshot by collecting data about the IV and DV at the same time. Because data are collected at one time, it is difficult to establish cause and effect using cross-sectional designs. For example, a researcher is studying the effect of self-efficacy on condom use in adolescents. If a cross-sectional design is used, it would be difficult to determine whether increased self-efficacy caused increased condom use or increased condom use resulted in a sense of increased self-efficacy.

Use of a strong theoretical framework can guide the researcher when speculating about the relationships of the variables being studied with a cross-sectional design. It is important not to confuse cross-sectional studies with other designs. For example, a researcher who is interested in subjects' cardiovascular responses to stress may start by measuring blood pressures, exposing subjects to a stressful video clip, and then remeasuring blood pressures during and immediately after the video. Although data are collected in the immediate present, data about the IV and DV are not collected at the same point in time. Therefore, this is an example of an experimental design rather than a cross-sectional design.

Cohort comparison studies are a specific type of nonexperimental cross-sectional design where more than one group of subjects is studied at the same point in time. Cohort comparison designs allow researchers to draw conclusions about variables over time even though data were collected at only one point in time. In the example of condom use, a cohort design could be used to study the factors associated with condom use among high school freshmen as well as high school sophomores, juniors, and seniors. The variables related to condom use in each group could be analyzed and compared to see if the same variables applied across the groups or to find out at which grade level the variables changed. Because following the same subjects as they progress through high school would take 4 years, gathering data from different subjects at each grade saves time. The advantages of cross-sectional designs are that they are easier to manage and are more economical. Because data are collected only one time from each subject, the threats of mortality, maturation, and testing are minimized. A limitation of cross-sectional designs is that it is difficult for researchers to make claims about cause and effect.

Longitudinal Designs

Longitudinal designs are used to gather data about subjects at more than one point in time. These may be either experimental or nonexperimental designs. Longitudinal designs are sometimes called *prospective designs*, which are studies that begin in the present and end in the future. Nonexperimental, prospective designs are commonly used in epidemiological studies where researchers begin by identifying presumed causes and then follow subjects into the future to determine whether the hypothesized effects actually occur.

KEY TERMS

cohort comparison: Nonexperimental cross-sectional design in which more than one group is studied at the same time so that conclusions about a variable over time can be drawn without spending as much time

longitudinal designs: Designs used to gather data about subjects at more than one point in time

prospective designs: Studies over time with presumed causes that follow subjects to determine whether the hypothesized effects actually occur

In *panel designs*, the same subjects are used to provide data at multiple points in time. The observational study component of the well-known Women's Health Initiative (WHI) is an example of a prospective, nonexperimental, panel design (National Heart, Lung, and Blood Institute [NHLBI], 2010). In the WHI, researchers funded by the NHLBI gathered data over an 8-year period from postmenopausal women between 50 and 79 years of age. The purpose of the study was to determine reliable estimates of the extent to which known risk factors predict heart disease, cancer, and fractures in older women. Women who joined the panel study were asked at different points in time to provide data about their health behaviors. They were not required to change any of their health habits—only to report them.

Trend studies use nonexperimental designs to gather data about the variables of interest from different samples from the target population across time. An example of this is the Youth Risk Behavior Surveillance System (YRBSS) conducted by the Centers for Disease Control and Prevention (http://www.cdc.gov/HealthyYouth/yrbs). Since 1992, the YRBSS has surveyed representative samples of students in grades 9–12. Repeated every 2 years, surveys provide data regarding the prevalence of risk behaviors among high school students. By using different samples of teens, researchers are able to determine whether the rates of risky behaviors are increasing, decreasing, or staying the same over time.

Another type of longitudinal design is the *follow-up* study. Researchers use this design to follow subjects into the future. These may be either experimental or nonexperimental designs. Nonexperimental follow-up studies differ from panel studies in that the samples are not drawn from the general population (e.g., not from all postmenopausal women or all teens in high school), but instead samples are selected because they have a specific characteristic or condition that researchers are interested in studying. An example of a nonexperimental follow-up design is a study involving the breastfeeding behaviors of new mothers. The researcher would select a sample of new mothers and follow them for a period of months to determine variables associated with their continuing or discontinuing breastfeeding.

Follow-up studies may also be experimental in design. A researcher may design a supportive educational intervention to increase new mothers' confidence in breastfeeding. The researcher would randomly assign mothers to either the new educational intervention group or the standard of care group. Mothers would be followed over the next few months to determine whether the educational intervention made a difference in the length of time that mothers breastfed their infants. The hormone replacement component of the WHI Clinical Trial and Observational Study (http://www.nhlbi.nih.gov/whi/ctos.htm) is another example of an experimental follow-up study. In this study, women were randomly assigned to either a treatment or placebo group and then followed for 8 years to determine the effect of hormone replacement therapy on the prevention of coronary heart disease and osteoporotic fractures.

Crossover designs are a type of longitudinal study in which subjects receive more than one experimental treatment and are then followed over time. Subjects act as their own control group. Researchers manipulate the IV by randomizing the order in which the treatments are provided. An example of a crossover design is one in which the researcher is interested in determining whether relaxation techniques or exercise has a greater effect on reducing blood pressure. Some subjects would be randomly assigned to receive training in relaxation techniques first while others would be given instructions about exercise first. As subjects enter the study, baseline measures of blood pressure would be obtained. They would then do either the exercise or relaxation procedures for a set time period and would have their blood pressure measured at different points in time. Subjects would then be asked to stop the intervention and resume their normal habits while blood pressures are measured again. At a later time, subjects would receive instructions about the experimental treatment they had not done initially. Again, subjects would be followed for a set period of time with their blood pressures being measured. At the end of the study, the researcher would be able to determine which intervention produced the greatest reduction in blood pressures. One problem with crossover studies, however, is the possibility of a carryover effect. Even though subjects are asked to stop performing the first intervention, sometimes they may continue to use it during the second phase of the study.

Gathering data at multiple points in time does not necessarily make a study longitudinal. Usually the term *longitudinal* is reserved for studies in which data are gathered over extended periods of time rather than in just a few hours or days. In some nursing situations, data may be repeatedly gathered but only for a relatively short period of time. For example, a researcher is studying the effects of music therapy on blood pressure of patients who are admitted to the intensive care unit. Although blood pressure is measured every hour for a 24-hour period, this study would not be described as a longitudinal study.

Longitudinal designs provide important information about the chronological relationships that exist between the IV and DV by determining changes over time. Another advantage is that this type of design can be used to test cause and effect. One disadvantage of longitudinal studies is

> **KEY TERM**
>
> **crossover designs:** Experimental designs that use two or more treatments; subjects receive treatments in random order

their cost in following subjects over an extended period of time. The threat of mortality is increased; thus, researchers need to make special plans to encourage subjects to complete the studies. Maturation is another threat inherent in longitudinal designs because changes of subjects are inevitable. Because longitudinal studies involve repeated measurements, the threat of testing is often increased.

TEST YOUR KNOWLEDGE 6-3

True/False

1. In retrospective designs, also known as ex post facto designs, the researcher manipulates the IV.

2. Cohort comparison studies can save time because more than one group of subjects is studied.

3. The threat of mortality is greater in cross-sectional designs than in longitudinal designs.

4. Any study that involves collecting data at multiple points in time is a longitudinal study.

How did you do? 1. F; 2. T; 3. F; 4. F

6.4 Keeping It Ethical

At the end of this section, you will be able to:

< Discuss ethical issues related to internal and external validity

Researchers are obligated to conduct well-constructed studies. If a study does not have adequate controls in place, then the researcher has wasted valuable resources such as time, money, and subject volunteerism. Furthermore, failure to control threats to study validity jeopardizes the integrity of the findings. When findings are flawed, patient safety could be affected when practice is changed based on the evidence. Researchers should make every effort to implement strategies that enhance control and manipulation while reducing bias.

FYI

Researchers are obligated to conduct well-constructed studies. If a study does not have adequate controls in place, then the researcher has wasted valuable resources such as time, money, and subject volunteerism.

Implementing strategies needs to be balanced with protecting the rights of human subjects. For example, when individuals are recruited for a study that involves two or more groups, they often express a desire to choose their group assignment. Allowing subjects to select their group assignment introduces the threat of selection bias. Most researchers would opt to randomly assign subjects to groups to reduce this threat. Therefore, it would be important for the researcher to inform subjects during the recruitment process that they will not be allowed to choose their own groups. Doing so allows individuals to make informed decisions about participating.

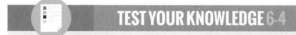

TEST YOUR KNOWLEDGE 6-4

True/False

1. Researchers should design studies that are easy for subjects to participate in regardless of how much control over extraneous variables is achieved.

2. Nursing's body of knowledge is dependent on the quality of research findings that are disseminated.

How did you do? 1. F; 2. T

RAPID REVIEW

»   Quantitative designs are used to describe phenomena, explain relationships, predict relationships, and explain causality.

»   Nurses must consider elements of design when appraising quantitative studies.

»   There are three major categories of quantitative designs: experimental, quasi-experimental, and nonexperimental.

»   Causality refers to a relationship that exists between a cause and its effect. The IV must occur prior to the DV in order to claim a cause-and-effect relationship. Because outcomes can have multiple causes, probability assertions leave open the possibility for multicausality.

»   In quantitative designs, researchers control, manipulate, and randomize to control for extraneous variables.

»   Randomization is used in two ways to control for extraneous variables. Random sampling is the process of selecting a sample whereby each element in the population has an equal chance of being selected. Random assignment to groups means that all subjects in the sample have an equal chance of being assigned to either the intervention or control group.

»   Researchers use within-groups designs to examine how subjects in the same group change over time. Between-groups designs involve comparisons of subjects of one group to subjects in another group.

»   There are two major types of validity: internal and external. Internal validity is the degree to which one can conclude that it was the IV, not extraneous variables, that produced the change in the DV. External validity refers to the confidence one has that findings can be generalized across different types of people, settings, and times.

» There are seven threats to internal validity: selection bias, history, maturation, testing, instrumentation, mortality, and statistical conclusion validity.

» There are five threats to external validity: construct validity, selection, interaction of treatment with selection of subjects, interaction of treatment and setting, and interaction of treatment and history.

» Quantitative studies can be classified as follows according to the timing of data collection: retrospective, cross-sectional, longitudinal, and prospective.

Apply What You Have Learned

Consider the designs used by Chun, Kim, and Park (2015) and Fakhry, Hannah, Anderson, Holmes, and Nathwain (2012). Identify any threats to internal and external validity, and discuss strategies researchers used to minimize these threats.

REFERENCES

Campbell, D. T., & Stanley, J. C. (1966). *Experimental and quasi-experimental designs for research*. Chicago, IL: Rand McNally.

Chun, H., Kim, K., & Park, H. (2015). Effects of hand hygiene education and individual feedback on hand hygiene behavior, MRSA, acquisition rate, and MRSA colonization pressure among intensive care unit nurses. *International Journal of Nursing Practice, 21*, 709–715.

Cook, T. D., & Campbell, D. T. (1979). *Quasi-experimentation: Design and analysis issues for field settings*. Boston, MA: Houghton Mifflin.

Fakhry, M., Hannah, G. B., Anderson, O., Holmes, A., & Nathwain, D. (2012). Effectiveness of an audible reminder on hand hygiene adherence. *American Journal of Infection Control, 40*, 320–323.

Gallo, R. C., & Montagnier, L. (2003). The discovery of HIV as the cause of AIDS. *New England Journal of Medicine, 349*, 2283–2285.

Kempthorne, O. (1961). The design and analysis of experiments with some reference to education research. In R. O. Collier & S. M. Elan (Eds.), *Research design and analysis* (pp. 97–126). Bloomington, IN: Phi Delta Kappa.

Mayo, E. (1933). *The social problems of an industrial civilization.* New York, NY: Macmillan.

National Heart, Lung, and Blood Institute. (2010). Women's health initiative. Retrieved from http://www.nhlbi.nih.gov/whi/index.html

At the end of this chapter, you will be able to:

< Explain the three essential components of experimental designs
< Identify major experimental designs
< Discuss the advantages and disadvantages of various experimental designs
< Discuss the key difference between quasi-experimental and experimental designs
< Identify major quasi-experimental designs
< Discuss the advantages and disadvantages of various quasi-experimental designs
< Describe the purpose of nonexperimental designs
< Identify major nonexperimental quantitative designs
< Discuss the advantages and disadvantages of various nonexperimental designs
< Define translational research, community-based participatory action research, and health services research
< Discuss ethical issues related to quantitative designs

community-based participatory research
comparative designs
correlational designs
covary
crossover designs
descriptive correlational designs
descriptive designs
experimental designs
exploratory designs
factorial designs
health services research

model testing
multiple experimental groups designs
nonequivalent control group pretest-posttest design
nonequivalent-groups posttest-only designs
nonexperimental designs
one-group posttest-only designs
one-group time series design

predictive correlational design
preexperimental
quasi-experimental designs
Solomon four-group design
survey designs
translational research
two-group posttest-only designs
two-group pretest-posttest design

CHAPTER 7

Quantitative Designs: Using Numbers to Provide Evidence

Rosalind M. Peters

7.1 Experimental Designs

At the end of this section, you will be able to:

‹ Explain the three essential components of experimental designs
‹ Identify major experimental designs
‹ Discuss the advantages and disadvantages of various experimental designs

Quantitative designs can provide evidence that describes a phenomenon, explain relationships and differences among variables, predict relationships and differences among variables, or determine causality (Campbell & Stanley, 1966; Cook & Campbell, 1979). *Experimental designs* provide the best evidence for claiming that a cause-and-effect relationship exists. This type of design often includes the terms *pretest* and *posttest*. These terms refer to the point in time when data collection is taking place. Sometimes these are labeled "before" and "after" designs because pretest means data are collected prior to or before the intervention group receives the treatment, and posttest refers to data collected after the intervention is completed. Experimental designs look for differences between treated and untreated subjects. Therefore, there must

CRITICAL THINKING EXERCISE 7-1

Remember an experiment you conducted in your chemistry class. Identify the three essential components of an experiment and tell how each was accounted for in your example.

KEY TERM

experimental designs: Designs involving random assignment to groups and manipulation of the independent variable

be a minimum of two groups. To be considered a true experimental design, three features must be present: randomization, control, and manipulation.

Essential Components of Experimental Designs

Randomization in experimental designs is used in two ways. One way requires researchers to randomly select subjects from the target population. The other way is to randomly assign subjects to groups. Because random selection of the sample usually is not possible in nursing research, random assignment to groups is considered to be sufficient to meet the criterion of randomization for an experiment.

The second component of experimental designs is control, which is related to randomization. A control group, for comparison to the experimental group, is one strategy researchers use to control for extraneous variables. In addition to a control group, other ways researchers control for extraneous variables are by exerting the highest level of control over the selection of subjects, the definitions of the variables, and the environment in which the experiment is conducted.

Manipulation is the third essential component. Researchers must be able to manipulate the independent variable (IV) for a design to be considered experimental. This is accomplished by consistently administering the intervention.

True Experimental Designs

When creating an evidence-based practice (EBP), experimental designs are most valued. When appraising quantitative research studies, you may see the term *randomized controlled trial* (RCT), a term used to describe an experimental study that is conducted in healthcare settings. The RCT designation refers to the fact that the study is "clinical" in nature rather than a specific type of design. Regardless of the specific experimental design used, RCTs are characterized by the following considerations: (1) they involve a large number of subjects, often from diverse geographic areas; (2) there are strict guidelines for including subjects in a study; (3) subjects are randomly assigned to either the intervention or control group; (4) subjects in each group must be comparable (equivalent) on key characteristics at baseline; (5) the intervention is consistently implemented to all subjects in the experimental group following a very rigidly defined protocol for implementation; and (6) all subjects in both groups are measured on the dependent variable (DV) using the same method of measurement at the same points in time.

FYI

Experimental designs look for differences between treated and untreated subjects. The untreated group is the control group.

There are six types of true experimental designs commonly reported in the scientific literature. These include: (1) two-group pretest-posttest, (2) two-group posttest-only, (3) Solomon four-group, (4) multiple experimental groups, (5) factorial, and (6) crossover designs.

Two-Group Pretest-Posttest Designs

The *two-group pretest-posttest design* is considered to be the "classic" experimental design. Subjects are randomized to either the experimental group receiving the intervention or the control group. They are measured before and after the intervention is implemented (see **Table 7-1**). This design allows researchers to examine within-subjects results as well as between-subjects results. For example, a researcher wants to test a new teaching strategy for diabetic patients.

KEY TERM

two-group pretest-posttest design: Subjects are randomly assigned to the experimental or control group and are measured before and after the intervention; classic or true experiment

TABLE 7-1	Experimental Designs			
Two-Group Pretest-Posttest (Classic)				
Experimental Group	R	O_1	X	O_2
Control Group	R	O_1		O_2
Two-Group Posttest-Only				
Experimental Group	R		X	O_1
Control Group	R			O_1
Solomon Four-Group				
Experimental Group 1	R	O_1	X	O_2
Experimental Group 2	R		X	O_2
Control Group 1	R	O_1		O_2
Control Group 2	R			O_2
Crossover (Randomization of Treatment Order)				
Experimental Group 1	$O_1\ O_2$ R $X_1\ O_3\ O_4$ (–X) $O_5\ O_6\ X_2\ O_7\ O_8$			
Experimental Group 2	$O_1\ O_2$ R $X_2\ O_3\ O_4$ (–X) $O_5\ O_6\ X_1\ O_7\ O_8$			

Note: R = randomization; O = observation or measurement; X = treatment or intervention; –X = treatment withdrawn.

Patients in a diabetic clinic are randomly assigned to either the computerized learning module group or the standard of care group. Knowledge about diabetes is measured before and after teaching for all subjects. One way the researcher can determine the efficacy of the intervention is to compare the pretest and posttest scores of subjects in the intervention group to see if learning occurred. Another way to evaluate the intervention would be to compare posttest scores from the two groups to determine whether one teaching method increased posttest scores more than another did.

A potential disadvantage of the two-group pretest-posttest design is that threats to internal validity are introduced from repeated testing. In the previous example, the threat of testing could be reduced by providing subjects with alternate forms of the diabetic knowledge test. Mortality is another threat because subjects are measured more than once and some subjects may drop out before the study is completed. Also, if the intervention or data collection is burdensome, subjects may be more likely to withdraw from studies.

Two-Group Posttest-Only Designs

In experimental *two-group posttest-only designs*, researchers randomly assign subjects to either an intervention group or a control group. In nursing studies, the intervention is conducted with the experimental group (see Table 7-1), while the control group receives the usual standard of care. After the intervention is completed, the DV is measured at the same point in time in both groups. This type of design is used when it is not possible or practical to measure the DV before the intervention is implemented. For example, a researcher is interested in examining the effect of music therapy on pain levels of patients undergoing invasive procedures. Because patients have no pain prior to invasive procedures, it would be impossible to determine whether the intervention decreased levels of pain. Therefore, the only way a researcher can determine whether music therapy effectively reduced pain would be to use a between-subjects design. Pain levels from subjects who used music therapy would be compared to the pain levels of subjects who did not. Because subjects are measured only once, threats of testing and mortality are minimized. A disadvantage of the two-group posttest-only design is that it is susceptible to the threats of selection bias. One cannot assume that the two groups are equivalent, because there was no measurement at baseline. Selection bias should be minimized because subjects are randomly assigned to groups. The characteristics of subjects that might affect the DV should be equally distributed between the two groups through the use of random assignment.

Solomon Four-Group Designs

As the name implies, there are four groups of subjects involved in the *Solomon four-group design*. Two groups of subjects receive the intervention, and two

KEY TERMS

two-group posttest-only designs: Experimental designs when subjects are randomly assigned to an experimental or control group and measured after the intervention

Solomon four-group design: An experimental design with four groups—some receive the intervention, others serve as controls; some are measured before and after, others are measured only after the intervention

groups of subjects receive the usual standard of care or a placebo. One experimental group and one control group are measured before and after the intervention, while the other experimental and control groups are measured only after the intervention (see Table 7-1). Researchers select this four-group design over the two-group pretest-posttest design to reduce the threat of testing. This design is also superior to the two-group posttest-only design because selection bias is minimized. Consider the diabetic teaching intervention example again. Suppose the researcher is concerned that subjects will learn information by taking the diabetic knowledge test. By adding two more groups that do not take the pretest, the researcher can compare posttest scores from subjects who took the pretest to scores of subjects who did not take the pretest. If testing is a threat, the researcher can expect that the pretest groups will have higher posttest scores than those who did not take the pretest.

Although the Solomon four-group design is a strong design, it has limitations. Because there are more groups, sample sizes must be large. This means that subjects must be available, recruitment of subjects will take longer, and costs will be increased.

Multiple Experimental Groups Designs

It is possible for researchers to use either the posttest alone or the pretest-posttest design with *multiple experimental groups designs*. To conduct this type of study, researchers would have multiple experimental groups and one control group. In the example of interventions to reduce pain during invasive procedures, the researcher might be interested in testing two different interventions. The researcher could randomly assign subjects to experimental group 1, which would receive music therapy. Other subjects would be randomly assigned to experimental group 2, where they would receive therapeutic touch. Other subjects would be randomly assigned to the control group for the usual standard of care. The advantage of the multiple-groups design is that it allows researchers to compare the effect of different interventions on the DV. A major disadvantage of this design is that a large number of subjects is needed to detect differences across multiple groups.

Factorial Designs

In the previously discussed designs, only one intervention has been manipulated. Even in multiple-groups experiments, each experimental group receives only one intervention. *Factorial designs* allow researchers to manipulate more than one intervention during the same experiment. Researchers may compare multiple interventions (e.g., music *and* therapeutic touch combined) or multiple levels of interventions (e.g., music with therapeutic touch for 10 minutes, 15 minutes, or 20 minutes). For example, a researcher is interested in increasing

| TABLE 7-2 | Factorial Design | | |

		Website Intervention	
		YES	**NO**
Home Visit Intervention	**YES**	Both home visit and website	Home visit alone
	NO	Website alone	No intervention control group

self-care behaviors of people with high blood pressure. The researcher hypothesizes that home visits and an interactive website will be effective in lowering blood pressures. Two experiments could be used to test each intervention separately, or a factorial design could be used to test both interventions separately, while testing the effects of a combined intervention for controlling high blood pressures. **Table 7-2** depicts the 2 × 2 factorial design for this example. Note that there are three intervention groups (home visit alone, website alone, and combined home visit and website) and one control group that receives neither the home visits nor the interactive website.

Because of its complex nature and sophisticated data analysis, more experienced researchers tend to use this type of design. Like Solomon four-group designs, sample sizes need to be large because there are a minimum of four groups. However, time and effort are saved by not having to conduct multiple studies.

Crossover Designs

In the discussion of longitudinal designs, *crossover designs* were mentioned. Although only one group of subjects is used, crossover designs include the three essential components of an experiment (see Table 7-1). Independent variables are manipulated by the researcher, and the order in which the interventions are administered to subjects is randomized. Because subjects serve as their own control group, the criterion of control is met because it is assumed that each subject will remain stable on the extraneous variables during the study.

Smaller sample sizes are needed because only one group of subjects is required, and subjects serve as their own controls. A disadvantage is that subjects may continue to engage in the first intervention after moving to the second.

KEY TERM

crossover designs: Experimental designs that use two or more treatments; subjects receive treatments in a random order

7.2 Quasi-Experimental Designs

At the end of this section, you will be able to:

‹ Discuss the key difference between quasi-experimental and experimental designs
‹ Identify major quasi-experimental designs
‹ Discuss the advantages and disadvantages of various quasi-experimental designs

Quasi-experimental designs are similar to experimental designs in that they involve manipulation of the IV, but they do not meet one of the other essential components of experimental designs (Campbell & Stanley, 1966; Cook & Campbell, 1979). They either lack randomization or a control group, which makes claims of cause and effect weaker than in experimental designs. Because of this, studies using quasi-experimental designs are ranked lower as sources of evidence than are studies using experimental designs. However, there are many situations involving the study of human health when it is not feasible or ethical to conduct an experiment. Therefore, quasi-experimental designs serve an important function in providing beginning evidence of causality. There are three commonly used quasi-experimental designs: (1) nonequivalent control group pretest-posttest, (2) one-group time series, and (3) preexperimental designs (see **Table 7-3**).

Nonequivalent Control Group Pretest-Posttest Designs

The *nonequivalent control group pretest-posttest design* differs from the classic experimental design in that researchers are unable to randomly assign subjects to groups. Because researchers are unable to randomize in these

KEY TERMS

quasi-experimental designs: Research designs involving the manipulation of the independent variable but lacking either random assignment to groups or a control group

nonequivalent control group pretest-posttest design: A quasi-experimental design where two groups are measured before and after an intervention

TABLE 7-3	Quasi-Experimental Designs					
One-Group Pretest-Posttest (No Randomization)						
Group 1	O_1	X	O_2			
Nonequivalent Control Group Pretest-Posttest (No Randomization)						
Experimental Group	O_1	X	O_2			
Comparison Group	O_1		O_2			
One-Group Time Series (No Randomization)						
Group 1	O_1	O_2	O_3	X	O_4	O_5
One-Group Posttest-Only (No Randomization, No Pretest)						
Group 1		X	O_1			
Nonequivalent Control Group Posttest-Only (No Randomization, No Pretest)						
Experimental Group		X	O_1			
Comparison Group			O_1			

Note: O = observation or measurement; X = treatment or intervention.

designs, the nonintervention group is referred to as a comparison group rather than a control group. Researchers are able to measure both groups on the DV prior to and after the intervention (see Table 7-3). For example, the faculty of a nursing college is considering changing a nursing research course offered to junior students. In one semester, a professor administers a pretest measuring knowledge about nursing research. The professor then teaches the course content in the usual lecture style. At the end of the semester, the final exam is used as a posttest to measure students' knowledge of research. The next semester, another group of students enter the research course. They are given the same pretest, but the instruction is online with no class lectures. At the end of the semester, the same comprehensive final exam is administered. The faculty would then be able to compare students' knowledge pre- and postintervention and make a determination regarding the effect of the different teaching methods on students' knowledge about research. Because students were unable to be randomly assigned to a teaching method, this is not an experimental design. Without randomization, it is possible that the students are not equivalent on important factors that may affect how they learned the course materials. This contributes to selection bias and weakens the design. Threats to internal validity as a result of testing, maturation, and mortality can exist.

One-Group Time Series Designs

The second most common quasi-experimental design is the *one-group time series design*. This type of design may be used when neither randomization nor a comparison group is possible. Researchers may opt to study one group over a prolonged period of time prior to administering the intervention and then make multiple observations after the intervention is conducted. For example, the faculty decides to change the pass rate on exams from 75% to 80%. They could compare the number of student nurses passing at 75% for four semesters to the number who pass at 80% over four semesters. Although many factors contribute to pass rates among student nurses, following the data for an extended period of time helps faculty to determine the effect of a policy change.

Preexperimental Designs

One-group posttest-only and *nonequivalent-groups posttest-only designs* are often referred to as *preexperimental* rather than quasi-experimental. The difference between pre- and quasi-experimental designs is that quasi-experimental designs, while lacking some elements of an experiment, use other strategies to control for extraneous variables. With preexperimental studies, many threats to internal validity can be found because these are posttest-only designs. An example of a one-group posttest-only study is when a researcher implements an educational intervention to teach new mothers the benefits of breastfeeding. After the intervention, the mothers' knowledge of breastfeeding was tested. Without a pretest to determine the mothers' previous knowledge and without any information about their prior history of breastfeeding, it would be almost impossible to determine what effect the intervention had on the breastfeeding outcome. One-group posttest-only designs provide a low level of evidence, and no change in nursing practice should be made based on this type of design.

Adding a comparison group slightly increases the quality of evidence found in posttest-only designs. A nonequivalent-groups posttest-only design involves manipulation of the IV and two or more groups of subjects who are compared on the DV. For example, a researcher works in an agency where the policy is that all new mothers will receive the breastfeeding educational intervention. Because randomization of mothers is not possible, the researcher decides to compare breastfeeding knowledge of mothers from a hospital requiring the educational intervention to breastfeeding knowledge of mothers from a hospital that does not offer that intervention. Because this is a nonequivalent-groups posttest-only design, it is impossible for the researcher to have any information about breastfeeding knowledge of the mothers in either group prior to the intervention. It is impossible to determine the equivalence of the two groups because the researcher does not have any pretest information. If the results of the study indicated that the mothers in the intervention group knew more about breastfeeding than the mothers in the comparison group, can the researcher conclude that the intervention was the cause of the increased knowledge? It is possible there were other factors, such as previous positive experiences with breastfeeding, increased family support, and encouragement to breastfeed by nursing staff, that were more influential in determining the results. Given that there could be many threats to internal validity, nurses should be cautious about changing practice based on data from preexperimental designs.

TEST YOUR KNOWLEDGE 7-2

1. Quasi-experimental designs include which of the following essential components?
   a. Randomization, control group, and manipulation of the IV
   b. Randomization and control group
   c. Manipulation of the IV
   d. Randomization and manipulation of the IV
2. Experimental designs have control groups. Quasi-experimental designs have which of the following?
   a. Control groups
   b. Comparison groups
   c. Extraneous groups
   d. Peer groups
3. Rank the evidence generated from the following designs from lowest to highest.
   a. Experimental designs
   b. Nonequivalent control group pretest-posttest
   c. One-group posttest-only
   d. Nonequivalent-groups posttest-only

How did you do? 1. c; 2. b; 3. c, d, b, a

7.3 Nonexperimental Designs

At the end of this section, you will be able to:

< Describe the purpose of nonexperimental designs
< Identify major nonexperimental quantitative designs
< Discuss the advantages and disadvantages of various nonexperimental designs

Although experimental designs are considered to provide the strongest quantitative evidence, that is not the only type of evidence needed for nursing practice. Nurses are concerned with the whole person in interaction with the environment, and as such, they need information that is not always available from experimental studies. Information about personal phenomena such as patients' thoughts, beliefs, and subjective experiences, especially related to health care, is often most appropriately obtained using either qualitative or quantitative *nonexperimental designs*, which are descriptive in nature (Campbell & Stanley, 1966; Cook & Campbell, 1979). Nonexperimental designs also are important when there is little information known about a particular phenomenon, when it would be unethical to manipulate the independent variable, or when it is not practical to conduct an experiment (e.g., lack of resources or excessive burden to the subjects). The primary difference between nonexperimental and other quantitative designs is that researchers do not actively manipulate the IV. Even though the IV is not being manipulated, it is important for quantitative researchers to exert as much control as possible to avoid threats to internal and external validity. Researchers still need to protect against bias when conducting these quantitative studies. Bias can be controlled with carefully selecting the sample, having an adequate sample size to ensure sufficient statistical power, clearly defining conceptual and operational variables, using reliable and valid instruments to measure the variables of interest, and exerting control over the conditions under which the data will be collected.

Nonexperimental designs can be used for the purposes of: (1) describing a phenomenon in detail, (2) explaining relationships and differences among variables, and (3) predicting relationships and differences among variables. Because the IV is not manipulated, researchers using quantitative nonexperimental designs cannot make claims about cause and effect. Although nonexperimental designs can be categorized in many ways, they fall into two general categories: descriptive and correlational.

Descriptive Designs

The purpose of *descriptive designs* is to describe in detail a phenomenon of interest. Descriptive designs provide a picture of a situation as it is naturally happening without manipulation of any of the variables. This type of design allows researchers to identify and document the different characteristics of phenomena and describe the frequency with which they occur. Because there is no manipulation of variables and no attempt to establish causality, the terms *IV* and *DV* should not be used with descriptive designs. Instead, the term *research variable* is more appropriate. Researchers use descriptive designs for a variety of

> **KEY TERMS**
>
> **nonexperimental designs:** Research designs that lack manipulation of the independent variable and random assignment
>
> **descriptive designs:** Designs that provide a picture of a situation as it is naturally happening without manipulation of any of the variables

> **FYI**
>
> Nonexperimental designs are descriptive in nature and can be used to describe phenomena in detail, explain differences among variables, and predict relationships and differences among variables.

purposes. These designs are often used to assess current practice. They can also be used in the early stages of theory development. Conceptual and operational definitions of the variables and possible theoretical relationships among the variables can emerge from descriptive studies. Although most descriptive designs tend to be cross-sectional, they can be conducted in any of the time dimensions as discussed previously.

Descriptive designs are often called by a variety of names, such as *exploratory*, *comparative*, and *survey designs*. The term *exploratory* is used because descriptive designs are used when little is known about a phenomenon, so exploration is required. For example, an exploratory design could be used to determine factors associated with nurses' willingness to discuss sexual concerns with their patients. The term *comparative* is used if the purpose of the study is to describe phenomena by comparing two or more groups or two or more variables. For example, a researcher could use this type of design to describe nurses' willingness to discuss sexual concerns with patients and compare oncology nurses to cardiology nurses. Another approach a researcher might take could be to study oncology nurses and compare their willingness to discuss sexual concerns with patients to variables such as the nurses' ages, levels of education, and years of experience. The term *survey* is used to indicate that data are obtained through subjects' self-report about variables such as their attitudes, perceptions, and behaviors. Surveys and questionnaires are popular methods used to collect descriptive data. They can be completed face to face, through the mail, online, or through telephone interviews.

A well-controlled descriptive study offers a number of advantages over other types of quantitative designs. Descriptive designs have flexibility in the methods that can be used to collect data, often leading to more rapid collection of data and cost savings. The major disadvantage of this type of design is the inability to establish causality.

Correlational Designs

Correlational designs are used when researchers are interested in establishing relationships between two or more variables. When reviewing the evidence from correlational studies, it is important for nurses to remember that correlation does not prove causality. Because correlational designs do not involve manipulation of the IV, no causal statements can be made. For example, for some individuals there is a correlation between their symptoms of arthritis and changes in the weather. Before a change in weather, individuals may experience joint pain. However, one cannot conclude that joint pain causes the weather to change even though there is a strong correlation between the two phenomena. The best way to interpret a correlation is to understand that correlations simply mean that the variables *covary*—that is, when there is a change in one variable,

KEY TERMS

exploratory designs: Nonexperimental design type used when little is known about a phenomenon

comparative designs: Descriptive design type that compares two or more groups or variables

survey designs: Descriptive design type involving data obtained through subjects' self-report

correlational designs: Nonexperimental designs used to study relationships between two or more variables

covary: When change in one variable is associated with change in another variable

there will be an associated change in the other. Evaluating statistical data provides information about the strength of the relationship, the direction of the relationship (positive or negative), and whether the relationship is statistically significant. There are three types of correlational designs commonly reported in the literature: (1) descriptive correlational, (2) predictive correlational, and (3) model-testing.

Descriptive Correlational Designs

Descriptive correlational designs build on comparative descriptive designs. Comparative descriptive designs simply describe the phenomena as they occur in two or more groups or among two or more variables associated with the phenomena. Descriptive correlational designs are used when researchers are interested in explaining the degree and characteristics of relationships that exist among the variables or groups. For example, in the case of nurses' willingness to discuss sexual concerns with their patients, the researcher can use a descriptive correlational design to determine the extent to which level of education or years of experience is related to the nurses' comfort with discussing sexual issues.

Predictive Correlational Designs

Sometimes there is insufficient empirical or theoretical literature for researchers to assume the degree or direction of the relationships among the variables. Researchers use descriptive correlational designs to test nondirectional hypotheses. Like descriptive studies, there is no IV or DV, and the variables are simply referred to as "research" variables. In other situations, researchers have sufficient evidence to predict the expected direction of relationships that will be found among the variables. When this is the case, a *predictive correlational design* is used. Researchers hypothesize which variables are predictors and which are outcomes. Although researchers may be able to predict a statistically significant relationship, the design is still correlational and causality cannot be assumed. Therefore, even though it is common to see the terms *IV* and *DV* used with this type of design, this is not technically correct. The variables should be referred to as predictor and outcome.

There are two major aims of predictive designs. First, and most commonly seen in nursing, researchers attempt to determine the amount of variance in an outcome variable that can be explained by multiple predictor variables. For example, a researcher is interested in determining which factors are most likely to predict the quality of life (QOL) in patients receiving dialysis treatments. The researcher could conduct a study to determine the relationship between the hypothesized predictor variables of emotional distress, functional status, marital status, employment status, age, and length of time on dialysis. The researcher could then use statistical tests to determine the amount of variance

KEY TERMS

descriptive correlational designs: Correlational design type used to explain the relationship among the variables or groups using a nondirectional hypothesis

predictive correlational design: Correlational design when researchers hypothesize which variables are predictors or outcomes

in QOL scores that could be predicted by this group of predictor variables. Suppose the researcher finds that emotional distress accounts for a large portion of QOL scores, and employment status accounts for only a small portion of QOL scores. Using this evidence to determine best practice, nurses should recognize that interventions directed toward alleviating emotional distress would have a greater influence on dialysis patients' perceptions of QOL than would interventions directed toward altering employment status.

Sometimes researchers want to know how accurately a group of predictor variables can determine group membership. Determining group membership is the second aim of predictive correlational designs. For example, this type of design could be used if a researcher wanted to determine to what degree the predictor variables of age, self-efficacy, level of education, and level of general stress predict whether a woman will smoke during pregnancy. Data will allow the researcher to calculate the odds that a woman will be a smoker versus the odds that she will be a nonsmoker. The outcome variable is the group membership because women are either predicted to be in the group of smokers or in the group of nonsmokers. Although correlational studies are considered to produce a lower level of evidence, odds ratios are growing in popularity as a way to inform practice.

Model-Testing Correlational Designs

A third type of correlational design is *model testing*. Researchers use this type of design to test a hypothesized theoretical model. All related variables are identified, and specific hypothesized relationships are stated. Researchers create graphic representations or paths to show the relationships among the variables. For example, **Figure 7-1** is a graphic resulting from a study (Tomake, Morales-Monks, & Shamaley, 2013) conducted to determine the relationships among variables related to alcohol problems in college students. Statistical analysis is done to test all of the relationships at one time. The analysis determines how well the data collected actually "fit" the hypothesized model. The better the fit of the model to the analysis, the more likely it is that the predicted theoretical relationships are true in reality.

Often the term *causal modeling* is used for model-testing designs, but this is misleading. Although model-testing designs provide a rigorous test of predicted relationships among multiple variables based on theory, they can only provide a suggestion of causality, not true evidence of causality. Model testing and predictive designs, although they establish predictive links between variables, do not allow researchers to say that variable *X* causes variable *Y*. True causality can be established only with an experimental design. However, because in nursing it is often unethical to manipulate IVs, model-testing designs provide the strongest nonexperimental evidence regarding the relationships among variables.

KEY TERM

model testing:
Correlational design to test a hypothesized theoretical model; causal modeling or path analysis

FIGURE 7-1   Diagram of a Structural Equation Model

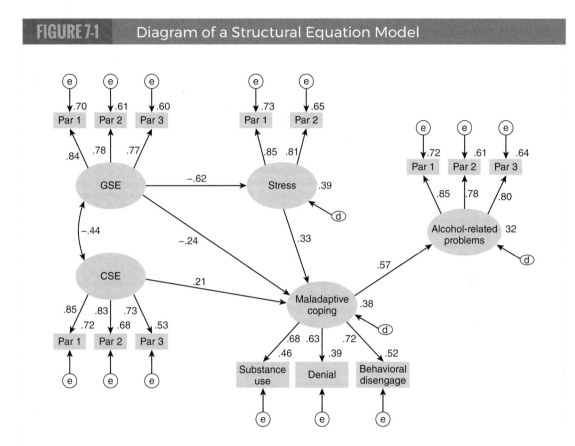

Reproduced from Tomaka, J., Morales-Monks, S., & Shamaley, A.G. (2013). Stress and coping mediate relationships between contingent and global self-esteem and alcohol-related problems among college drinkers. *Stress and Health, 29*(3), 205–213.

TEST YOUR KNOWLEDGE 7-3

True/False

1. In nonexperimental designs, researchers manipulate the IV to determine cause-and-effect relationships.

2. Nonexperimental designs can be used to develop and test theories.

3. The purposes of nonexperimental designs are to describe, explain, and predict relationships.

4. Descriptive data are usually cross-sectional and can be collected through surveys and questionnaires.

5. Researchers use correlations to determine if there are differences between two groups.

How did you do? 1. F; 2. T; 3. F; 4. T; 5. F

7.4 Specific Uses for Quantitative Designs

At the end of this section, you will be able to:

‹ Define translational research, community-based participatory research, and health services research

Quantitative designs are often used in translational research, community-based participatory research, and health services research. Because there are commonalities among these types of research, a study may fit in more than one of these categories.

Translational research "transforms scientific findings or discoveries from basic laboratory, clinical, or population studies into new clinical tools, processes, or applications" (Grady, 2010, p. 164). There are two areas of translation: one involves moving knowledge from basic, laboratory research into clinical studies, and the second involves translating best practices identified in those clinical trials to adoption in the broader community. The purpose of this type of research is to link basic research to the point of care, ultimately improving patient outcomes.

Like EBP, translational research is the study of how nurses and other healthcare providers can apply scientific findings to address real clinical problems (Grady, 2010; Woolf, 2008). Recall the cycle of scientific development. Translational research occurs when research findings are disseminated and subsequently applied. For example, if a cure for the common cold were discovered through basic research, translational research could be used to determine the best way to distribute the treatment to individuals. Application of findings provides feedback for further development of theory and research. For example, if the cure is distributed and side effects are identified, additional research may be indicated to improve the product.

Funding for translational research is increasing because of the recognition that failure to adopt new innovations thwarts the cycle of science. The Agency for Healthcare Research and Quality (AHRQ), committed to the support of translational research, is the federal agency accountable for disseminating research findings for clinical decision making (AHRQ, 2016).

An alternative to traditional research approaches is *community-based participatory research* (CBPR)

(National Institutes of Health, Office of Behavioral and Social Sciences Research, 2017). CBPR is based on a philosophy that when users of research are involved from the start of the research process, findings that are practical and relevant to community needs are more likely to result. Critical principles for CBPR include engaging in collaborative, equitable partnerships; building on resources and goals present in the community; creating long-term sustainable partnerships; and using dynamic processes where ideas flow between researchers and community members. CBPR aims to combine knowledge from community members and researchers with a goal for action and social change to improve community health and often reduce health disparities (National Institutes of Health, Office of Behavioral and Social Sciences Research, 2017).

For example, if nurses wanted to improve the health of immigrants in an urban area using a CBPR model, the nurses would first meet with community leaders to determine the needs, priorities, strengths, and desired outcomes. The research team and community members would mutually agree upon the purpose and methods to be used. By working together, they could create an intervention that fit with the community's culture and would be sustainable when the research was completed. However, CBPR, if done with marginalized or vulnerable populations such as immigrants, may present ethical issues during the research process that may not have been identified during the institutional review board review process. Researchers need to be sensitive to those issues and address them when reporting findings (Campbell-Page & Shaw-Ridley, 2013).

The goals of *health services research* are to determine strategies to effectively organize, manage, finance, and deliver high-quality care. Research topics include ways to reduce medical errors and improve patient safety (AHRQ, n.d.). Studies often involve multidisciplinary teams. For example, a study might be conducted to determine how Internet communications can be used to connect healthcare providers practicing in rural areas to specialists around the world.

> **KEY TERM**
>
> **health services research:** Research involving phenomena, such as cost, political factors, and culture, related to the delivery of health care

CRITICAL THINKING EXERCISE 7-2

A researcher is interested in studying the effect of different medications on the pain of fractures in children admitted to the emergency department. The researcher wants to compare intravenous morphine, oral ibuprofen, and oral acetaminophen with codeine. What kind of design do you think the researcher should use? Why?

1. A researcher is conducting a study to determine whether a radio advertisement about the importance of early detection for colorectal cancer increases the attendance of middle-aged men at a free screening. Which type of research is this an example of? (Select all that apply.)

   a. Basic research

   b. Community-based participatory research

   c. Health services research

   d. Translational research

How did you do? 1. c, d

7.5 Keeping It Ethical

At the end of this section, you will be able to:

< Discuss ethical issues related to quantitative designs

When researchers plan studies using quantitative designs, they must incorporate mechanisms to safeguard the rights of subjects. In nursing and other health research, no subject can receive less than what is considered to be the usual standard of care. Even if subjects withdraw from studies, they must continue to receive standard care. Providing standard care protects subjects' rights to fair treatment. For example, in a study testing the effects of several educational programs on patient outcomes, it would be unethical for subjects in the control group to receive no education because the usual standard of care is to provide all patients with education about their care. When studies involve the use of placebos, decisions about their use must be scrutinized carefully because it is unethical to withhold treatment while testing a new intervention.

To protect the autonomy of individuals, they must be made aware of the benefits and risks of participating in a study so that they can make informed decisions about participating. All institutional review boards require that a description of benefits and risks be provided on consent forms. Most researchers also provide verbal explanations of the benefits and risks when recruiting subjects.

When designing quantitative studies, researchers must assess the associated benefits and risks of any intervention or test that they plan to use.

To protect subjects from harm, the goal is to maximize the benefits while minimizing the risks. For example, suppose a researcher is testing radiation doses in women with breast cancer. Ideally, the researcher should select the dose of radiation that obtains the desired effect with the least amount of side effects. It would be unethical to irradiate women with unusually large doses of radiation, even though it could be hypothesized that larger doses are more effective, because there are known complications associated with high doses. Consideration must be given to potential psychological harm as well. For example, suppose a researcher plans to interview women shortly after their miscarriages. Because miscarriage is an emotional incident for most women, the researcher must use sensitive language in consent forms and during interviews. Referring to the product of conception as a baby may cause undue emotional stress for some subjects.

> **FYI**
>
> When designing quantitative studies, researchers must assess the associated benefits and risks of any intervention or test that they plan to use. To protect subjects from harm, the goal is to maximize the benefits while minimizing the risks.

In some studies, the risk of harm remains high regardless of strategies incorporated by researchers. For example, a researcher is testing a new medication for a serious condition. Regardless of whether subjects are assigned to the control or experimental groups, they are at risk for harm. When it is identified that one treatment is better than another, all subjects should be offered the best intervention. At times, unanticipated adverse reactions to interventions occur. When researchers discover that subjects are having adverse reactions, they should report the reactions immediately. Careful consideration should be given to discontinuing a study if this occurs.

Researchers have an obligation to minimize subject burden—that is, to place as few demands as possible on subjects. For example, a researcher is studying the effects of diet on cholesterol. Careful consideration should be given to the length of the study and the number of times subjects need to have blood samples drawn. If subjects perceive their participation in a study to be too burdensome, there is greater likelihood that they will not complete the study.

Although it is important to exert control to reduce threats to validity, researchers must ensure that strategies used are sensitive to the rights of subjects. When recruiting subjects, care must be taken to follow selection criteria to reduce selection bias. Sometimes subjects express a desire to be placed in a particular treatment group. Researchers cannot be swayed by these requests, and they must adhere to protocols about assigning subjects to groups. When subjects are enrolled in studies, it can be tempting to coerce subjects to remain in a study to limit threats related to mortality, but this is unethical. Subjects must feel free to withdraw at any time without consequences.

TEST YOUR KNOWLEDGE 7-5

Which of the following situations is unethical?

1. A researcher tells a subject that he will not receive as high quality care if he withdraws from the study.

2. A research assistant carefully explains in English, without using an interpreter, the benefits and risks of being in a study to a woman who speaks only Spanish.

3. After discovering that subjects are experiencing adverse reactions to an intervention, researchers agree to discontinue the study.

How did you do? 1. Unethical; 2. Unethical; 3. Ethical

Apply What You Have Learned

You've come a long way in your understanding of how studies are designed and evidence is reported. Review Chun, Kim, and Park (2015) and Fakhry, Hannah, Anderson, Holmes, and Nathwain (2012). Also read Huis et al. (2013) and Al-Hussami, Darawad, and Almhairat (2011). Cite these in APA style, and complete the intervention and comparison columns of the grid. Look at the examples to see what information is needed to complete these columns.

RAPID REVIEW

» Experimental designs provide the best evidence of cause-and-effect relationships. These types of designs must include three features: randomization, control, and manipulation. There are six types of experimental designs: two-group pretest-posttest, two-group posttest-only, Solomon four-group, multiple-experimental groups, factorial, and crossover designs.

» Quasi-experimental designs involve manipulation of the IV but do not meet one of the other criteria for experimental designs. Three common quasi-experimental designs are nonequivalent control group pretest-posttest, one-group time series, and preexperimental designs.

» In nonexperimental designs, the IV is not manipulated; therefore, cause and effect cannot be established. These types of designs are used to explore phenomena when the information is scant. Descriptive designs and correlational designs are two major types of nonexperimental designs.

» Researchers must consider maintaining standards of care and the benefits and risks of study participation when designing quantitative studies.

» Quantitative designs can be used in translational research, community-based participatory research, and health services research.

REFERENCES

Agency for Healthcare Research and Quality. (n.d.). Quality and patient safety. Retrieved from http://www.ahrq.gov/qual/

Agency for Healthcare Research and Quality. (2016). AHRQ profile. Retrieved from https://www.ahrq.gov/cpi/about/index.html

Al-Hussami, M., Darawad, M., & Almhairat, I. I. (2011). Predictors of compliance handwashing practice among healthcare professionals. *Healthcare Infection, 16,* 79–84.

Campbell, D. T., & Stanley, J. C. (1966). *Experimental and quasi-experimental designs for research.* Chicago, IL: Rand McNally.

Campbell-Page, R. M., & Shaw-Ridley, M. (2013). Managing ethical dilemmas in community-based participatory research with vulnerable populations. *Health Promotion Practice, 14,* 485–490.

Chun, H., Kim, K., & Park, H. (2015). Effects of hand hygiene education and individual feedback on hand hygiene behavior, MRSA, acquisition rate, and MRSA colonization pressure among intensive care unit nurses. *International Journal of Nursing Practice, 21,* 709–715.

Cook, T. D., & Campbell, D. T. (1979). *Quasi-experimentation: Design and analysis issues for field settings.* Boston, MA: Houghton Mifflin.

Fakhry, M., Hannah, G. B., Anderson, O., Holmes, A., & Nathwain, D. (2012). Effectiveness of an audible reminder on hand hygiene adherence. *American Journal of Infection Control, 40,* 320–323.

Grady, P. A. (2010). Translational research and nursing science. *Nursing Outlook, 58,* 164–166.

Huis, A., Schoonhoven, L., Grol, R., Donders, R., Hulscher, M., & van Achterber, T. (2014). Impact of a team and leaders-directed strategy to improve nurses' adherence to hand hygiene guidelines: A cluster randomized trial. *International Journal of Nursing Studies, 50,* 464–474.

National Institutes of Health, Office of Behavioral and Social Sciences Research. (2017). Community-based participatory research program. Retrieved from https://obssr.od.nih.gov/

Tomaka, J., Morales-Monks, S., & Shamaley, A. G. (2013). Stress and coping mediate relationships between contingent and global self-esteem and alcohol-related problems among college drinkers. *Stress and Health, 29*(3), 205–213.

Woolf, S. H. (2008). The meaning of translational research and why it matters. *Journal of the American Medical Association, 299*(2), 211–213.

CHAPTER OBJECTIVES

At the end of this chapter, you will be able to:

- Define epidemiology
- Describe the use of epidemiology in nursing practice
- Discuss infectious disease using the epidemiologic triangle
- Describe transmission
- Describe the steps to an outbreak investigation
- Describe count data, ratios, proportions, and rates
- Define and compute prevalence
- Define and compute incidence
- Explain descriptive characteristics of person, place, and time when examining the distribution of disease in a population
- Describe descriptive study designs, including case reports and series, ecologic studies, and cross-sectional studies
- Construct a 2 × 2 data table
- Calculate a prevalence ratio for a cross-sectional study design
- Describe analytic study designs, including case-control studies, cohort studies, and intervention studies
- Calculate an odds ratio for a case-control study design
- Calculate relative risk for a cohort study design
- Define screening
- Calculate sensitivity, specificity, and positive predictive value
- Explain the relationship between sensitivity and specificity
- Describe the use of epidemiologic designs in evaluating health outcomes and health services in evidence-based practice
- List ethical concerns related to epidemiology

KEY TERMS

aggregate data
analytic epidemiology
case-control
case reports or series
cohort studies
count data
cross-sectional
descriptive epidemiology
determinants
distribution
ecologic fallacy
ecologic studies

endemic
epidemic
epidemiology
etiology
exposure
false negative
false positive
incidence
intervention study
odds ratio
pandemic
period prevalence

point prevalence
positive predictive value
prevalence
proportion
rate
ratio
relative risk
screening
sensitivity
specificity
temporal ambiguity

CHAPTER 8

Epidemiologic Designs: Using Data to Understand Populations

Amy C. Cory

8.1 Epidemiology and Nursing

At the end of this section, you will be able to:

‹ Define epidemiology
‹ Describe the use of epidemiology in nursing practice

Epidemiology is the study of the distribution and determinants of disease in human populations. *Distribution* describes the pattern of disease occurrence in and among populations or subgroups. *Determinants* are factors that are "capable of bringing a change in health" (Friis & Sellers, 2009, p. 6). Determinants can be preventative or causal. For example, immunizations are a method of preventing disease in populations, while H1N1 is an infectious agent that causes influenza. Epidemiology is based on two fundamental assumptions: (1) disease does not occur at random, and (2) the determinants of disease can be identified through systematic investigation of populations or subgroups within populations (Hennekens & Buring, 1987).

The word *epidemiology* is derived from the Latin prefix of *epi* meaning "upon," the root *demos*, meaning "the people," and the suffix *logos*, meaning "the study of." Although epidemiology dates back to Hippocrates, the father of medicine, John Snow is considered the modern father of epidemiology as a result of his investigations into the 1854 cholera epidemic in London.

Epidemiologic principles provide the foundation for public health and are useful for supporting evidence-based practice. Principles of epidemiology are used to determine the effect and extent of disease in a population. Knowing these determinations is important for decision making regarding prevention, treatment, control, and research of disease in populations. Epidemiology is used to describe the natural history of disease and to identify the *etiology*, or cause of disease. Epidemiology is used in surveillance of disease. Disease surveillance is used to monitor the distribution of disease and evaluate the effectiveness of prevention and control programs.

There are two types of epidemiologic investigations: descriptive and analytic. *Descriptive epidemiology* examines the distribution of disease in a population in terms of person, place, and time. The purpose of descriptive epidemiology is to identify subgroups that may have the highest risk of disease or the outcome of interest. Epidemiologists also use this approach to find clues about the potential causes of disease and to generate hypotheses about the relationship between exposures and outcomes. *Analytic epidemiology* is used to investigate the determinants of disease. Differing from descriptive epidemiology, analytic epidemiology is hypothesis testing and is used to determine the etiology of disease or health-related outcomes. Special types of statistics are used to determine associations among determinants of disease.

Epidemiology is an exciting field by which nurses use *CSI*-like skills to investigate patterns of disease to best determine contributing factors with the goal of improving health outcomes. For example, a nurse in the pediatric intensive care unit might ask, "What factors are contributing to the increase in gunshot wounds in September as compared to March?" A family nurse practitioner might ask, "Why are more children affected by asthma in one county as compared with children in a neighboring county?" A nurse scientist might ask, "Why are women who cook over open flames more at risk for upper respiratory infections as compared to women who cook with gas or electricity?" By understanding findings from epidemiologic studies that result from questions such as these, nurses can identify strategies to improve health outcomes. Nurses can then implement various strategies to determine best practice.

TEST YOUR KNOWLEDGE 8-1

Indicate whether the following statements are true or false:

1. Epidemiology is the study of disease in populations rather than in individuals.
2. Descriptive epidemiology is used to investigate the determinants of disease.

How did you do? 1. T; 2. F

8.2 Infectious Diseases and Outbreak Investigations

By the end of this section, you will be able to:

‹ Discuss infectious disease using the epidemiologic triangle
‹ Describe transmission
‹ Describe the steps to an outbreak investigation

Because epidemiology is the study of the distribution and determinants of disease in human populations, epidemiologists are by nature concerned with infectious diseases. Their goal is to control infectious diseases and to eradicate them when possible. Endemic diseases, which are diseases that are localized to a particular geographic area, are controlled to prevent epidemics or pandemics. Eradication of a disease occurs when the infectious agent no longer exists in the human population. For a disease to be eradicated, there needs to be 3 years of data to support that the population is disease free with no newly occurring cases. Smallpox is the only disease that has been eradicated.

Epidemiologists view disease through the lens of the epidemiologic triangle (see **Figure 8-1**). The host is the human, the agent is the organism, and the environment is the world in which we live. Each one of these components contributes to the control of infectious diseases.

To better understand and control infectious diseases, nurses must understand the transmission cycle. Transmission of disease occurs through both direct and

FIGURE 8-1 The Epidemiologic Triangle

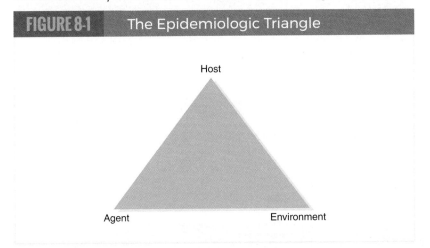

Host

Agent   Environment

indirect mechanisms. Direct transmission occurs from person to person; indirect transmission occurs through vehicles (e.g., water, food), vectors (e.g., mosquitoes), and airborne mechanisms (e.g., droplet, dust).

The purpose of an outbreak investigation is to stop the transmission of disease from the environment to the host, the host to the agent, or the agent to the environment. For example, the cycle of transmission of disease from the environment to the host can be stopped through hand washing, water chlorination, and food safety. The cycle of transmission of disease from the host to the agent can be broken with immunizations, isolation, and treatment. Finally, the cycle of transmission from agent to the environment can be stopped with insect and vector controls. In an outbreak investigation, nurses can follow steps to prevent further transmission of disease (see **Box 8-1**).

BOX 8-1   Steps of an Outbreak Investigation

1. Detect a possible outbreak.
2. Find cases in an outbreak.
3. Generate hypotheses through interviews.
4. Test hypotheses through analytic studies and laboratory testing.
5. Solve point of contamination and original source of outbreak vehicle.
6. Control outbreak through recalls, facility improvements, and industry collaboration.
7. Decide an outbreak is over.

Modified from Centers for Disease Control and Prevention. (2004, November 17). Steps in an Outbreak Investigation. Available at https://www.cdc.gov/foodsafety/outbreaks/investigating -outbreaks/investigations/index.html

CRITICAL THINKING EXERCISE 8-1

When you watch the news, what kinds of outbreaks are reported? Are any of these concerns for college students? Have you encountered patients diagnosed with a disease associated with an outbreak?

TEST YOUR KNOWLEDGE 8-2

1. All of the following are components of the epidemiologic triangle except:
   a. agent
   b. environment
   c. host
   d. population

How did you do? 1. d

8.3 Measures of Disease Frequency

At the end of this section, you will be able to:

< Describe count data, ratios, proportions, and rates
< Define and compute prevalence
< Define and compute incidence

Measures of disease frequency are used to quantify health outcomes to describe and compare populations. Several types of epidemiologic measures are used to calculate disease frequency. These include count data, ratios, proportions, and rates.

Epidemiologic Measures

The simplest measure used is count data. *Count data* refer to the raw number of health phenomena under investigation and would include health events such as births, cases of a disease, and deaths. Count data are not particularly useful when comparing populations of different sizes. For example, a country with a large population will have more births than will a country with a small population regardless of other factors associated with birth rate.

When populations differ in size, epidemiologists use ratios to compare and contrast health outcomes across populations. A *ratio* describes a mathematical relationship between two numbers. The formula is a/b, and the numerator and the denominator do not necessarily have to have a specified association. For example, of 1,000 patients with acute myocardial infarction (AMI), 600 were male and 400 were female. The sex ratio for AMIs is

$$\frac{\text{Number of male cases}}{\text{Number of female cases}} = \frac{600}{400} = 1.5:1 \text{ male to female}$$

Proportions and rates are all types of ratios. A *proportion* is a type of ratio in which the numerator is included in the denominator. The formula for calculating a proportion is $a/a + b$ multiplied by 1,000. In a proportion, the numerator and denominator have an association. The numerator is the number of cases, deaths, or events, and the denominator is the population being studied. Proportions are used in epidemiology to describe measures such as prevalence, cumulative incidence, case fatality rates, and attack rates. For example, of 300,000 children, 3,800 were diagnosed with an autism spectrum disorder and 296,200 were not. The proportion for children diagnosed with autism spectrum disorders is

$$\frac{a}{a+b} \times 1,000 = \frac{3,800}{3,800 + 296,200} \times 1,000 = \frac{3,800}{300,000} \times 1,0$$
$$= 0.01266 \times 1,000 = 12.66 \text{ per } 1,000 \text{ childrer}$$

KEY TERMS

count data: The raw number of health phenomena under investigation in epidemiology

ratio: The highest level of measurement that involves numeric values that begin with an absolute zero and have equal intervals; in epidemiology a mathematical relationship between two numbers

proportion: A type of ratio where the numerator is included in the denominator

The proportion of autism spectrum disorder in this population of children is 12.66 per 1,000 children.

A *rate* is a measure of disease frequency in a defined population over a specified period of time. Rates are used in epidemiology to describe measures such as incidence density, crude mortality rates, and fertility rates. When calculating rate, the numerator is the number of people affected and the denominator is the entire population. For example, of 6,182 babies born in Lake County in 2016, 52 babies died before reaching their first birthday. The infant mortality rate in 2016 was

$$\frac{\text{Number of infant deaths during time period}}{\text{Number of live births during time period}} \times 1,000 =$$

$$\frac{52}{6,182} \times 1,000 = 8.4 \text{ per 1,000 live births}$$

Prevalence and Incidence

In epidemiology two important rates are reported. These rates are named prevalence and incidence, and they describe the extent to which a disease is present in a population.

Prevalence describes the number of existing cases of disease in a population. It is an indicator of the extent of a health problem in a population and is used for planning healthcare needs for communities. Prevalence may be expressed as a number, percentage, proportion, or rate. Prevalence rate per 100,000 at a specified time is

$$\text{Prevalence} = \frac{\text{Number of existing cases of a disease}}{\text{Total population}} \times 100,000$$

For example, in 2016, of the 82,692,308 people younger than age 20 years, 215,000 people had diabetes. The prevalence of diabetes in the United States in 2016 in this age group was

$$\frac{\text{Number of existing cases}}{\text{Total population}} \times 100,000 =$$

$$\frac{215,000}{82,692,308} \times 100,000 = 0.0026 \times 100,000 = 260 \text{ per } 100,000$$

There are two different terms used to describe prevalence. *Point prevalence* describes the number of *existing* cases of disease in a population at a particular point in time. For example, one might calculate the point prevalence of flu on a college campus today and then compare that to the point prevalence of flu on the same day in the previous year. *Period prevalence* denotes the number of existing cases of disease in a population during a specified period of time. The time period might be a week,

KEY TERMS

rate: A measure of disease frequency in a defined population over a specified period of time

prevalence: The number of existing cases of disease present in the population

point prevalence: The number of existing cases of disease in a population at a particular point in time

a month, a year, or a number of years. For example, nurses at a campus health center may calculate the period prevalence of flu from the previous year's flu season to make decisions about how many flu shots to purchase for the current year.

Incidence describes the number of *new* cases of a disease in a population during a specified period of time. Incidence rate is a measure of disease occurrence and is used for investigating the causes of disease. Nurses use incidence rates to investigate risk of disease in populations or subgroups related to many factors such as age, gender, occupation, and exposures. Incidence is calculated by dividing the number of new cases that occur during a time period by the number of individuals who are at risk. It is important to understand that the population at risk is different from the entire population. This is because once people are diagnosed with a disease, they are no longer at risk for acquiring the disease. Therefore, to determine the population at risk, the number of known cases must be subtracted from the population. Incidence rates involve a multiplier (i.e., 1,000 or 100,000) that is relevant to the phenomenon.

> **FYI**
>
> Incidence rate is a measure of disease occurrence and is used for investigating the causes of disease. Nurses use incidence rates to investigate risk of disease in populations or subgroups.

> **KEY TERMS**
>
> **period prevalence:** The number of existing cases of disease in a population during a specified period of time
>
> **incidence:** The number of new cases of a disease in a population during a specified period of time

$$\text{Incidence} = \frac{\text{Number of NEW cases of a disease}}{\text{Total population at risk of developing that disease}} \times multiplier$$

For example, between 2000 and 2016, the prevalence of persons living with Lyme disease was 970. In 2016, of the 6,483,802 people living in Indiana, there were 81 confirmed new cases of Lyme disease. Because there were 970 people living with Lyme disease who were no longer at risk for developing that disease, those individuals must be subtracted from the 6,483,802 people living in Indiana. The population at risk is 6,482,832. The incidence of Lyme disease in Indiana in 2016 was

$$\frac{\text{Number of NEW cases}}{\text{Total population at risk}} \times 100{,}000 = \frac{81}{6{,}483{,}802 - 907} = \frac{81}{6{,}482{,}832}$$

$$= 0.000012 \times 100{,}000 = 1.25 \text{ per } 100{,}000$$

TEST YOUR KNOWLEDGE 8-3

Match the following:

1. Count data
2. Incidence
3. Prevalence
4. Rate

a. measure of disease frequency in a defined population over a specified period of time

b. the number of existing cases of disease in a population

c. the raw number of health phenomena under investigation

d. the number of new cases of disease in a population

How did you do? 1. c; 2. d; 3. b; 4. a

8.4 Descriptive Epidemiology

By the end of this section, you will be able to:

< Explain descriptive characteristics of person, place, and time when examining the distribution of disease in a population

The purpose of descriptive epidemiology is to identify subgroups in populations that may have the highest risk for a specific disease or outcome. Descriptive epidemiology is used to find clues about potential causes of disease so that nurses can generate hypotheses about the relationship between different exposures and diseases or other health-related outcomes. Descriptive epidemiology is used to measure disease frequency by person, place, and time to determine why disease occurs more frequently under certain conditions.

Person

Many descriptive characteristics of the person are factors that contribute to the frequency of diseases and health-related outcomes (see **Table 8-1**).

For example, nurses know that life expectancy varies with sex. Other characteristics such as race and ethnicity contribute to life expectancy. Consider the average life expectancy in the United States for 2011. For all races and both sexes, life expectancy was 78.7 years. But there are variations in life expectancy

TABLE 8-1	Examples of Descriptive Characteristics by Person	
Age		Alcohol
Diet/Exercise		Education
Ethnicity		Genetic markers
Marital status		Occupation
Parity		Race
Religion		Sex
Smoking		Socioeconomic status

TABLE 8-2	Examples of Descriptive Characteristics by Place	
Altitude		City
Country		County
Distance from exposure site		Latitude
Pollution		Rainfall
Rural		State
Sunlight		Urban
Zip code		

depending on race. For example, Hispanic females have a life expectancy of 83.7 years compared to non-Hispanic white females whose life expectancy is 81.1 years, while non-Hispanic black females have a shorter life expectancy at 77.8 years (Centers for Disease Control and Prevention [CDC], 2013a).

Place

A second way to examine descriptive characteristics is by place. These also contribute to the frequency of disease or other health-related outcome (see **Table 8-2**).

For example, obesity is an epidemic in the United States. The frequency of obesity can be examined by state to identify patterns, also called spatial clustering (see **Figure 8-2**). Nurses will note that in the South and in some Midwestern states the prevalence of adult obesity is reported to be between 30% and 35% (CDC, 2016).

Time

A third way that descriptive epidemiology is used is to investigate by time. Several temporal factors contribute to disease frequency and other health-related outcomes (see **Box 8-2**). Trends can be secular, cyclical, or short term.

Secular trends, changes in disease patterns that occur over a long period of time, are often difficult to interpret but can yield important information. For example, the CDC has trended diabetes over decades. The incidence of diabetes in adults, aged 18 to 79 years, in the United States has more than tripled from 493,000 in 1980 to more than 1.4 million in 2014 (CDC, 2015).

Cyclical trends, changes in disease patterns that are often predictable and that recur over time, are seen more readily in health care, particularly as they

FIGURE 8-2	Prevalence of Self-Reported Obesity Among U.S. Adults

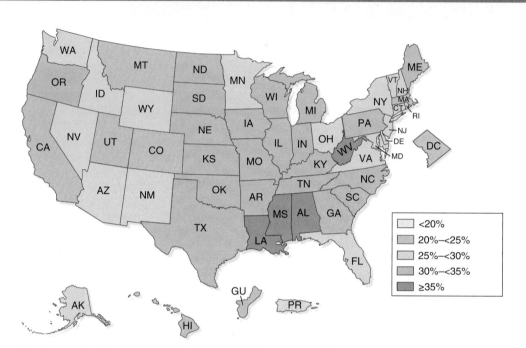

Prevalence estimates reflect BRFSS methodological changes started in 2011. These estimates should not be compared to prevalence estimates before 2011.

Reproduced from Centers for Disease Control and Prevention. (2017). Overweight & obesity: Adult obesity prevalence maps. Retrieved from https://www.cdc.gov/obesity/data/prevalence-maps.html

BOX 8-2	Examples of Descriptive Characteristics by Time

Secular

» Trends over years

Cyclical

» Seasonal trends

Short-term changes

» Epidemics

relate to infectious diseases. A common infectious disease with a seasonal trend is influenza. The CDC trends positive influenza test results reported each week. **Figure 8-3** shows that during the 2016–2017 influenza season, positive influenza test results peaked during the 8th week of 2017 (CDC, 2017).

FIGURE 8-3	Influenza Positive Tests Reported to CDC by U.S. WHO/ NREVSS Collaborating Laboratories, National Summary, 2016–2017

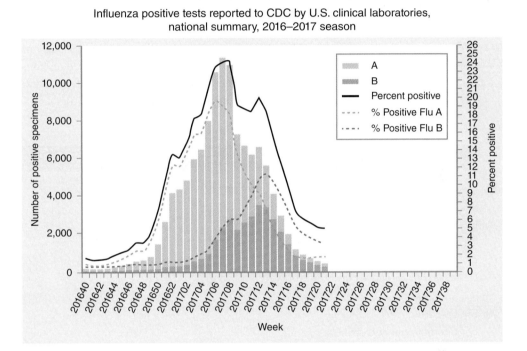

Influenza positive tests reported to CDC by U.S. clinical laboratories, national summary, 2016–2017 season

Reproduced from Centers for Disease Control and Prevention. (2017). Weekly U.S. influenza surveillance report. 2016-2017 Influenza season week 31 ending August 5, 2017. Retrieved from https://www.cdc.gov/flu/weekly/index.htm#whomap

Finally, the frequency of diseases may also be described by short-term trends, which are brief, unexpected changes in disease distribution. Short-term changes include epidemics and pandemics. To understand epidemic and pandemic, it is important first to understand the definition of *endemic*. *Endemic* describes the expected occurrence of a particular disease within a community or population. *Epidemic* is a widespread occurrence of a disease in a community or population that is in excess of what is expected. *Pandemic* is an epidemic that has spread worldwide. For example, in 2012 and 2013, Japan experienced an epidemic of rubella.

Until the early 2000s, rubella was endemic in Japan, with periodic epidemics approximately every 5 years and seasonal increases in the spring and summer. The number of reported rubella cases remained at record low levels until 2010 [n = 87], and in 2011 [n = 378], a few outbreaks were

KEY TERMS

endemic:
The expected occurrence of a particular disease within a community or population

epidemic: A widespread occurrence of a disease in a community or population that is in excess of what is expected

reported in the workplace among adult males. In 2012, the number of rubella cases sharply increased to 2,392, with the rise in cases continuing into 2013. From January 1 to May 1, 2013, a total of 5,442 rubella cases were reported. (CDC, 2013b)

These data demonstrated short-term trends in the number of reported cases of the rubella virus in Japan that were in excess of normal expectancy. As a result, health officials deemed that Japan was experiencing a nationwide rubella epidemic (CDC, 2013b). As a result of these findings, Japan initiated a country-wide education and immunization campaign focused on households with pregnant women to further protect this population from contracting rubella because of the risks to the unborn child (CDC, 2013b).

TEST YOUR KNOWLEDGE 8-4

1. Diseases that occur over long periods of time are known as:
   a. cyclical changes.
   b. intermittent trends.
   c. secular trends.
   d. short-term trends.
2. Diseases that spread around the world are known as:
   a. endemic.
   b. epidemic.
   c. international outbreak.
   d. pandemic.

How did you do? 1. c; 2. d

8.5 Descriptive Study Designs

By the end of this section, you will be able to:

< Describe descriptive study designs, including case reports and series, ecologic studies, and cross-sectional studies
< Construct a 2 × 2 data table
< Calculate a prevalence ratio for a cross-sectional study design

Descriptive study designs are hypothesis-generating and are used to examine different types of phenomena. These studies include case reports or series, ecologic studies, and cross-sectional studies.

Case Reports or Series

Case reports or series are used to describe rare diseases or outcomes. The purpose of these studies is generally to describe new diseases, explain a change in disease patterns, or alert the healthcare community to unusual signs and symptoms in an individual patient (case report) or rare findings among a few patients (case series). Here is an example of a case series:

> In the period October 1980–May 1981, 5 young men, all active homosexuals, were treated for biopsy-confirmed *Pneumocystis carinii* pneumonia at 3 different hospitals in Los Angeles, California. Two of the patients died. All 5 patients had laboratory-confirmed previous or current cytomegalo-virus (CMV) infection and candidal mucosal infection. . . . The diagnosis of *Pneumocystis* pneumonia was confirmed for all 5 patients antemortem by closed or open lung biopsy. The patients did not know each other and had no known common contacts or knowledge of sexual partners who had had similar illnesses. Two of the 5 reported having frequent homosexual contacts with various partners. All 5 reported using inhalant drugs, and 1 reported parenteral drug abuse. Three patients had profoundly depressed *in vitro* proliferative responses to mitogens and antigens. Lymphocyte studies were not performed on the other 2 patients. (AIDS.gov, n.d.)

This edition of the *Morbidity and Mortality Weekly Report* was the first official report of what later became known as the AIDS epidemic (AIDS.gov, n.d.).

The advantage of case reports is that this design can be used to describe unusual signs and symptoms so that healthcare providers may be able to identify commonalities among patients when a new disease appears in a population. Case reports also can be helpful in identifying when a current disease mutates. The disadvantage of case reports is the lack of a comparison group. Without a comparison group, there is no mechanism to test hypotheses.

Ecologic Studies

Correlational studies are used when the unit of analysis is a population, not an individual, and are known as *ecologic studies*. These studies are used to compare a summary measure of disease frequency across summary measures of exposure. Merriam-Webster defines *exposure* as "the condition of being subject to some effect or influence." As a result, the nurse is evaluating group-level rates of disease and exposures. When data from individuals are reported as group information, they are said to be *aggregate data*. For example, suppose a nursing administrator has to report salaries for staff nurses. Rather than telling each individual's salary, the nurse administrator would aggregate the data and report the average salary by unit or by shift. Reporting aggregate data in this manner preserves confidentiality.

Ecologic studies can be used to compare distribution and determinants of diseases across many different population units such as states, counties, zip codes, and even schools. For example, epidemiologists can use this type of design to make comparisons about disease frequency or death rates for different countries or to compare food consumption or exercise patterns in different states. Another example is a nurse examining the relationship between childhood obesity and physical education classes. By plotting the average weights and average number of hours students spent in physical education classes by schools, a nurse could determine the association between childhood obesity and physical education classes among schools.

Ecologic studies offer many advantages. They are expedient and relatively inexpensive because they often rely on secondary data, which are data that have already been collected. Ecologic studies can be used to examine a broad range of exposures and diseases. They are useful when generating hypotheses and may even be used to evaluate the effectiveness of population-level interventions, such as immunizations, smoking bans, and seat belts.

Ecologic studies have disadvantages as well. The single greatest disadvantage is that the nurse is unable to link exposure to disease with specific individuals. For example, in the study of childhood obesity and physical education classes, the nurse is unable to determine whether the student who participated the least number of hours in physical education classes is obese. Another disadvantage is when the pattern demonstrated in the population data is not the same as the pattern shown in the individual data. To take this example further, suppose the nurse finds an association between aggregate data of students' weights and aggregate data of hours spent in physical education classes in the schools she assessed. Based on this information, the nurse might assume that obese children spend fewer hours in physical education classes. However, if the nurse were to look at individual student data, the nurse would find that there is no association between weight and hours spent in physical education classes. When an observation is made at the group level and nurses make inferences at the individual level, it is known as the *ecologic fallacy*. Another disadvantage of ecologic studies includes situations when there are differences in data collection systems, disease definitions, treatment modalities, and survival across population units. These differences can make comparisons difficult and sometimes inappropriate. Also, inability to control for confounding variables and inability to determine whether the exposure truly occurred before the disease, called *temporal ambiguity*, can compromise the findings.

Cross-Sectional Studies

Cross-sectional studies, also called prevalence studies, measure exposure and disease as each exists in a defined population, or representative sample, at one specific point in time. These studies provide a snapshot of the current health status and behaviors, or exposures, of the population. Cross-sectional studies measure the prevalence

KEY TERMS

ecologic fallacy: When false assumptions are made about individuals based on aggregated data and associations from populations

temporal ambiguity: The inability to control for confounding variables and the inability to determine whether the exposure truly occurred before the disease

cross-sectional: Nonexperimental design used to gather data from a group of subjects at only one point in time; study design used to measure exposure and disease as each exists in a population or representative sample at one specific point in time of exposure and disease; therefore, the measure of association for cross-sectional studies is the prevalence ratio (PR). The PR estimates the magnitude of the association between the exposure and the disease. The PR does not inform the nurse that the exposure causes the disease because these data are collected at the same time.

It is important to review how data are organized in epidemiology. Data are put into a 2 × 2 table, also known as a contingency table. The 2 × 2 table categorizes subjects in a study based on exposure and disease status, where A equals the number of people with both the exposure and disease; B equals the number of people with the exposure, but not the disease; C equals the number of people with the disease, but not the exposure; and D equals the number of people with neither the disease nor the exposure. It is very important always to place the same information in the same cell; otherwise, the calculation will be incorrect.

	Disease	**No Disease**	**Total**
Exposure	A	B	A+B
No Exposure	C	D	C+D
Total	A+C	B+D	A+B+C+D

For example, the Texas Department of Health sent a questionnaire to 1,000 adults to inquire about their blood pressure and exercise patterns. Analysis of the surveys showed that 100 cases of hypertension (HTN) were reported among those who exercise more than three times per week, while 400 cases of HTN were found among those who reported no exercise. Of the 500 cases without HTN, 300 reported exercising more than three times per week and 200 reported no exercise. These data were entered into a 2 × 2 table as shown here.

	HTN	**No HTN**	**Total**
Exercise	100	300	400
No Exercise	400	200	600
Total	500	500	1,000

Using these data, a PR was calculated using the following formula:

$$PR = \frac{\dfrac{a}{a+b}}{\dfrac{c}{c+d}} = \frac{\dfrac{100}{400}}{\dfrac{400}{600}} = \frac{0.25}{0.66} = 0.38$$

In this study, the exposure of exercising more than three times per week provided a protective effect for HTN. With protective effects, the PR is subtracted from 1 and multiplied by 100 to derive the percentage of the reduced risk. People who exercised more than three times per week were 62% (1 − 0.38 = 0.62 × 100 = 62%) less likely to have HTN as compared to those people who did not exercise at all.

Cross-sectional studies have advantages and disadvantages. Cross-sectional studies can be used to explain current exposures and diseases in a given population. These studies are efficient and relatively inexpensive. They can also be used to examine a number of different phenomena, including behaviors, symptoms, diseases, and health status. The investigator is not limited to a single exposure and disease but can examine multiple exposures and diseases simultaneously. The major disadvantage of cross-sectional studies is temporal ambiguity. Because data about exposure and disease status are collected at the same time, an investigator is unable to ascertain if the exposure preceded the disease. Another disadvantage exists because cross-sectional studies measure prevalence. Because prevalence is a function of incidence and duration of time, it is difficult to distinguish determinants of the cause of the disease from determinants of survival with the disease. As a result, with a cross-sectional design, the investigator is not able to determine whether the specific exposures caused the specific diseases.

TEST YOUR KNOWLEDGE 8-5

Calculate the PR for the following 2 × 2 table

	Preterm Labor	No Preterm Labor	Total
Smoking	150	150	300
No Smoking	25	275	300
Total	175	425	600

How did you do? PR = 6.02

8.6 Analytic Study Designs

By the end of this section, you will be able to:

< Describe analytic study designs, including case-control studies, cohort studies, and intervention studies
< Calculate an odds ratio for a case-control study design
< Calculate relative risk for a cohort study design

Analytic study designs are hypothesis-testing and are used to test the association between exposure and disease. These studies include case-control studies, cohort studies, and intervention studies.

Case-Control Studies

Case-control studies are designed to sample a group of people with and a group of people without the disease or the outcome measure being studied. Individuals are asked to recall their past exposures to risk factors associated with the disease. Because individuals are recalling their past, these designs are retrospective designs. Individuals who have the disease are known as cases. Those individuals who do not have the disease of interest but who are at risk for developing the disease are known as controls. Cases are often asked to recall exposures up to 1 year prior to diagnosis. Controls are asked about their history of exposures up to the point of entry into the study.

In a case-control study, the investigator compares the probability of exposure for persons who have the disease to the probability of exposure for persons who do not have disease. The statistical test used for a case-control study is the *odds ratio* (OR). For example, the Mississippi Department of Health was interested in examining the relationship between smoking and heart disease. Investigators examined medical records at Jackson County Hospital and invited 500 patients who had experienced an AMI to join the case-control study. Then they contacted 500 people from Jackson County who did not have a history of heart disease but who were similar to the cases in all other demographic areas. The investigators asked the cases to recall their exposures 1 year prior to diagnosis and asked the controls to recall their exposures up to the date of the interview. The investigators found that 400 of the cases were current smokers compared to 150 controls who were smokers. In a 2 × 2 table, the data are expressed as follows:

FYI

Researchers use analytic study designs to test hypotheses and to test the association between exposure and disease. These types of studies include case-control studies, cohort studies, and intervention studies.

KEY TERMS

case-control: A type of retrospective study in which researchers begin with a group of people who already have the disease; studies that compare two groups: those who have a specific condition and those who do not have the condition

odds ratio: The statistic reported when epidemiologists conduct a case-control study

	AMI (Cases)	No AMI (Controls)	Total
Smoking	400	150	550
No Smoking	100	350	450
Total	500	500	1,000

The investigators, using the 1,000 participants, calculated an OR using the following formula:

$$OR = \frac{ad}{bc} = \frac{(400)(350)}{(150)(100)} = \frac{140,000}{15,000} = 9.33$$

The value of an OR is interpreted by comparing it to 1.0. When an OR is equal to 1.0, the probability of disease among the exposed and the nonexposed is identical; therefore, there is no association between the exposure and the disease. When an OR is greater than 1.0, there is a greater probability of disease among the exposed; therefore, there is an association between the exposure and the disease. An OR of less than 1.0 indicates there is decreased probability of disease among the exposed or a protective effect. In this example, the value of 9.33 shows that there is an association between smoking and having an AMI. Individuals who smoke were 9.33 times more likely to have an AMI compared to those who did not smoke.

Case-control studies can be advantageous. They are expedient, require a small sample size, and are relatively inexpensive. Case-control studies are used to examine rare diseases and situations that involve individuals who have had many exposures. Another advantage is that the risk of attrition is low because participants are asked to recall exposures and thus do not leave the study.

Case-control studies have disadvantages as well. They cannot measure incidence. These designs are able to examine only one disease rather than many. The design is not conducive to measuring rare exposures. Because of the retrospective design, recall bias is a threat. This bias can be especially significant when cases are searching for a reason to explain why they acquired the disease. They may be more likely to report potential causes and risk factors as well as exposures that may not have happened to them.

Cohort Studies

Cohort studies are natural experiments. One famous cohort study is the Nurses' Health Study that began in 1976. The primary goal of this study was to examine diet and lifestyle risk factors and their associations with cancer, heart disease, and other chronic diseases. The study was initiated in 1976 with 120,000 female nurses between the ages of 30 and 55 years. The population of the study was ethnically and racially diverse, although all had a higher education than the general population of women. Now in its third version, nurses continue to be followed and outcomes have been added (Nurses' Health Study, n.d.).

Unlike case-control studies where individuals are selected based on the presence or absence of disease, in cohort studies individuals are selected based on their exposure. The investigator selects a sample group that is representative of the target population. Once the sample has been selected, the investigator assigns individuals to groups based on their exposure status. Exposure status is hypothesized to be positively or negatively associated with risk of disease. Investigators can use either prospective or retrospective designs. Prospective designs follow individuals from the time they enroll in the study until they develop the disease. When investigators use retrospective designs, they determine

KEY TERM

cohort studies: Quasi-experimental studies using two or more groups; epidemiologic designs in which subjects are selected based on their exposure to a determinant

a historical exposure and then follow the sample forward to the present time to determine whether the disease is present.

In a cohort study, the investigator compares the probability of disease in individuals who are exposed to the probability of disease in individuals who are not exposed. The statistical test used for a cohort study is *relative risk* (RR). For example, consider the Mississippi Department of Health study that was previously described. Investigators were interested in examining the relationship between heart disease and smoking. In the previous example of a case-control study, the investigators sought individuals who had AMIs. In contrast, when using a cohort design, investigators select individuals based on whether or not they smoke. Therefore, medical records at Jackson County Hospital were examined and 1,000 patients were invited to join the cohort study. Of the 1,000 patients, investigators found 550 patients who smoked, and 450 patients who did not have a history of smoking but who were similar to the smokers in all other demographic areas. They followed these individuals to see who did and did not have an AMI. Of the 550 patients who smoked, 400 patients developed an AMI compared to only 100 patients who never smoked developing an AMI. These data are recorded in the 2 × 2 table as follows:

	AMI	No AMI	Total
Smoking (Cases)	400	150	550
No Smoking (Controls)	100	350	450
Total	500	500	1,000

An RR was calculated using the following formula:

$$RR = \frac{\frac{a}{a+b}}{\frac{c}{c+d}} = \frac{\frac{400}{550}}{\frac{100}{450}} = \frac{0.727}{0.222} = 3.27$$

The interpretation of an RR is the same as an OR. An RR equal to 1.0 indicates the probability of disease among the exposed and the nonexposed is identical; therefore, there is no association. An RR greater than 1.0 indicates there is a greater probability of disease among the exposed; therefore, there is an association. An RR less than 1.0 indicates there is decreased probability of disease among the exposed or a protective effect. For this example, the RR value indicates that smokers were 3.27 times more likely to have an AMI compared to nonsmokers.

KEY TERM

relative risk: The statistic reported by epidemiologists when they conduct a cohort study

KEY TERM

intervention study:
In epidemiology,
a study that has a
treatment that can
be manipulated by
the researcher

Cohort studies are advantageous because they can be used to measure incidence and to study many outcomes. Generally, cohort studies are quite large, so they are a good design to study rare exposures and can readily establish that an exposure preceded the disease. Cohort studies are less vulnerable to recall bias.

Cohort studies have disadvantages as well. They tend to be expensive because of the need for a large sample size and their longitudinal nature. They require a significant amount of time depending on the disease of interest and are impractical for rare outcomes. Because cohort studies are longitudinal, the threat of mortality is significant because subjects drop out, move, or even die during the course of the study. Exposures during the course of a cohort study may change. For example, a person may begin a study smoking two packs per day but during the study may cut back to half a pack per day or quit smoking entirely. These changes can be controlled if the investigator measures exposures more frequently throughout the study rather than simply at baseline.

Intervention Studies

A third design commonly used in epidemiology is an *intervention study*. The key feature of this design is that the investigator manipulates the exposure of interest and then assigns subjects to one or more exposure groups, including a placebo or a group receiving the standard of care. Like experimental designs, an intervention study has the hallmark feature of random assignment of individuals into treatment groups. Randomization is used to control for the effects of confounding variables. Like cohort studies, the statistical test used for intervention studies is the RR.

There are advantages and disadvantages of intervention studies. The advantages include control over the exposure, randomization to control for potential confounding variables, and blinding to reduce bias. Some disadvantages associated with intervention studies are costs and time. The study subjects may experience the Hawthorne effect. Because intervention studies are often time-consuming, subjects may become noncompliant or withdraw from the study, which biases outcomes. For ethical reasons, not all exposures are able to be manipulated, and therefore this design would not be appropriate.

 CRITICAL THINKING EXERCISE 8-2

When reading research reports, have you encountered any reports of incidence or prevalence? How about OR or RR?

TEST YOUR KNOWLEDGE 8-6

Match the following:

1. Case-control study   a. OR

2. Cohort study   b. RR

How did you do? 1. a, 2. b

8.7 Screening

By the end of this section, you will be able to:

< Define screening

< Calculate sensitivity, specificity, and positive predictive value

< Explain the relationship between sensitivity and specificity

In epidemiology, *screening* involves testing people without known disease to determine whether they have a disease. Screening is not a diagnostic tool. It is used to reduce morbidity and mortality in a population. Early detection of disease allows for early entry into the healthcare system with the idea that early treatment will lead to more favorable outcomes. For example, newborns are routinely screened for a variety of genetic diseases, such as phenylketonuria (PKU) and sickle cell disease.

In articles involving screenings, it is important to assess the validity of a screening test. Investigators often report measures for sensitivity, specificity, and positive predictive value of the test. *Sensitivity* describes the ability of the test to correctly identify people with the disease by positive test results. *Specificity* describes the ability of the test to correctly identify people without the disease by negative results. *Positive predictive value* is the probability that a person who screens positive actually has the disease.

To calculate sensitivity, specificity, and positive predictive value, investigators use a variation of the 2×2 table as follows:

	Disease	No Disease
Positive Screen	True positives (TP)	False positives (FP)
Negative Screen	False negatives (FN)	True negatives (TN)

KEY TERMS

screening: Testing people without known disease to determine whether they have a disease; used to reduce morbidity and mortality in populations

sensitivity: The ability of the test to correctly identify people with the disease by positive test results

specificity: The ability of the test to correctly identify people without the disease by negative results

Sensitivity measures the accuracy of the test for identifying who has the disease (TP and FN) and is calculated as follows:

$$\text{Sensitivity} = \frac{TP}{TP + FN}$$

Specificity measures the accuracy of the test for identifying who does not have the disease (FP and TN) and is calculated as follows:

$$\text{Specificity} = \frac{TN}{TN + FP}$$

Positive predictive value measures the proportion of positive screening test results that correctly identifies those patients who actually have the disease and is calculated as follows:

$$\text{Positive Predictive Value} = \frac{TP}{TP + FP}$$

So, what does this mean? If the sensitivity of a test is 80%, then the screening will correctly identify 80% of the people who have the disease. In other words, 80% of the people who have the disease will test positive, while 20% of the people who are screened will be missed, which is known as a *false-negative* result. If the specificity of a test is 95%, then the screening will correctly identify 95% of the people who do not have the disease and 5% of the people without the disease will have a *false-positive* result. A false-positive result means that individuals are told that they have the disease when in reality they do not.

These principles are evident in the reported estimates about mammography. The American College of Preventive Medicine (ACPM) and the U.S. Preventive Services Task Force reported estimates for the sensitivity and specificity for mammography. For all women, sensitivity estimates range from 75% to 95% with specificity ranging from 90% to 97% (AHRQ, 2016; Ferrini, Mannino, Ramsdell, & Hill, 1996). Positive predictive value for mammography was also distributed by age. For women younger than 50 years of age, the positive predictive value was about 20% compared to a range of 60% to 80% in women 50 to 69 years of age (Ferrini et al., 1996). With the positive predictive value for mammography being 20% in women younger than age 50 years, then 20% of the women in this age group who screened positive for breast cancer during mammography actually have breast cancer. If the positive predictive value for mammography was 70% in women 50 to 69 years of age, then 70% of the women in this age group who screened positive for breast cancer during mammography actually have breast cancer. Therefore, mammography is better at detecting breast cancer in older women than in younger women.

It is important to ascertain the psychological and financial costs to the population for the consequences of false-negative and false-positive screening results. False-negative screening results can lead to further progression of disease without treatment until symptoms become more apparent or the patient is rescreened. False-positive screening results have psychological effects as well as potential medical risks and inherent financial costs associated with further diagnostic assessment because individuals are receiving follow-up care for diseases they do not have. As a result, decisions must be made when establishing guidelines for positive and negative results in screenings. These decisions are based on the perceived costs of false-positive or false-negative screening test results.

CRITICAL THINKING EXERCISE 8-3

Suppose you were told that your stool smear for occult blood was positive. The physician orders a colonoscopy for you. After the procedure, you are told that your colon is healthy and that the smear must have produced a false-positive result. How would you feel about this situation?

TEST YOUR KNOWLEDGE 8-7

Indicate whether the following statements are true or false.

1. Screenings are done even when there is no treatment for the disease being screened.
2. Sensitivity describes the ability of the test to correctly identify people without the disease by negative results.
3. As sensitivity of a test increases, specificity of the test decreases.
4. A false positive is when individuals are told they have the disease when in reality they do not.

How did you do? 1. F; 2. F; 3. T; 4. T

8.8 Evaluating Health Outcomes and Services

By the end of this section, you will be able to:

‹ Describe the use of epidemiologic designs in evaluating health outcomes and health services in evidence-based practice

Epidemiologic designs provide sound methodology for nurses to investigate patterns of disease to best determine contributing factors to improve health outcomes and services. Nurses can measure the frequency of disease in clinics, hospitals, and communities and describe diseases by person, place, and time. They can examine the cost-benefit of screening initiatives by examining the sensitivity, specificity, and positive predictive value of screening tests. Outbreaks can be investigated when there appears to be an excess of disease. By analyzing best practice with case-control and cohort studies, nurses can evaluate evidence-based practice interventions using epidemiologic designs and measures.

TEST YOUR KNOWLEDGE 8-8

1. Diseases can be described by all of the following except:
   a. dimension.
   b. person.
   c. place.
   d. time.

How did you do? 1. a

8.9 Keeping It Ethical

At the end of this section, you will be able to:

‹ List ethical concerns related to epidemiology

Ethical concerns in epidemiology are similar to those associated with quantitative designs. For ethical reasons, not all exposures can be manipulated in intervention studies. For example, it would be highly unethical for an investigator to assign individuals to a smoking intervention knowing the inherent risks associated with this behavior.

Risk-benefit ratios must be carefully considered while conducting intervention studies. Investigators must make informed decisions regarding the potential need to terminate a study if either the risks or benefits become clearer during the course of the study.

Risk-benefit must also be considered when setting guidelines for screenings. Screening individuals without the ability to provide follow-up is unethical for two reasons. First, screening conditions for which there is no treatment is a waste of time and money. Furthermore, undue stress may result for individuals who are made aware of untreatable conditions. Additionally, this can also result in needless false positives and false negatives. Best practice dictates that nurses must be wise consumers of limited healthcare resources and sensitive to the impact that misdiagnosis can have on the mental health of individuals.

TEST YOUR KNOWLEDGE 8-9

Indicate whether the following statements are true or false.

1. There are no ethical concerns related to false negatives.
2. It would be unethical to expose individuals to asbestos to study the disease pattern.

How did you do? 1. F; 2. T

RAPID REVIEW

» Epidemiology is the study of disease in populations.

» Nurses use epidemiology to determine the effect and extent of disease in a population.

» The epidemiologic triangle consists of agent, environment, and host. If one relationship can be altered, then the spread of infectious disease can be reduced or eliminated.

» Direct transmission of disease is spread person to person. Indirect transmission involves vehicles, vectors, and airborne mechanisms.

» When an outbreak occurs, nurses can follow seven steps to prevent further transmission of disease.

» Epidemiology involves data that can be expressed as count data, ratios, proportions, and rates.

» Prevalence is the number of existing cases of disease that are present in the population.

» Incidence is the number of new cases of disease that are present in the population during a specified period of time.

» Characteristics of person, place, and time are important when examining the distribution of disease in a population.

» Descriptive study designs include case reports, ecologic studies, and cross-sectional studies.

» Epidemiologic data are often expressed in a 2 × 2 data table that compares the exposed and unexposed cases to whether or not a disease is present.

» Epidemiologists calculate a PR when they use a cross-sectional study design.

» Analytic study designs include case-control studies, cohort studies, and intervention studies.

» Epidemiologists calculate an OR for a case-control study design. They calculate an RR when conducting a cohort study.

» Screenings are tests to identify symptoms of disease and are not diagnostic. Screenings involve testing people without known disease to determine whether they have a disease. They are used to reduce morbidity and mortality in a population.

» Sensitivity, specificity, and positive predictive value are measures used to describe the validity of a screening test.

» When the sensitivity of a test increases, the specificity of the test will decrease. When the sensitivity decreases, specificity will be increased.

» Epidemiologic designs can be used to investigate patterns of disease and evaluate cost-benefit of screening initiatives.

» False-positive and false-negative results from screenings can have ethical implications related to psychological and financial costs.

Apply What You Have Learned

As committee members have been reviewing the evidence, they are finding that some studies use epidemiological approaches to examine data. For example, Chhapola and Brar (2015) examined the impact of their handwashing intervention on times when hand hygiene is indicated. Look at Table 1, on page 489, to see the relative risk (RR) values for each of the five observations. When the intervention is used, at which observation are HCWs 1.25 times more likely to comply with hand hygiene guidelines?

REFERENCES

Agency for Healthcare Research and Quality. (2016). Screening for breast cancer with digital tomosynthesis. Retrieved from www.uspreventiveservicestaskforce.org/Home/GetFile/1/16477/dbt-screen-tomo-finalevidrev/pdf

AIDS.gov. (n.d.). A timeline of AIDS. Retrieved from https://www.aids.gov/hiv-aids-basics/hiv-aids-101/aids-timeline/

Centers for Disease Control and Prevention. (n.d.). Steps of an outbreak investigation. Retrieved from https://www.cdc.gov/foodsafety/outbreaks/pdfs/steps-in-oubreak-investigation-508c.pdf

Centers for Disease Control and Prevention. (2013a). Death in the United States, 2011. NCHS Data Brief No. 115. Retrieved from http://www.cdc.gov/nchs/data/databriefs/db115.htm

Centers for Disease Control and Prevention. (2013b). Nationwide rubella epidemic—Japan, 2013. *Morbidity and Mortality Weekly Report, 62*(23), 457–462. Retrieved from http://www.cdc.gov/mmwr/preview/mmwrhtml/mm6223a1.htm?s_cid=mm6223a1_w

Centers for Disease Control and Prevention. (2016). Adult obesity facts. Retrieved from http://www.cdc.gov/obesity/data/adult.html

Centers for Disease Control and Prevention. (2017). Long-term trends in diabetes. Retrieved from https://www.cdc.gov/diabetes/statistics/slides/long_term_trends.pdf

Centers for Disease Control and Prevention. (2017). Seasonal influenza: 2016–2017 influenza season week 39 ending September 29, 2012. Retrieved from https://www.cdc.gov/flu/weekly/index.htm#whomap

Chhapola, V., & Brar, R. (2015). Impact of an educational intervention on hand hygiene compliance and infection rate in a developing country neonatal intensive care unit. *International of Nursing Practice, 21*, 486–492.

Ferrini, R., Mannino, E., Ramsdell, E., & Hill, L. (1996). *Screening mammography for breast cancer: American College of Preventive Medicine practice policy statement.* Retrieved from http://c.ymcdn.com/sites/www.acpm.org/resource/resmgr/policy-files/polstmt_breast.pdf

Friis, R. H., & Sellers, T. A. (2009). *Epidemiology for public health practice* (4th ed.). Sudbury, MA: Jones and Bartlett.

Hennekens, C. H., & Buring, J. E. (1987). *Epidemiology in medicine.* Boston, MA: Little, Brown.

Nurses' Health Study. (n.d.). *History: Nurses' health study.* Retrieved from http://www.channing.harvard.edu/nhs/?page_id=70

At the end of this chapter, you will be able to:

< Define qualitative research
< Describe sampling techniques in qualitative research
< Discuss the three major sources of qualitative data
< Explain analysis and interpretation methods with qualitative data
< Describe techniques used to meet the four elements of evaluation
< Distinguish among the four major types of qualitative research
< Discuss the philosophical underpinnings of four major types of qualitative research
< Explain the focus of phenomenological inquiry
< Give an example of grounded theory used in nursing
< Name a major nurse contributor to the advancement of ethnographic research
< List two hypothetical examples of historical research in nursing
< Discuss how qualitative studies can be used to create evidence-based practice (EBP)
< Discuss ethical considerations that are unique to qualitative methods

KEY TERMS

audit trail
bracketing
case studies
confirmability
credibility
data reduction
data saturation
dependability
emic
ethnography
ethnonursing

ethnoscience
etic
fieldwork
focus groups
gatekeeper
grounded theory
historical
informants
key informants
lived experience
member checks

memoing
participant observation
participants
peer debriefing
persistent observation
phenomenology
purposive
referential adequacy
snowball sampling
strategic sampling
transferability

CHAPTER 9

Qualitative Designs: Using Words to Provide Evidence

Kristen L. Mauk

9.1 What Is Qualitative Research?

At the end of this section, you will be able to:

‹ Define qualitative research
‹ Describe sampling techniques in qualitative research
‹ Discuss the three major sources of qualitative data
‹ Explain analysis and interpretation methods with qualitative data
‹ Describe techniques used to meet the four elements of evaluation

Qualitative research was first used by disciplines such as the social and psychological sciences. It is used to answer questions related to the hows and whys of behavior that are not easily explained through quantitative methods, to investigate topics about which little is known, or to generate theory. Nursing, although using qualitative research since the 1970s, has only recently begun to embrace qualitative methods as an equally valuable means to explore certain topics while advancing the science and providing foundational evidence for best practice. Unfortunately, in the evidence-based practice (EBP) process, qualitative research is still considered to be far less compelling than quantitative research is because of the subjective nature of data analysis and interpretation.

In contrast to quantitative research, qualitative research focuses on words instead of numbers, on understanding and giving meaning to a phenomenon or an event. Data often stem from telling stories, describing events, analyzing case studies, and examining context, all of which emphasize words versus numbers and statistics (Anthony & Jack, 2009). Qualitative research is more exploratory and inductive, while quantitative research aims to reach conclusions by deduction and hypothesis testing. In deciding whether qualitative methods would be appropriate to the topic being studied, Patton (2003) suggested a checklist such as the one found in **Box 9-1**.

With qualitative studies, researchers often discover those important aspects of inquiry that would be easily missed if the researchers had relied completely on quantitative data. Qualitative research is often the most appropriate method of inquiry for subjects that have been scarcely studied and for those topics about which the researcher wishes to obtain a different viewpoint. For example, if a nurse was interested in exploring the healthcare practices of a culture different from his or her own, and one that had not been referenced in the research literature, a type of qualitative research method would be the logical place to begin. The nurse would not expect to be able to develop an appropriate questionnaire or instrument to measure healthcare practices in a culture about which

---

BOX 9-1 Example of a Qualitative Evaluation Checklist

1. Determine the extent to which qualitative methods are appropriate given the evaluation's purposes and intended uses.
2. Determine which general strategic themes of qualitative inquiry will guide the evaluation. Determine qualitative design strategies, data collection options, and analysis approaches based on the evaluation's purpose.
3. Determine which qualitative evaluation applications are especially appropriate given the evaluation's purpose and priorities.
4. Make major design decisions so that the design answers important evaluation questions for intended users. Consider design options, and choose those most appropriate for the evaluation's purposes.
5. When fieldwork is part of the evaluation, determine how to approach fieldwork.
6. When open-ended interviewing is part of the evaluation, determine how to approach the interviews.
7. Design the evaluation with careful attention to ethical issues.
8. Anticipate analysis—design the evaluation data collection to facilitate analysis.
9. Analyze the data so that the qualitative findings are clear and credible and they address the relevant and priority evaluation questions and issues.
10. Focus the qualitative evaluation report.

Patton, M. Q. (2003). Qualitative evaluation checklist. Retrieved on March 3, 2017, from http://citeseerx.ist.psu.edu/viewdoc/summary?doi=10.1.1.135.8668.

nothing had been previously written or studied. So, qualitative methods are useful to answer descriptive and exploratory questions.

The Basics of Qualitative Research

Before nurses can apply findings from qualitative studies to nursing practice, they must have the ability to critically appraise and evaluate qualitative studies. Understanding the basics of sampling, collecting data, analyzing and interpreting data, and evaluating findings is necessary so that nurses can ensure that qualitative evidence is trustworthy.

Sampling

In qualitative research, the volunteers who participate in a study are called *participants* rather than subjects. Participants are also known as *informants*. The sampling method used is *purposive* rather than random, which is preferred in quantitative methods, because in qualitative methods, the researchers wish to obtain information from specific persons who could provide inside information about the subject being studied. Such people are sometimes referred to as *key informants* because they have intimate knowledge of the subject being investigated and are willing and able to share this with the researcher. A purposive sample is one selected intentionally, yet it includes volunteers who are willing to tell their stories.

Another type of sampling often used alone or in combination with purposive is called *snowball sampling*. This refers to the accumulation of participants based on word of mouth or referrals from other participants. For example, if a researcher interviewed a participant in his home and he mentioned that he attended a support group with others who might wish to talk with the researcher, this referral to the support group could be an additional source of participants for the study. If those in the support group suggest others who might be included in the study, the number of participants snowballs by referrals from the existing sample. Qualitative researchers often find this to be an effective way to identify key informants.

The number of participants in a qualitative research study is also different from the numbers involved in quantitative methods. Generally, a smaller number is involved (often 6 to 10 participants in many studies). Instead of being determined by the number of variables the researchers might include in a quantitative study, in qualitative designs sample size is determined by the information being provided by the participants. Data collection stops when no new information is being obtained and repetition of information is consistently heard. This is called *data saturation*.

KEY TERMS

participants: Individuals in a qualitative study; informants

informants: Individuals in a qualitative study; participants

purposive: Sampling method to recruit specific persons who could provide inside information

key informants: Individuals who have intimate knowledge of a subject and are willing to share it with the researcher

snowball sampling: Recruitment of participants based on word of mouth or referrals from other participants

data saturation: In qualitative research, the time when no new information is being obtained and repetition of information is consistently heard

FYI

Researchers in nursing have only recently begun to embrace qualitative methods as equal in value to quantitative research to advance the science and provide foundational evidence for best practice. However, qualitative research is still gaining acceptance in the EBP process because of the subjective nature of data analysis and interpretation.

Collecting Data

There are three main sources of data in qualitative research: (1) in-depth interviews, (2) direct observation, and (3) artifacts such as written documents, photographs, and physical objects. Each of these sources of data provides rich information for researchers. The data come from *fieldwork*, which is a term used to describe the time researchers spend interacting with participants through interviews, observations, and sessions during which detailed records are created. These records include field notes, methodological logs, and reflective journals. Field notes include notations made before, during, and after contacts with participants to record observations about such details as the participant's mood, environment, and others in the setting. Methodological logs are used to document the researcher's decisions about the study, such as changing an interview question or coding data. Researchers also use a reflective journal to record personal feelings and insights as studies progress. These records are important mechanisms for keeping the researcher true to the data. The researcher must continually refer back to the data in these records as analysis and interpretation progress.

The interview is often the key source of data in qualitative research. Generally, interview questions are open ended, allowing the participant to respond freely and provide the most information possible. The researcher may use an unstructured interview and then follow up with questions as the informant leads. However, most researchers compile a set of questions that arise from the literature review or previous interviews, and these questions guide the discussion with interview participants. The skill of the researcher as an interviewer is important in qualitative research. A common saying is "in qualitative inquiry the researcher is the instrument" (Patton, 1990, p. 14). This means that the qualitative researcher should be skilled in the art of communication and be able to pick up on key words, phrases, thoughts, or ideas informants mention during the interview. Researchers use themselves as tools to solicit information from key informants to obtain the most accurate and useful data for the study.

Researchers should avoid common pitfalls of qualitative research (Easton, McComish, & Greenberg, 2000). They should pay attention to seemingly simple details such as bringing backup batteries for the tape recorder, having plenty of space on the video recorder to complete an interview that runs longer than expected, being sure there is a power source available if using electricity, and the like. A quiet place where the interview can be conducted without interruption is essential. The investigators must anticipate every problem and have a plan in place. The normal interruptions of daily life make it difficult enough to conduct an interview, even without common problems interfering.

Recruiting volunteers who are willing to be interviewed can present a challenge. Nurse scientists may find participants by advertising in newspapers or newsletters, visiting support groups, using the media such as television or radio, posting fliers in places where potential participants might be, or partnering with a healthcare facility that services patients who may volunteer. For example, a nurse who wishes to recruit older people for a study about their attitudes toward living arrangements might find participants in independent living homes, church groups, senior centers, long-term care facilities, intergenerational care centers, and even the grocery store. In addition, snowball sampling may work well with this population. Whichever method of recruiting participants is used, it is essential that the researcher maintain integrity, obtain informed consent, and have institutional review board (IRB) approval to protect the rights of participants and maintain scientific rigor.

Interviews are generally audio- or videotaped as unobtrusively as possible. The interview must be sufficiently long to allow participants to share all essential information. A typical interview may last between 30 and 90 minutes. Open-ended responses and direct quotations are basic sources of data. The researcher also keeps notes during or immediately after the interview to record thoughts, ideas, and reflection on the interview itself. This provides additional contextual data from which to view the results.

The researcher continuously compares information obtained from various interviews, documents, or other sources. Unlike in quantitative research, the interview questions may even change over time as the researcher collects additional data that prompt exploration in other directions. The researcher must keep in mind that the purpose of the interview is to obtain as much pertinent information as possible about the phenomenon being studied and that the person with this information is the participant.

After an interview is complete, it is transcribed verbatim and printed for review. Simple mistakes during transcription can change the meaning of a phrase, even making it read the opposite of what the participant actually said. Although most researchers have support personnel who assist with transcribing, if the transcriber is unfamiliar with the jargon or slang used by the participant, common errors can occur. The researcher is ultimately responsible for the tapes being correctly transcribed. Researchers typically read over the line-by-line transcriptions many times prior to analysis and interpretation. When researchers use software to help with data analysis, they must also be careful to continually revisit the data throughout all stages of analysis. Waiting until later stages of data analysis to perform queries in the software program can result in inconsistencies in the results (Bergin, 2011).

Participant observation is the term most often used to describe the role of the researcher in qualitative data collection (Spradley, 1979). Entire books have been written on this subject because of its importance to the data collection process. The researcher is not merely an observer but also a participant during

KEY TERM

participant observation: Role of the researcher in qualitative methods when the researcher is not only an observer but also a participant during data collection

data collection. Because researchers are considered to be tools for obtaining information, they cannot be merely a detached observer in most cases. For example, a nurse scientist studying how prostate cancer survivors cope with urinary incontinence after surgery might choose to sit in on a support group for these patients. As a participant observer, the nurse might ask questions of the group while keeping notes on patient interactions and the main topics of concern. The nurse would be a part of the support group for that day rather than a nonparticipating attendee. The members of that support group may even later become key informants to the nurse's study of this subject. The role of participant observer takes on an even greater meaning if the researcher has personally experienced the phenomenon being studied. In the preceding case, if the researcher had experienced surgery for prostate cancer and suffered the complication of urinary incontinence, he might participate within such a group at a deeper level. In such a case, however, the researcher must be careful not to allow the bias of personal experience to cloud the results that arise from the data collected from others.

Artifacts provide an additional source of data in qualitative research. This is particularly true in historical research when the main source of data is governmental reports, journals, books, memos, photographs, letters, or diaries. It is important for researchers to remember when using these sources that they can provide only a snapshot in time. Furthermore, the researcher must determine the authenticity of these sources of evidence. There is always room for discussion about the interpretation of findings (Marshall & Rossman, 2011).

Analyzing and Interpreting Data

Although data analysis techniques may vary somewhat depending on the type of qualitative method used, some general comments can be made. Data analysis in qualitative research involves description, data reduction, analysis, and interpretation. Unlike quantitative methods where analysis occurs only after data collection is completed, qualitative data analysis occurs as data are collected. *Immersion* refers to the data collection process in which the researcher "lives" with the data over time. The researcher should constantly reflect on the data and make comparisons with existing data as new information is obtained. Reading and rereading the text that has been transcribed verbatim are essential. The researcher should live with the data for a significant time, comparing every piece of data with the others.

> **KEY TERM**
>
> **memoing:** A technique used in qualitative research to record ideas that come to researchers as they live with the data

Researchers use a technique called ***memoing*** to record ideas that come to them as they live with data. Researchers must keep paper and pencil or their tape recorder handy because ideas may occur at any moment. It is important to memo ideas as they occur because it is difficult to re-create them after a period of time. Researchers use self-reflection to explore personal feelings and experiences to minimize their biases. This is important because analysis and interpretation are inherently subjective in qualitative research. *Bracketing* is a strategy used by researchers to set aside their personal interpretations to avoid bias.

Data reduction occurs when the researcher begins to simplify the large amounts of data obtained from interviews and/or other sources. Terms, ideas, or quotations from transcribed interviews are identified to help the researcher focus on the common themes and patterns that will emerge. The researcher attaches meanings to certain portions of the data that seem to best represent what the majority of participants have reported. Data segments may be coded and indexed by identifying categories in the data. Repeated words or common ideas are noted. Computer software may be of great assistance in managing these data and helping to assign codes, numbers, colors, or other distinguishing marks to sets of data as the researcher attempts to group the data into meaningful segments.

After the data have been reduced in some fashion, the researcher identifies themes, patterns, and relationships. Essential to analysis and interpretation is that the themes, categories, or patterns that are ultimately chosen to represent the data do just that—represent what most of the participants in the study said. In qualitative research, one must be "true to the data" and build in continuous checks and rechecks to be certain that the labels assigned to various themes or patterns reflect what participants have told the researcher. Often, words used by the study participants form the basis for categories assigned.

The final phase of managing the data is interpretation. Interpretation is critical because it brings the message of the participants to the public for reading and application. The researcher uses interpretation to provide meanings that can be used in EBP. Interpretation is open to subjectivity because it is likely that no two researchers would interpret the meaning of the data in exactly the same way. Cassidy (2013) cautioned qualitative researchers to beware of hubris, defined as overconfidence and exuberance for one's interpretations of the data that could potentially influence or cloud the accuracy of conceptual development. However, in spite of the inherent difficulties of defending the results and analysis of qualitative research, Sandelowski (2010) concluded that "qualitative descriptive research is still interpretive" (p. 79). To establish scientific rigor, other nurse scientists should be able to follow the paper trail and the researcher's analysis and to agree that the interpretation and results reported are true to the data obtained from the participants.

KEY TERMS

bracketing: A strategy used by qualitative researchers to set aside personal interpretations to avoid bias

data reduction: The simplification of large amounts of data obtained from qualitative interviews or other sources

FYI

The interview is frequently used as the key source of data in qualitative research. Interview questions are generally open ended, allowing the participant to respond freely and provide the most information possible so that there is an abundance of data from which to draw interpretations.

KEY TERMS

credibility: One of four criteria for establishing a trustworthy qualitative study; refers to the truth or believability of findings

transferability: One of four criteria for a trustworthy qualitative study that relates to whether findings from one study can be transferred to a similar context; application of findings to a different situation

dependability: One of four criteria for a trustworthy qualitative study that relates to consistency in the findings over time; auditability; findings are reflective of data

confirmability: One of four criteria for a trustworthy qualitative study that relates to the rigorous attempts to be objective and the maintenance of audit trails to document the research process; findings can be substantiated by participants

In some types of qualitative research, theory development is an expected outcome. In this case, the researcher must identify concepts and find links or relationships among them to form a theory. The theory is then shared with participants to ensure that it reflects or captures what they experienced or felt. Remember that theories just provide a blueprint or framework from which to view a phenomenon and that they need to be tested and refined.

Evaluation

Guidelines have been established for evaluating qualitative research. Because qualitative methods are so different from quantitative methods, terms such as *validity* and *reliability* are not useful.

However, checklists have been developed to help evaluate the results of qualitative research (Boeije, van Wesel, & Alisic, 2011; Patton, 2003). Lincoln and Guba (1985) provided what remains the standard for evaluation of qualitative research. There are four essential elements of evaluation: *credibility, transferability, dependability,* and *confirmability.* Credibility is the qualitative equivalent of validity in quantitative research. It refers to the truth or believability of the findings (Leininger, 1985). Credibility is established through many strategies that are built into qualitative research. Strategies include *persistent observation, peer debriefing, referential adequacy,* and *member checks.*

Persistent observation means that the researcher has spent a good deal of quality time with the participants while attempting to describe and capture the essence of the phenomenon being studied. The nature of qualitative research requires prolonged engagement. Thus, it is not considered to be a quick form of research.

Peer debriefing is when the researcher enlists the help of another person who is educationally prepared at a similar level to the researcher and who would be considered a peer. Throughout the study the researcher meets on at least several occasions with the peer debriefer, who has consented to assume this role. The researcher and peer debriefer discuss the data and findings, as well as the researcher's reflections, feelings, and struggles. The peer debriefer provides another pair of eyes to examine the consistency of the researcher's interpretation of the data, thus holding the researcher accountable during this process. This is an excellent strategy for new researchers, particularly doctoral students, in that it provides support as well as validation for the student.

Referential adequacy and member checks are additional ways to establish credibility of qualitative research (Lincoln & Guba, 1985). Referential adequacy is satisfied when a researcher can refer to other sources of data, such as photos or journals, for comparison and have the results hold true when referencing these other data. Member checks involve the researcher going back to study participants either during or after the study, or both, and sharing the results with them to be sure that the end product reflects what the participants said.

Transferability relates to whether the findings from one study can be transferred to a similar context. The goal of qualitative research is to understand a particular phenomenon (Leininger, 1985) rather than generalizing to a population as in quantitative methods. Transferability is accomplished through techniques such as eliciting thick descriptions, executing adequate sampling, and achieving data saturation. Thick descriptions involve rich, written comments and narrative related to the situation being studied. Journals and mementos that help to enlighten the process can be kept. Deep and detailed description is needed to establish the scientific rigor of the study. Therefore, researchers must maintain an *audit trail* that can demonstrate the researcher's decision making throughout the study. Adequate sampling means that the researcher took enough time to be sure that data saturation was reached. That is, enough subjects were interviewed so that consistent patterns and themes emerged prior to stopping data collection. When no new information is being obtained, data saturation is said to have been achieved.

The criterion of dependability is satisfied when the researcher has established sufficient audit and paper trails through accurate and detailed journaling and logs. Record keeping and reflective writing are essential in this type of research. Other people, such as peer debriefers, should be able to look at the researcher's writings and see that the theory or results accurately reflect the data.

Confirmability means that the researcher made rigorous attempts to be objective and that audit trails were kept to document the research process. Evaluating interview questions to ensure that they are open ended and not leading is important for ensuring confirmability. The reader must be satisfied that the researcher has revealed that data were confirmed with the participants through member checks. The researcher's written records should reveal a detailed review of the data, careful analysis and coding, and detailed logs and field notes.

KEY TERMS

persistent observation: When the researcher has spent sufficient quality time with participants while attempting to describe and capture the essence of the phenomenon

peer debriefing: A technique used in qualitative research in which the researcher enlists the help of another person, who is a peer, to discuss the data and findings

referential adequacy: A technique used in qualitative research in which multiple sources of data are compared and the findings hold true

CRITICAL THINKING EXERCISE 9-1

Which of the three types of data collection would you use to answer each of the following questions? How would you defend your choice of data collection method for each of these items? Would a combination of methods be appropriate for any of the questions below? If so, why?

1. What factors influence a student nurse's decision in choosing his or her first job after graduation?

2. How did Florence Nightingale choose elements to focus on when she began to formalize nursing as a profession?

3. What influences whether a nurse reports a medication error to his or her supervisor?

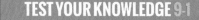

TEST YOUR KNOWLEDGE 9-1

1. Which of the following terms are associated with qualitative sampling? (Select all that apply.)
   a. Snowball
   b. Random
   c. Purposive
   d. Subjects
2. Which of the following are techniques for maintaining scientific rigor in qualitative studies? (Select all that apply.)
   a. Achieving saturation
   b. Thick descriptions
   c. Peer debriefing
   d. Generalizing to populations

How did you do? 1. a, c; 2. a, b, c

9.2 The Four Major Types of Qualitative Research

At the end of this section, you will be able to:

‹ Distinguish among the four major types of qualitative research
‹ Discuss the philosophical underpinnings of four major types of qualitative research
‹ Explain the focus of phenomenological inquiry
‹ Give an example of grounded theory used in nursing
‹ Name a major nurse contributor to the advancement of ethnographic research
‹ List two hypothetical examples of historical research in nursing
‹ Discuss how qualitative studies can be used to create evidence-based practice

KEY TERM

member checks: A strategy used in qualitative studies when the researcher goes back to participants and shares the results with them to ensure the findings reflect what participants said

There are four major types of qualitative research: *phenomenology*, *grounded theory*, *ethnography*, and *historical*. Each of these types of research has distinguishing characteristics, so it is important for a researcher to select a method appropriate to the question. **Table 9-1** provides a comparison of these four major types.

Phenomenological Research: Studying the Lived Experience

Phenomenology is the method used when one wishes to study *lived experience*. The general question being asked is, "What is the meaning of. . .?" The goal is to achieve understanding of an experience from the perspective of the participants.

TABLE 9-1	Comparisons of Qualitative Methods

Type of Qualitative Research	Focus	Example Question
Phenomenology	Lived experience	What is the lived experience of a woman dying from breast cancer?
Grounded theory	Process	What is the process of recovery following breast cancer?
Ethnography	Culture	What are the self-breast-exam practices of Amerasian women?
Historical	The past	What were the ancient Romans' basic beliefs regarding diseases of the breast?

Philosophical Underpinnings

Phenomenology has its roots in the human sciences. Edward Husserl and Martin Heidegger were philosophers whose work inspired current phenomenology. Husserl was a German philosopher credited with moving from naturalistic science to philosophical reduction by separating the researcher's preconceived notions to reveal a true lived experience. "Husserl's phenomenology emphasized a way of coming to know through the actual experience of a phenomenon (experiential epistemology) with a goal of describing the experience of the phenomenon. Thus methodology inspired by Husserl is often called *description methodology*" (Converse, 2012, p. 29).

Heidegger's philosophy was influential in the development of the use of phenomenology in nursing today. He supported the idea that the researcher needs to know about the history of an individual in order to have proper context for investigation. Heidegger (1962) believed "that the meaning of being is an important way of understanding human existence" (Pratt, 2012, p. 12). The concepts of "time" and "being" were essential to helping researchers have a context to explore the lived experience of others. Phenomenology focuses on the human experience and causes the nurse to ask *why* a particular phenomenon has occurred. In addition, Heidegger saw nurses' experience

KEY TERMS

audit trail: The documentation of the research process and researcher's decision making in qualitative studies

phenomenology: A type of qualitative research that describes the lived experience to achieve understanding of an experience from the perspective of the participants

grounded theory: A type of qualitative research that examines the process of a phenomenon and culminates in the generation of a theory

ethnography: A type of qualitative research that describes a culture

historical: A type of qualitative research used to examine events or people to explain and understand the past to guide the present and future

lived experience: The perspective of an individual who has experienced the phenomenon

as a valuable part of the research process. "When conducting research using the Heideggerian perspective, researchers can draw on their backgrounds as nurses" (Pratt, 2012, p. 13).

Method

Using purposive sampling, phenomenological studies more than likely will have small sample sizes, depending on the phenomenon being studied. For example, in Su and Chen's (2006) study of women terminating treatment after in vitro failure, the sample size was 24. Women were selected from a common area and clinics because they were likely to have shared similar experiences. *Case studies* can also provide a description of the lived experience. For example, Marshall, Kitson, and Zeitz (2012) examined the views about patient-centered care based on 10 patients on a surgical unit in Australia. The case study was a unit of persons with like experiences. It is important to keep in mind that one person's experience may be unique and not totally reflective of the experiences of others.

Data Collection and Management

Most of the data for phenomenological research are obtained from fieldwork, particularly interviews with people who have experienced the phenomenon being examined. Marshall and Rossman (2011) described phenomenological interviewing as an in-depth type of interviewing that discovers how experiences are put together to develop a worldview. Interviews are transcribed verbatim and read multiple times by the researchers. Significant statements are identified; items are coded and analyzed for themes and patterns. Statements may link together to form common themes. The researcher identifies broad themes with categories and subcategories that are consistent among participants. There may be several core themes or one broad theme with associated categories.

Benner (1984) described three interpretive research steps of phenomenology: thematic analysis, analyzing exemplars, and identifying paradigms. During thematic analysis, the reasons, feelings, and thoughts of participants are explored. Meanings of the categories are analyzed and integrated into a theme or themes. Step 2 involves analyzing exemplars. This is when researchers repeatedly read data for possible new categories, corrections of thematic or categoric assignments, and analysis of differences among the data. Last, according to Benner, the researcher identifies paradigms, checking the themes and categories to be sure that they are representative of the responses from all participants.

Examples of Nursing Research Using Phenomenology

There are many examples of nursing research using phenomenology. Some of the better-known nursing theories coming from this type of research are Parse's (1991) theory of human becoming and Watson's (1989) theory of human caring. Probably the best-known research of this type is Benner's (1984) work *From Novice to Expert* in which she identified five stages of nursing competence that are still used to guide practice. Dr. Benner based her work on dialogue with nurses who were interviewed individually or in small groups. Her research offers examples of excellence in nursing practice and a framework demonstrating the development of nurses as they move through five stages: novice, advanced beginner, competent, proficient, and expert. This is indeed an example of how qualitative research translates into EBP as nurses all over the world study ways in which nurses develop into expert clinicians. In many healthcare facilities, professional promotion and clinical ladders are based on this model.

Lapidus-Graham (2012) examined the lived experiences of nursing students who participated in a student nurse organization. The sample was 15 nursing students who had graduated from schools in Long Island. The themes that emerged from the data were "(1) leadership: communication, collaboration and resolving conflict; (2) mentoring and mutual support; (3) empowerment and ability to change practice; (4) professionalism; (5) sense of teamwork; and (6) accountability and responsibility" (p. 4). The author concluded that student nurse associations (SNAs) were important to the development of future nurses and that instructors should integrate SNA activities into the existing curricula to foster leadership behaviors.

Grounded Theory Research: Creating Theory Through Induction

Grounded theory is the method of choice when the researcher wants to discover the process of something. The general question being asked is, "What is the process of. . .?" This method is most commonly used in areas where there is little or no previous research. The grounded theory method was originated by Glaser and Strauss in 1967 when they looked at the way people approach the process of dying. The researchers specified a systematic set of procedures that is used to inductively create a theory that is grounded in the data about a phenomenon (Strauss & Corbin, 1990). These theories can be useful in explaining and predicting phenomena (Glaser & Strauss, 1967).

Philosophical Underpinnings

Grounded theory was developed as a way of conceptualizing research information. Although grounded theory was developed by two social scientists, Glaser and Strauss (1967), its philosophical underpinnings are from a variety of paradigms, including positivism, postpositivism, and constructivism. Positivism focuses on deductive reasoning and logical thinking, suggesting that the world is ordered in an organized fashion. Postpositivism contends that true reality may exist, but we can never truly know it. The constructivist view is that the researcher and the inquiry are linked. This suggests that humans do not truly discover knowledge, but rather they create or construct it through their interactions (Hall, Griffiths, & McKenna, 2013). One can clearly see the influence of each of the epistemologies on the development of grounded theory.

Method

A few characteristics make grounded theory different from other qualitative methods. The most important difference concerns the review of literature. In most research methods, an extensive review of literature is done prior to beginning the study to shed light on the phenomenon in question and identify gaps in the literature. In grounded theory, just enough literature is examined to identify the gaps in the literature, but a more extensive review of literature is done only after the research is completed (Glaser, 1978). The purpose of this approach is to avoid bias because a grounded theory must emerge from the data and never be forced by preconceived notions. Writing in a reflective journal is an effective strategy for raising self-awareness, thus reducing bias. After the theory has been generated, a thorough review of the literature is done, and the researcher compares the theory with other research. This is known as comparative analysis, and Glaser and Strauss (1967) listed the following steps: (1) obtaining accurate evidence, (2) making empirical generalizations, (3) specifying a concept, (4) verifying theory, and (5) generating theory. Grounded theory is dynamic and subject to change as new data become available. One could almost say that a grounded theory is never really finished but that it can be constantly validated and refined.

Data Collection and Management

Data are gathered mainly through interviews. As with other qualitative methods, the face-to-face interviews are video- or audiotaped and are conducted using open-ended questions. The researcher keeps detailed field notes and methodological logs to record observations and reflections. The interview questions may become more focused as the study progresses so the researcher can discover the major processes taking place.

Another unique aspect of grounded theory is that researchers may use the literature as data. Both the technical and nontechnical literature can be used for this purpose (Glaser, 1992; Strauss & Corbin, 1990). Technical literature includes research reports or theoretical/philosophical papers of a scholarly nature. Nontechnical literature may include biographies, diaries, reports, newsletters, and records. Literature could be used as primary data or to supplement data gathered from interviews.

There is no set sample size for grounded theory. The researcher obtains data until data saturation is reached. This may be as few as 10 interviews or more than double that, depending on the data obtained. The use of *focus groups*, a strategy often employed in qualitative research, lends itself well to grounded theory. Focus groups are useful to generate ideas and help formulate interview questions to be used later with key informants. Generally, a focus group consists of six to eight people with a common interest but who do not know each other well. The researcher may act as a facilitator by using open-ended questions to begin the discussion and guide the group to provide sought-after information. Or the researcher may be a participant observer in a focus group, such as attending a breast cancer support group to gain insight. Focus groups have the added benefit of being an excellent way to identify key informants for one-on-one interviews later (Easton, 1999b).

Another difference between grounded theory and other qualitative methods is the use of constant comparison. Comparisons are continuously made among the data. In this way, both data gathering and analysis occur somewhat simultaneously. The researcher records ideas, thoughts, possible emerging themes and patterns, questions for follow-up, and potential categories for data coding. As data are coded and clustered, the researcher continues to explore commonalities as interviewing and data collection continue. Negative case examples and conflicting information are also noted. All of these data form the basis for the final categories that are generated to reflect the process described by participants. As more interviews are conducted, the emerging theory is confirmed and refined as the researcher asks more focused questions (Cooney, 2011). In addition, new subconcepts may be added or deleted to further refine the categories identified.

Examples of Nursing Research Using Grounded Theory

Folden (1994) used a grounded theory approach to describe how stroke survivors managed multiple functional deficits produced by stroke. The process was labeled "ensuring forward progress" (p. 81). Folden indicated that each person defined recovery "as the accomplishment of personal goals" (p. 81). Her

> **KEY TERM**
>
> **focus groups:** A strategy to obtain data from a small group of people using interview questions

findings were consistent with other findings in the stroke literature at the time, adding credibility to her work. Although Folden's work added much to nursing knowledge about stroke, the published articles stopped short of proposing a complete theory with assumptions and relational statements.

Using the same population, stroke survivors, Mauk, who published earlier as Easton, sought to answer the question: What is the process of stroke recovery? (Easton, 1999a). From her research, a grounded theory emerged for poststroke recovery that was labeled the poststroke journey: from agonizing to owning. Mauk used writings and videotapes from stroke survivors to identify concepts and generate a theory. She then conducted face-to-face interviews with 18 stroke survivors to refine the theory. The end result of this grounded theory research showed that stroke survivors reported six major phases in the process of recovery: agonizing, fantasizing, realizing, blending, framing, and owning (Mauk, 2001, 2006). Nursing interventions targeted to each phase of recovery are being developed and explored but have yet to be tested.

More recently, Gallagher (2011) developed a grounded theory that focused on the emotional process of stroke recovery. In a sample of nine stroke survivors, she found three key themes related to emotional recovery: "1) recognizing that stroke will not go away, 2) choosing to work on recovery, 3) working on being normal" (p. 24). Interestingly, many of these themes are similar to what Mauk found in examining the overall process of stroke recovery.

These three studies illustrate that grounded theory can be used by nurses to explore a phenomenon about which little is known. In the previous examples, the process of stroke recovery was one that had to be discovered from survivors themselves. Theories can be used to develop practice guidelines. By listening to, documenting, and explaining the process that patients go through, nurses can provide better care because they are sensitized to patients' situations.

Ethnographic Research: Understanding Culture

Spradley (1979), considered to be a leading expert in ethnography, defined the method as "the work of describing a culture" (p. 3). He further stated that instead of just studying people, ethnography involves learning from people. Spradley (1980) suggested three basic aspects of human experience that researchers needed to discover: cultural behavior (what people do), cultural knowledge (what people know), and cultural artifacts (what people make and use). "The goal of inquiry is rounded, not segmented understanding. It is comprehensive in intent" (Hughes, 1992, p. 443). Ethnographic research involves studying groups and making collective observations. It is the method of choice for studying cultures.

Additional related methods that grew out of ethnography, *ethnoscience* and *ethnonursing*, warrant mention here. Ethnoscience is a method used in anthropology to discover nursing knowledge. Ethnonursing is the systematic study and classification of nursing care beliefs, values, and practices in a particular culture (Leininger, 1985; Welch, 2002). Cultural representatives share knowledge acquired through their language, experiences, beliefs, and value systems regarding nursing phenomena such as care, health, and environment. Because the focus is on nursing, studies using these methods are usually not as broad in scope and depth as studies conducted to explain an entire culture. Therefore, obtaining information may not require one to live in the culture for an extended period of time. These methods were used by Madeleine Leininger (1985), founder of transcultural nursing. Leininger, a noted professor and prolific author and theorist, earned a doctorate in cultural and social anthropology, which influenced her research related to nursing. She derived her theory of culture care diversity and universality from work in anthropology and nursing. Leininger firmly believed that quantitative methods had limited use in studying cultures and health and that ethnographic methods provided the clearest information when researching other cultures.

> ### KEY TERMS
>
> **ethnoscience:** A method used in anthropology to discover nursing knowledge
>
> **ethnonursing:** Systematic study and classification of nursing care beliefs, values, and practices in a particular culture

Philosophical Underpinnings

Ethnography, whether general or focused, grew out of the idea that researchers learn about people by learning from them (Roper & Shapira, 2000). Ethnography originated from the discipline of anthropology with social scientists such as Margaret Mead. However, early ethnographers were often considered "professional strangers" (Cruz & Higginbottom, 2013, p. 37), unwanted by the people whom they studied, and whose writings often mispresented the culture and beliefs of the people because of the influence of the day's political loyalties. The philosophical roots of ethnography are in naturalism, which emphasizes or focuses on setting and environment of subjects. Participant observation is still considered a key method in ethnography, though many researchers have used more broad qualitative methods to conduct ethnographic research. Today, ethnography is used by nurse researchers not only to study other cultures but also to study specific areas or "cultures" in nursing such as nurse triaging in the emergency room (Fry, 2012).

Method

A few techniques distinguish ethnographic research from the other methods previously discussed in this chapter. Because participant observation is a key strategy in this type of research, gaining access to a group, particularly if it is one to which the researcher is not attached, has unique challenges. Gaining access to a particular group often requires that the researcher go through a *gatekeeper*. This is a person who facilitates the entry of the researcher into the particular group being studied. For example, if a Caucasian researcher wished to study the culture of a particular tribe of Native Americans, the researcher might first need to identify a person from that tribe who would invite the researcher to be a participant observer because it is highly unlikely that the researcher would gain access without assistance. The gatekeeper is generally a person with some authority in the group.

When obtaining information from key informants, the researcher strives to discover the *emic* perspective, or the informant's perspective (i.e., the "inside" scoop; Boyle, 1994). Conversely, the researcher has an *etic*, or outside, perspective. In ethnography, discovering the emic perspective is essential. The researcher needs to record and observe both what key informants say and what they do, looking for consistencies or inconsistencies between the emic and etic perspectives.

Data Collection and Management

Researchers using ethnographic methods study people in their natural environments over long periods of time to gain a comprehensive view of the culture (Leininger, 1995). There is direct personal involvement with the study of participants over time, usually several months to years (Boyle, 1994). This method takes prolonged engagement and patience.

Along with participant observation, the researcher conducts in-depth interviews with key informants. As with any method that uses interviews, the skill of the researcher largely influences the quality and credibility of the results. Interviews should begin with open-ended questions that allow the informant to provide as much information as possible and that support the grand tour question, or the major question that the researcher is trying to answer.

Spradley (1979) believed that the ethnographic interview should be like sharing a friendly conversation. He identified three important elements to the interview: (1) explicit purpose, (2) ethnographic explanations, and (3) ethnographic questions. First, the researcher must make the purpose of the interview perfectly clear and gradually take the lead in directing the questions and conversations to discover the knowledge of the informant. Throughout interviews the researcher must also give repeated explanations to the informant about information that needs to be obtained. Informants may need to be reminded to speak from their own perspective and not "translate" for the researcher. Interviews are usually conducted over weeks during numerous encounters so that the researcher can gradually guide the informant toward providing relevant information. Spradley listed more than 30 kinds of ethnographic questions that could be used during an interview (see **Table 9-2**). Easygoing conversation should be interspersed with questions that the researcher wishes to have answered.

TABLE 9-2	Examples of Ethnographic Questions	

Type of Question	Focus	Example
Descriptive	Sample of language	Could you describe a typical day at the mill?
Structural	How participants organize	What are all the activities you do at the mill?
Contrast	For a participant to explain differences or relationships	You mentioned earlier that _____ is a habit that only a "millrat" does. Would a _____ do that? Would _____ do that? Who wouldn't do that?

Modified from Spradley, J. P. (1979). *The ethnographic interview.* Orlando, FL: Harcourt, Brace, Jovanovich College Publishers.

One can see from this style of interviewing that the researcher needs to gain skill through practice and experience to be able to conduct such interviews effectively. **Box 9-2** summarizes some key points for ethnographic interviewing. In this method, as with many others, keeping detailed field notes is essential along with in-depth ethnographic interviews. The researcher should also collect artifacts or symbols of the culture, employ maps and diagrams, and obtain family trees and the like to help understand the culture. The importance of language cannot be overemphasized. Words convey various meanings in context, so the meanings of words and the situations in which they are used are essential to record and understand. Body language, vocal inflection, and tone in the context of the situation should be recorded and analyzed. Slang or jargon should be noted and explored.

As with grounded theory, the constant comparison method is often used so that data collection and data analysis may occur somewhat simultaneously. Thick descriptions are used in each area of data collection. The researcher may log an example of a typical day within the group, focus on specific unique events, or develop a story with a plot and characters (Marshall & Rossman, 2011). Several logs or journals may be kept to organize data and observations.

The data are coded and grouped according to their meanings. Patterns and categories are identified. When presenting the findings, the researcher often uses a more personal reporting style. Researchers must strive to have objectivity when analyzing and interpreting the data (Fetterman, 2010). Bias can occur as a result of the closeness that the researcher typically gains with the culture when living among the people. The ultimate goal is to present a detailed picture of a culture that an outsider could read to obtain a better understanding and gain empathy for a specific group. Ethnographic research is an excellent way to increase sensitivity to those whose culture is different from researchers' and readers'.

| **BOX 9-2** | Suggestions for Ethnographic Interviewing |

Explain the purpose of the interview clearly.

Obtain informed consent and ensure confidentiality and anonymity.

Gain entry into the culture through a gatekeeper.

Identify key informants.

Develop a rapport with the participants.

Practice and study techniques related to ethnographic interviewing.

Allow sufficient time for prolonged engagement to observe and participate in the culture.

Keep detailed field notes, records, and reflective journals.

Collect significant artifacts.

Keep in mind the grand tour question.

When interviewing, begin with open-ended questions and progress to more focused questions over time and in repeated interviews.

Be sure all equipment is working and that you have a plan for malfunctions of tape recorders, etc.

Keep interviews conversational and friendly even when trying to elicit specific information.

Pay special attention to the language of the participants and the use of key words.

Clarify the meanings of terms using contrast questions.

Constantly compare and contrast data with each other during the collection process.

Record all interviews and transcribe them verbatim.

Be true to the data.

Modified from Spradley, J. P. (1979). *The ethnographic interview*. Orlando, FL: Harcourt, Brace, Jovanovich College Publishers.

Examples of Nursing Research Using Ethnography

Nurses have used ethnography in many unique ways to understand cultures related to health or the health practices of other cultures (Roper & Shapira, 2000). For example, Rosenbaum (1990) used Leininger's theory of culture care as a framework to uncover the cultural care needed for older Greek Canadian widows. The sample contained 12 key informants and 30 general informants, and the researcher collected data using participant observation and interviews. Rosenbaum found that for these widows, health meant a state of well-being, ability to perform activities in their role, and avoidance of pain and illness. These findings could stimulate future nursing interventions for EBP related to caring for widows in this culture and perhaps others.

Another example of nurses using ethnography is a study by Shambley-Ebron and Boyle (2006) that explored self-care and mothering in African American women with HIV/AIDS. The researchers studied 10 African American mothers and found themes related to disabling relationships, strong mothering, and redefining self-care, with a cultural theme of creating a life of meaning. The researchers concluded that their study pointed out the strengths of African American women and helped to generate theory that will promote better care for this population.

In a meta-ethnography about older persons' views on risk for falls, the researchers selected 11 qualitative articles from 7 databases to gain a conceptual understanding about how elders view falls and their needs for fall prevention interventions. Researchers examined the culture of falls in elderly adults. The researchers found six key concepts that explained how older adults appraised their risk for falls and how they coped with fall risk interventions. The six key concepts identified were: (1) beyond personal control, (2) rationalizing, (3) salience, (4) life change and identity, (5) taking control, and (6) self-management (McInnes, Seers, & Tutton, 2011). By synthesizing findings using meta-ethnography, the researchers were able to identify a culture unique to older adults who experience falls.

Street (1992) conducted a study that became a book titled *Inside Nursing: A Critical Ethnography of Clinical Nursing Practice*. She studied nurses and the culture of nursing at a large hospital in Australia. Street's background was social theory and feminism rather than nursing. Nonetheless, her work provided great insight into the politics, power struggles, and frustrations reported by nurses that challenged the traditional view of nursing at the time.

These studies demonstrate that culture does not have to be merely defined in terms of one's ethnic group, but that culture embodies the feelings, beliefs, attitudes, values, and behaviors of a group of people and ethnography can be conducted on a variety of topics in different settings. Today's nurse researchers "would be well-served by describing specific cultural patterns in order to develop targeted interventions to best meet increasingly diverse patient needs" (Oliffe, 2005, p. 397).

Historical Research: Learning from the Past

Historical research is based on documentation of sources that are used to retrospectively examine events or people. "Historical methods are concerned with uncovering and generating evidence and with interpreting that evidence in the historical context in which it was created" (Fealy, Kelly, & Watson, 2013, p. 1882). The questions being asked are "Who are we?" "Where did we come from?" "Why did we do this?" and "How did we get to this point?" The goal of this type of research is to explain and understand the past with the hope of guiding the present and future.

Philosophical Underpinnings

The philosophy of historical nursing research is grounded in the idea that historical documents and recordings can be used as research data. In 1948, Professor Allan Nevis described "the oral history method as the process of recording the expressed memories of the authorized persons" (Firouzkouhi, Zargham-Boroujeni, Nouraei, Yousefi, & Holmes, 2013, p. 226). This method has been useful in qualitative research because it allows persons to share their mementos, feelings, diaries, photographs, and other data with researchers to learn more about a phenomenon.

Historical studies have been defined as studies containing narratives using rigorous historical methods and/or studies that synthesize previous historical knowledge (Fealy et al., 2013). In examining the history of nursing through published articles in the *Journal of Advanced Nursing* from 1976 to 2011, the authors believed that "for a discipline like nursing, the relevance of historical scholarship is its ability to demonstrate the particular and distinct contribution that nursing has made to society through its role in the development of systems of health care" (Fealy et al., 2013, p. 1882).

Method

One unique type of sampling used in this method is called *strategic sampling*. This is when the researcher locates a small group of people who were either witnesses to or participants in the phenomenon being studied. In such a sample, often no restrictions on age or gender are made except as delineated by the phenomenon being studied. There is no set sample size, but an accumulation of facts continues until no new data are obtainable. For example, Harmon (2005) studied nursing in a state hospital between 1950 and 1965. This researcher used oral history methods to describe the experiences of eight American nurses who worked in psychiatric hospitals before and during the introduction of antipsychotic medications.

Data Collection and Management

The major sources of data in historical research are eyewitness accounts and documentation. Although interviews with participants are possible, participants would be reflecting on past events, and data would be based on their recollections. A common criticism of the method is that data may not always be reliable because data are based on the memories of the participants. Accurate and detailed documentation on the part of the researcher is needed to maximize credibility. Some of the documentation sources that nurses might use in historical research include government reports, professional journals, oral evidence, books, memos, photographs, letters, newsletters, newspapers, diaries, journals, videos, films, official publications, written responses to surveys, and memorabilia.

After the researcher has obtained all sources of data, including the verbatim transcription of personal accounts or oral histories, central themes are identified from "disciplined reflection" (Galvin, Todres, & Richardson, 2005, p. 3). The analysis and interpretation should be logical and easy to follow, flowing smoothly from the data. Most historical research tells a story of events over time. The usefulness to nursing lies in allowing the past to illuminate and positively influence the future. The following examples of historical research in nursing provide thought-provoking ways nurses can examine the evidence on which we base our practice.

Examples of Nursing Research Using Historical Research

Lusk (2005), one of the proponents of nurses using historical research, used this method to study nurses who cared for patients with cancer between 1920 and 1950. She used primary sources from U.S. archives, nursing procedure books, annual reports, and even minutes from meetings. Her secondary sources included textbooks and journal articles. Lusk chronicled the development of cancer as a specialty in nursing and revealed the discomfort nurses experienced when hiding a cancer diagnosis from patients.

The Careful Nursing Philosophy, a model for professional nursing, was derived from historical research. The author (Meehan, 2012) derived a model from examining the practices of 19th-century Irish nurses. Twelve Irish nurses were appointed to work closely with Florence Nightingale to develop a system for nursing that became widely used in Europe. Using historical nursing research as a method, the author used content analysis of historical documents to discover the thinking and practice of these early nurses. Meehan's (2006) work on this model spanned many years, and she developed a practice model based on an in-depth scrutiny and thematic analysis of historical writings in context. Her results revealed 4 major concepts with 18 dimensions. The major concepts for practice were "therapeutic milieu, practice competence and excellence, management of practice and influence in health systems and professional authority" (Meehan, 2012, p. 2905). Meehan believed that our present nursing system could be improved and enhanced by revisiting our successful roots within these four major areas. This research shows how identifying past behavior can be used as a basis to inform decisions about nursing practice in the present and future.

CRITICAL THINKING EXERCISE 9-2

Consider a time when you may have been exposed to a new culture. What were the emic perspectives? How did these compare to your etic perspectives?

TEST YOUR KNOWLEDGE 9-2

1. Which method would you choose to answer the question, What process do older adults use when they quit smoking?
   a. Ethnography
   b. Historical
   c. Phenomenology
   d. Grounded theory

2. Match the following terms with one of the four types of qualitative methods:
   a. Constant comparison
   b. Strategic sampling
   c. Lived experience
   d. Emic

How did you do? 1. d; 2. a. grounded theory b. historical c. phenomenology d. ethnography

9.3 Keeping It Ethical

At the end of this section, you will be able to:

‹ Discuss ethical considerations that are unique to qualitative methods

Qualitative researchers are held to the same ethical standards as are researchers using other methods. Participants have the same rights as individuals who volunteer for research involving quantitative measures. Researchers must obtain informed consent, protect privacy, allow volunteers to withdraw from the study at any time, and avoid harm to individuals who participate. Because of their noninvasive nature, most qualitative studies qualify for exempt status from the institutional review board review.

Some ethical considerations, however, are unique to qualitative research. These considerations fall into two major categories: those that have to do with

CRITICAL THINKING EXERCISE 9-3

Review Table 9-1. Devise one research question for each of the four methods that could be answered by appropriately applying phenomenological, grounded theory, ethnographic, or historical research.

the relationship between the researcher and participant and those that involve procedures to handle the data.

When conducting qualitative research, the researcher spends a prolonged time in contact with participants, and relationships are formed. It is not uncommon for researchers and participants to move from a formal (stranger) relationship to one that is more personal (friend) (Leininger, 1985, 1995). For example, a participant may share information in the context of a friendship, never expecting it to be study data. Other consequences of prolonged engagement may include the difficulty of ensuring ongoing informed consent or allowing a participant to withdraw from the study if indicated. Another dilemma can occur when the subject matter is emotional for participants. They may become upset and begin to cry during an interview while sharing their experiences. When this occurs, the appropriate response for the researcher is to ask if the tape recorder should be turned off until the participant regains composure. Researchers must examine the appropriateness of responding with therapeutic use of self versus maintaining the role of researcher. In addition, researchers must avoid taking advantage of a friendship. For example, the researcher may be tempted to prolong the length of an interview past the agreed-upon time or to ask for a second interview when this was not included in the original plan. Researchers are obligated to report suspicions of abuse, neglect, or criminal activity if this is revealed. Therefore, it is essential that the consent form indicates to participants that this is the case.

Spradley (1979) listed ethical principles that must be considered when working with participants. These are summarized in **Box 9-3**. Some important strategies must be implemented when handling qualitative data to safeguard participants' rights. When audiotapes are transcribed, all identifying information such as name, address, place of employment, and phone numbers must be replaced with fictitious information. Participants are often assigned gender-appropriate code names that progress alphabetically. Audio- and videotapes must be treated as confidential and kept secured until the conclusion of the study when they are destroyed. If a participant withdraws from the study, the researcher may

FYI

Some ethical considerations are unique to qualitative research. These fall into two major categories: the relationship between the researcher and participant and the procedures to handle the data.

still use the data, provided that the participant agrees to this. A unique feature of qualitative research is that sharing findings with participants is expected as part of the research process. It is appropriate to share categories, themes, and theories with participants; however, transcripts, audio- and videotapes, and participant names must never be shared.

BOX 9-3   Ethical Principles for Consideration with Participants

Protect the participants' rights and interests.

Put participants' interests first.

Clearly communicate the goals of the research.

Obtain informed consent.

Ensure privacy.

Avoid exploitation.

Share results and reports.

Modified from Spradley, J. P. (1980). *Participant observation*. Orlando, FL: Harcourt, Brace, Jovanovich College Publishers.

TEST YOUR KNOWLEDGE 9-3

Indicate whether the following statements are true or false:

1. Qualitative researchers do not have to adhere to the usual protection of human subjects because most studies are noninvasive.
2. Qualitative findings must be shared with participants.
3. When a nurse researcher suspects abuse, it is unethical to report it because this information was obtained during a research interview.
4. Fictitious names should be used when transcribing data so that actual participants remain unknown to others.

How did you do? 1. F; 2. T; 3. F; 4. T

Apply What You Have Learned

The EBP committee has found another qualitative study about hand hygiene compliance. Read Jackson et al. (2014). Enter the citation, and place N/A in the intervention and comparison columns. Why? Because qualitative studies do not have interventions. See the example about Salmon and McLaws (2015) provided in the grid. Reflect on this article to determine how consistent the authors were with qualitative methods regarding the following:

» Sampling method and size

» Data collection methods

» Analysis and interpretation

» Strategies used to maintain scientific rigor

» Ethical considerations

RAPID REVIEW

» Qualitative research focuses on words instead of numbers to give meaning to a phenomenon or events.

» Qualitative research uses induction to inquire about topics with little evidence and/or to develop a theory.

» Individuals who volunteer for qualitative studies are known as participants. Purposive sampling is used to obtain a sample.

» Sampling continues until data saturation is achieved. Typically, sample sizes are small in qualitative studies.

» The three main sources of data in qualitative research are in-depth interviews, direct observation, and artifacts.

» Data come from fieldwork and can involve participant observation.

» Analysis and interpretation are conducted simultaneously with data collection.

» The four essential elements of evaluation are credibility, transferability, dependability, and confirmability.

» Strategies to maintain scientific rigor include bracketing, persistent observation, peer debriefing, referential adequacy, member checks, and audit trails.

» The four major types of qualitative research are phenomenology, grounded theory, ethnography, and historical.

» Phenomenology describes the lived experience and has provided the foundation for some nursing theories.

» Grounded theory uses constant comparison to create theories about processes.

» Ethnography is the method of choice when studying a culture. Ethnoscience and ethnonursing are methods used to study cultural interpretations of nursing phenomena such as care, health, and environment.

» The emic perspective provides the "inside" scoop, while the etic perspective is the outsider's viewpoint.

» Historical research examines past events or people with the purpose of guiding the present and future. Strategic sampling can be used to obtain participants.

» Findings from qualitative studies contribute to EBP by sensitizing nurses to patient experiences and providing theories to explain various processes.

» Qualitative researchers are held to the same ethical standards as are researchers using other methods; however, some unique ethical considerations are associated with qualitative methods.

REFERENCES

Anthony, S., & Jack, S. (2009). Qualitative case study methodology in nursing research: An integrative review. *Journal of Advanced Nursing, 65*(6), 1171–1181.

Benner, P. (1984). *From novice to expert: Excellence and power in clinical nursing practice.* Menlo Park, CA: Addison-Wesley.

Bergin, M. (2011). NVivo 8 and consistency in data analysis: Reflecting on the use of a qualitative data analysis program. *Nurse Researcher, 18*(3), 6–12.

Boeije, H. R., van Wesel, F., & Alisic, E. (2011). Making a difference: Towards a method for weighing the evidence in a qualitative synthesis. *Journal of Evaluation in Clinical Practice, 17*(4), 657–663. doi:10.1111/j.1365–2753.2011.01674.x10.1111/j.1365–2753.2011.01674.x

Boyle, J. S. (1994). Styles of ethnography. In J. M. Morse (Ed.), *Critical issues in qualitative research methods.* Thousand Oaks, CA: Sage.

Cassidy, S. (2013). Acknowledging hubris in qualitative data analysis. *Nurse Researcher, 20*(6), 27–31.

Converse, M. (2012). Philosophy of phenomenology: How understanding aids research. *Nurse Researcher, 20*(1), 28–32.

Cooney, A. (2011). Rigour and grounded theory. *Nurse Researcher, 18*(4), 17–22.

Cruz, E. V., & Higginbottom, G. (2013). The use of focused ethnography in nursing research. *Nurse Researcher, 20*(4), 36–43.

Easton, K. L. (1999a). The post-stroke journey: From agonizing to owning. *Geriatric Nursing, 20*(2), 70–75.

Easton, K. L. (1999b). Using focus groups in rehabilitation nursing. *Rehabilitation Nursing, 24,* 212–215.

Easton, K. L., McComish, J., & Greenberg, R. (2000). The pitfalls of qualitative data collection and transcription. *Qualitative Health Research, 10*(5), 703–707.

Fealy, G., Kelly, J., & Watson, R. (2013). Legitimacy in legacy: A discussion paper of historical scholarship published in the *Journal of Advanced Nursing, 1976–2011. Journal of Advanced Nursing, 69*(8), 1881–1894. doi:10.1111/jan.12048

Fetterman, D. M. (2010). *Ethnography step by step.* Thousand Oaks, CA: Sage.

Firouzkouhi, M., Zargham-Boroujeni, A., Nouraei, M., Yousefi, M. H., & Holmes, C. A. (2013). The wartime experience of civilian nurses in Iran-Iraq war, 1980–1988: An historical research. *Contemporary Nurse, 44*(2), 225–231.

Folden, S. L. (1994). Managing the effects of a stroke. *Rehabilitation Nursing Research, 3*(3), 79–85.

Fry, M. (2012). An ethnography: Understanding emergency nursing practice belief systems. *International Emergency Nursing, 20*(3), 120.

Gallagher, P. (2011). Becoming normal: A grounded theory study on the emotional process of stroke recovery. *Canadian Journal of Neuroscience Nursing, 33*(3), 24–32.

Galvin, K., Todres, L., & Richardson, M. (2005). The intimate mediator: A carer's experience of Alzheimer's. *Scandinavian Journal of Caring Science, 19,* 2–11.

Glaser, B. G. (1978). *Theoretical sensitivity: Advances in the methodology of grounded theory.* Mill Valley, CA: Sociology Press.

Glaser, B. G. (1992). *Emergence vs. forcing: Basics of grounded theory analysis.* Mill Valley, CA: Sociology Press.

Glaser, B. G., & Strauss, A. L. (1967). *The discovery of grounded theory.* Chicago, IL: Aldine.

Hall, H., Griffiths, D., & McKenna, L. (2013). From Darwin to constructivism: The evolution of grounded theory. *Nurse Researcher, 20*(3), 17–21.

Harmon, R. B. (2005). Nursing care in a state hospital before and during the introduction of antipsychotics, 1950–1965. *Issues in Mental Health Nursing, 26,* 257–279.

Heidegger, M. (1962). *Being and time.* New York, NY: Harper & Row.

Hughes, C. C. (1992). Ethnography: What's in a word—Process? Product? Promise? *Qualitative Health Research, 4,* 439–450.

Jackson, C., Lowton, K., & Griffiths, P. (2014). Infection prevention as "a show": A qualitative study of nurses' infection prevention behaviours. *International Journal of Nursing Studies, 51,* 400–408.

Lapidus-Graham, J. (2012). The lived experience of participation in student nurse associations and leadership behaviors: A phenomenological study. *Journal of the New York State Nurses Association, 43*(1), 4–12.

Leininger, M. M. (1985). Ethnography and ethnonursing: Models and modes of qualitative data analysis. In M. M. Leininger (Ed.), *Qualitative methods in nursing* (pp. 33–71). New York, NY: Grune & Stratton.

Leininger, M. M. (1995). *Transcultural nursing: Concepts, theories, and practice*. Columbus, OH: McGraw-Hill College Custom Series.

Lincoln, Y. S., & Guba, E. G. (1985). *Naturalistic inquiry*. Newbury Park, CA: Sage.

Lusk, B. (2005). Prelude to specialization: U.S. cancer nursing, 1920–1950. *Nursing Inquiry, 12*(40), 269–277.

Marshall, A., Kitson, A., & Zeitz, K. (2012). Patients' views of patient-centred care: A phenomenological case study in one surgical unit. *Journal of Advanced Nursing, 68*(12), 2664–2673. doi:10.1111/j.1365–2648.2012.05965.x

Marshall, C., & Rossman, G. B. (2011). *Designing qualitative research*. Thousand Oaks, CA: Sage.

Mauk, K. L. (2001). *The post-stroke journey: From agonizing to owning*. Unpublished doctoral dissertation, Wayne State University, Detroit, MI.

Mauk, K. L. (2006). Nursing interventions within the Mauk model for post-stroke recovery. *Rehabilitation Nursing, 31*, 259–267.

McInnes, E., Seers, K., & Tutton, L. (2011). Older people's views in relation to risk of falling and need for intervention: A meta-ethnography. *Journal of Advanced Nursing, 67*(12), 2525–2536. doi:10.1111/j.1365–2648.2011.05707.x

Meehan, T. C. (2006). *Careful nursing model, theoretical bases of nursing module*. Dublin, Ireland: University College Dublin.

Meehan, T. C. (2012). The careful nursing philosophy and professional practice model. *Journal of Clinical Nursing, 21*, 2905–2916. doi:10.1111/j. 1365–2702.2012.04214.x

Oliffe, J. (2005). Why not ethnography? *Urologic Nursing, 25*, 395–399.

Parse, R. R. (1991). Parse's theory of human becoming. In I. E. Goertzen (Ed.), *Differentiating nursing practice: Into the twenty-first century* (pp. 51–53). Kansas City, MO: American Academy of Nursing.

Patton, M. Q. (1990). *Qualitative evaluations and research methods*. Newbury Park, CA: Sage.

Patton, M. Q. (2003). Qualitative evaluation checklist. Retrieved from http://citeseerx .ist.psu.edu/viewdoc/summary?doi=10.1.1.135.8668

Pratt, M. (2012). The utility of human sciences in nursing inquiry. *Nurse Researcher, 19*(3), 12–15.

Roper, J. M., & Shapira, J. (2000). *Ethnography in nursing research*. Thousand Oaks, CA: Sage.

Rosenbaum, J. N. (1990). Cultural care of older Greek Canadian widows within Leininger's theory of culture care. *Journal of Transcultural Nursing, 2*(1), 37–47.

Sandelowski, M. (2010). What's in a name? Qualitative description revisited. *Research in Nursing and Health, 33*, 77–84.

Shambley-Ebron, D. Z., & Boyle, J. S. (2006). Self-care and mothering in African American women with HIV/AIDS. *Western Journal of Nursing Research, 28*(1), 42–69.

Spradley, J. P. (1979). *The ethnographic interview*. Orlando, FL: Harcourt, Brace, Jovanovich College Publishers.

Spradley, J. P. (1980). *Participant observation*. Orlando, FL: Harcourt, Brace, Jovanovich College Publishers.

Strauss, A., & Corbin, J. (1990). *Basics of qualitative research: Grounded theory procedures and techniques*. Newbury Park, CA: Sage.

Street, A. (1992). *Inside nursing: A critical ethnography of clinical nursing practice*. Albany, NY: University of New York Press.

Su, T. J., & Chen, Y. C. (2006). Transforming hope: The lived experience of infertile women who terminated treatment after in vitro fertilization failure. *Journal of Nursing Research, 14*(1), 46–54.

Watson, J. (1989). Watson's philosophy and theory of human caring in nursing. In J. Riehl-Sisca (Ed.), *Conceptual models for nursing practice* (3rd ed., pp. 219–236). Norwalk, CT: Appleton & Lange.

Welch, A. Z. (2002). Madeleine Leininger: Culture care: Diversity and universality theory. In A. M. Tomey & M. R. Alligood (Eds.), *Nursing theorists and their work* (pp. 501–526). St. Louis, MO: Mosby.

At the end of this chapter, you will be able to:

- Identify factors that should be considered when planning for data collection
- Discuss reasons for piloting data collection
- Describe various methods to measure and collect quantitative data
- Discuss advantages and disadvantages to data collection methods
- Identify levels of measurement
- Examine strategies used to address issues associated with quantitative data collection methods
- Identify types of random and systematic measurement errors
- Define validity and reliability

- Name strategies that researchers use to establish reliability and validity of various measures
- Recognize questions used to appraise quantitative data collection methods
- Identify the researcher as the most important data collection instrument
- Describe various methods used to collect qualitative data
- Discuss the advantages and disadvantages of qualitative data collection methods
- Recognize questions used to appraise qualitative data collection methods
- Discuss the importance of protecting human subjects during data collection

KEY TERMS

alternate form
case studies
categorical data
concurrent validity
construct validity
content validity
content validity testing
continuous data
convergent testing
correlation coefficient
criterion-related validity
Cronbach's alpha
dichotomous
direct observations
divergent testing
equivalence
face validity
factor analysis

focus groups
hypothesis testing
internal consistency
interrater reliability
interval
interviews
item to total correlation
known group testing
Kuder-Richardson coefficient
levels of measurement
Likert scales
measurement error
methodological
multitrait-multimethod testing
nominal
observation

ordinal
parallel form
physiological measures
predictive validity
psychometrics
questionnaires
random error
ratio
reliability
scales
split-half reliability
stability
storytelling
systematic error
test-retest reliability
unstructured observations
validity
visual analog scale

CHAPTER 10

Collecting Evidence

Jan Dougherty

10.1 Data Collection: Planning and Piloting

At the end of this section, you will be able to:

‹ Identify factors that should be considered when planning for data collection

‹ Discuss reasons for piloting data collection

Data collection is a key component in all research studies. Just as it is essential to use a theoretical or conceptual model to ask the important research questions, there must be a solid plan for collecting and managing the data to study and ultimately to answer research questions. Many nurses may be intimidated as they read the methods section of a research article. Words describing study designs, such as *double-blind*, *quasi-experimental*, and *ethnography*, can be overwhelming for those with limited research background. Additionally, terms discussing reliability, validity, and level of significance may further intimidate or overwhelm nurses (Granger et al., 2013). Many readers may be tempted to skim this information or to bypass it completely. However, because practice decisions will be made based on the findings of the data, it is important for nurses to be able to understand and critically evaluate methods used by researchers. Accurate data collection methods are more likely to yield valid findings. These findings provide or support the evidence that nurses can trust when making evidence-based practice (EBP) decisions. In EBP, quantitative studies are considered to produce the strongest evidence. Yet, in health care, many clinical and cultural phenomena are better studied using qualitative research. Many nursing and health research studies draw upon both quantitative and qualitative measures. In both types of methods, it is imperative that the same rigor be employed when collecting data.

Planning for Data Collection

Researchers are often very excited to begin collecting data. Most often they have spent months working on their overall framework and/or research questions and have organized pertinent literature to further support the study at hand. They have also carefully selected and developed data collection methods. This requires that researchers detail the data collection plan from the time consent from subjects is obtained to the actual completion of the data collection period. A timeline should be included along with a comprehensive budget that accounts for costs such as salaries of research staff, mileage, meals, data collection materials and instrumentation, fees related to the recruitment of subjects, and data input and interpretation. A plan for how data will be managed should also be included. A haphazard approach to collecting data, planning the timeline and budget, and managing data can lead to serious problems for researchers. Therefore, when appraising research studies, it is important for nurses to carefully read and determine whether the data collection methods support the framework and are appropriate for the study questions. If appropriate data collection methods are not used, the findings can easily be challenged and the evidence may not support the desired changes in practice (Havens, 2001).

Researchers begin by determining the type of data that need to be collected. This includes when and how data will be collected, who will collect the data, and what type of data collection methods, devices, or instruments will be used. Many factors affect data collection. Such factors may include availability and access to preexisting instruments, mobile devices (including personal digital assistants [PDAs], tablets, phones, laptops, or netbooks) or data collection sites, personnel needed to collect data, the amount of data to be collected, and the sample size. Budget considerations are key because researchers are accountable to stay within the planned budget. Data collection can be one of the most costly parts of conducting a research project. With the growing use of technology for data collection, the researcher must also consider the capabilities of mobile devices such as connectivity, mobility, and software compatibility. Care must also be taken to secure data (Drayton, 2013).

Piloting Data Collection Methods

Many researchers conduct a pilot study using a scaled-back version of the data collection method. This is very helpful to evaluate the instruments, devices, and process so that unexpected problems can be identified. Additionally, a pilot study helps confirm the study's feasibility and allows for revisions to be made. Researchers do not want to get midway into projects only to find that the instruments are flawed, the projected sample size is unachievable, a need for additional research assistants arises, or the study cannot be completed within the budget. All of these issues can cause serious problems and ultimately jeopardize the study.

TEST YOUR KNOWLEDGE 10-1

1. Factors to consider when planning data collection include which of the following? (Select all that apply.)
   a. Time frame
   b. Budget
   c. Training of personnel
   d. Availability of preprinted questionnaires
2. A pilot:
   a. is a small version of the study.
   b. confirms feasibility of the study.
   c. critiques the conclusions from a study.
   d. is the small stipend that subjects receive for participating in a study.

How did you do? 1. a, b, c, d; 2. a, b

10.2 Collecting Quantitative Data

At the end of this section, you will be able to:

< Describe various methods to measure and collect quantitative data
< Discuss advantages and disadvantages to data collection methods
< Identify levels of measurement
< Examine strategies used to address issues associated with quantitative data collection methods

Collecting Numbers

Quantitative methods are used to test stated hypotheses and call for researchers to use formal, objective, and systematic procedures and instruments that produce numerical data (Havens, 2001). Data from quantitative studies are the highest level of evidence on which clinicians can base EBP decisions. For example, studies involving meta-analyses of multiple randomized controlled

TABLE 10-1	Quantitative Research Designs and Data Collection Methods

Quantitative Research Design	Data Collection Methods
Exploratory/descriptive (answers *what* questions; describes frequency of occurrence)	Questionnaire Scales
Correlational (examines relationships among variables)	Questionnaire Scales Biophysiological
Quasi-experimental (examines why certain effects occur)	Questionnaire Scales Biophysiological
Experimental/clinical trial (examines causes of certain effects)	Questionnaire Scales Biophysiological

trials (RCTs) are considered to be the strongest level of evidence, whereas those based on case reports and opinions of experts and authorities are considered to be the lowest level of evidence (Myers & Meccariello, 2006). In quantitative studies, research questions and hypotheses are derived from theories. The study design reflects the objectives of the study. Researchers must decide how each variable will be operationalized and what types of data will need to be gathered. The main methods used in quantitative research include questionnaires, observation, scales, and physiological measures. **Table 10-1** provides an overview of data collection methods that are associated with various quantitative research designs.

Questionnaires

Questionnaires are commonly used in quantitative research and can provide an inexpensive way to gather numerical data from a potentially large number of respondents. Although questionnaires may be inexpensive to administer, when compared to other data collection methods, they can be expensive in terms of design time and interpretation. It is essential that each question is monitored for clarity, sensitivity to the respondent, reading level, and absence of bias (Sinkowitz-Cochran, 2013).

KEY TERM

questionnaires: Printed instruments used to gather numerical data

FIGURE 10-1	Example of Easy, Consistent Survey Design

1. Nursing research is interesting to me.	Yes_____	No_____
2. I have to study a lot in my nursing research course.	Yes_____	No_____
3. I understand how evidence can be used to improve practice.	Yes_____	No_____

The formatting and length of the questionnaire are important details. The questionnaire should include only essential questions because shorter questionnaires are more likely to be completed. Whenever possible, the questions using numbered answers should be either circled or checked and should use a consistent pattern throughout (**Figure 10-1**). There should be a balance between positive and negative questions to decrease biased responses in subjects (Sinkowitz-Cochran, 2013). Each research subject is assigned a research identification number that should be on each page of the questionnaire in case the pages get separated.

Questionnaires can be administered in person; on computers and handheld devices; and via telephone, interactive voice response, mail, and, increasingly, email. Confidentiality is necessary to ensure that respondents not only participate in the study but also answer questions honestly and without fear of reprisal. It is desirable to have a good response rate, which is the percentage of questionnaires that are returned. Return rates can be increased when a cover letter is included. The cover letter can provide an explanation or brief description of the purpose of the research because respondents may be more likely to participate if they perceive benefit to self or society. The letter can also provide some brief instructions about how to complete the survey (Meadows, 2003).

E-questionnaires are growing in popularity and may be used as a strategy to enhance response rates (Hunter, 2012). Low response rates can lead to bias because samples may not be representative. A variety of factors can influence whether subjects complete a questionnaire. Not all subjects are able to respond to questionnaires. For example, young children, people who are blind, and many elders who are frail or cognitively impaired may have difficulty completing questionnaires. Questionnaires that are long, hard to understand, or time consuming are not likely to be completed. Using appropriate colors, fonts, and white space can improve the likelihood that individuals will complete a questionnaire. Thanking respondents for their participation at the end of the questionnaire/survey is important, along with providing them contact information if they have additional questions/concerns (Meadows, 2003).

Observation

Structured observations provide a way to quantify an explicit feature of the phenomenon under *observation*. For example, a researcher could count the number of people who wash their hands after using a public restroom. Researchers serve as objective observers and follow systematic methods using specific directions during a scheduled period of time. In the hand washing example, the researcher may observe individuals during dinner time at a popular restaurant. Not only do researchers outline what observations are made but they also note how observations are recorded and coded. The researcher in this example may record tallies under three columns: no hand washing, water only, or soap and water. Establishing a detailed protocol is extremely important if researchers use research assistants.

Scales

Scales are used to assign a numeric value or score along a continuum. They are frequently incorporated into a questionnaire or interview. Numerous types of scales have been developed to measure social and psychological concepts specific to nursing. Researchers choose scales based on the scales' ability to measure identified concepts. Ideally, it is best to choose scales that have already been tested. If a scale does not exist, researchers can develop and test a new scale (Meadows, 2003). Scales can be designed to measure either a single or multidimensional concept. For example, the Marwit-Meuser Caregiver Grief Inventory is a 50-item multidimensional scale that measures grief reactions by current caregivers of people with progressive dementias (Marwit & Meuser, 2002). Because three subscales compose the total grief score, it is a multidimensional scale. Each subscale measures a specific part of the caregiving experience as detailed in the Caregiver Grief Model (Meuser & Marwit, 2001).

You may already be familiar with *Likert scales*, which are frequently used to collect data. A Likert scale consists of statements placed on a continuum of seven points and to which respondents indicate whether they agree or disagree. Seven points allow for a neutral opinion. Some researchers find a neutral response hard to interpret. Therefore, researchers may adapt the scale to eliminate the neutral point by having an even number of points. Scales containing fewer than seven points are known as Likert-type scales (see **Figure 10-2**).

Another type of scale is the *visual analog scale (VAS)* (see **Figure 10-3**). Researchers use this type of scale to measure the intensity of sensations and

FIGURE 10-2 Example of Likert-Type Scale

When several Likert scales are used in a questionnaire, the positive numbers or indicators should
consistently be in the same position, for example
1 = strongly disagree, 2 = disagree, 3 = neutral,
4 = agree, 5 = strongly agree.

FIGURE 10-3 Example of a VAS to Measure Pain

Line length = 100 mm

No pain   Worst pain

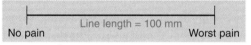

CRITICAL THINKING EXERCISE 10-1

A nurse researcher is interested in testing an intervention on the quality of life of individuals
with lung cancer. What methods do you think the nurse researcher should use to collect data?

feelings. The VAS is a 100-mm line that is anchored on each end with words or
symbols. Subjects mark a line across the VAS to indicate the intensity of their
feelings or attitudes along the continuum represented. In nursing, VAS scales
are frequently used to collect data about pain, fatigue, quality of life, and health
status. This type of scale can be completed easily and quickly and is understood
by most people. To score the VAS, researchers measure the distance of the
mark from the end of the scale in millimeters. Usually the low end of the scale
is used as the zero point.

Physiological Measures

Physiological measures provide a wide range of biological, chemical, and
microbiological data. Measures of blood pressure, cardiac output, and weight
are examples of biological variables. Chemical measures include electrolytes,
hormones, and cholesterol, while microbiological measures include the bacte-
rial counts obtained from urine and blood cultures. There are many advantages
to using these objective measures because they tend to be accurate. Some

KEY TERM

**physiological
measures:** Data
obtained from
biological, chemical,
and microbiological
phenomena

physiological data are typically accessible in most healthcare settings, allowing for ease of data collection with minimal or no cost to the researcher. Researchers must specify measurement protocols that include specific equipment used for measurement, frequency and methods for calibration of equipment, training for data collectors, specific times to obtain measurements, procedures for measuring and recording data, and any special storage or handling considerations (Merchant & Mateo, 1993).

Issues in Quantitative Data Collection

Regardless of how the data are collected, researchers must consider a variety of issues to ensure a high-quality study. They must have a written plan that outlines the process for data collection, particularly when additional data collectors are employed. Research assistants must be trained to collect data in a very consistent manner (i.e., instruments should be administered in the same order for all subjects, in the same context and setting, using the same set of directions). Interrater reliability must also be established when more than one person is involved in making observations. Interrater reliability is the extent to which two or more individual raters agree. Although it is necessary for multiple observers or raters to achieve interrater reliability, this may slow the process of observational methods. Interrater reliability should be monitored periodically throughout the study to increase the degree of confidence in the data (Casey, 2006). Researchers may choose to prepare a code book to organize the raw data prior to collection and to assign numerical values to data obtained during data collection. For example, researchers may assign a numerical value of 1 to females and 2 to males (Wolf, 2003).

Data collection plans should detail a time frame. It is not uncommon for researchers to encounter unplanned obstacles when gathering data. Frequently data collection requires at least twice as long as the researcher anticipates. Issues such as slow enrollment of consented subjects, heavy workloads, and staff turnover are common causes of delay. Plans should include strategies to manage attrition of subjects as a result of death, dropout, or relocation. Plans also must address decisions about missing data. For example, subjects may fail or refuse to respond to particular questions.

Many studies are funded by federal grants, state grants, or private foundation monies. A budget is necessary to consider all of the factors involved in data collection, including any delays that may be anticipated. Time extensions may be requested by researchers because of delay, and this subsequently requires researchers to account for any changes in budgeting. If the project is cut back as a result of delays or exceeding the budget, the research can be seriously compromised (Anastasi, Capili, Kim, & Chung, 2005).

KEY TERMS

nominal: The lowest level of measurement whereby data are categorized simply into groups; categorical data

ordinal: A continuum of numeric values where the intervals are not meant to be equal

interval: A continuum of numeric values with equal intervals that lacks an absolute zero

Levels of Measurement

Measurement is the process of assigning numbers using a set of rules. Four categories are used to describe measurements: *nominal*, *ordinal*, *interval*, and *ratio*. These categories are more commonly known as *levels of measurement*. When researchers collect data, they must know which level of measurement is used to select appropriate statistical tests for analyzing data (Trochim, 2000).

Nurses must be able to identify levels of measurement correctly to appraise evidence. Nominal measurement is the weakest level of measurement. The word *nominal* is derived from the word *name*. Researchers use nominal measurement to classify or categorize variables, also referred to as *categorical data*. The numbers assigned to each category are just labels and do not indicate any value. For example, responses of "yes" and "no" on a survey are often assigned numbers 1 and 2. The value of these numbers has no meaning because one cannot claim that a "no" response is higher than a "yes" response. The arbitrary numbers are assigned for the purpose of coding, recording, and entering data for collection and analysis. Questionnaires often utilize nominal measures to record a variety of categorical data and/or closed-ended questions with fixed responses such as gender, race, and diagnosis (see **Figure 10-4**). *Dichotomous*

KEY TERMS

ratio: The highest level of measurement that involves numeric values that begin with an absolute zero and have equal intervals; in epidemiology a mathematical relationship between two numbers

levels of measurement: A system of classifying measurements according to a hierarchy of measurement and the type of statistical tests that is appropriate; levels are nominal, ordinal, interval, and ratio

categorical data: Lowest level of measurement whereby data are categorized simply into groups; nominal data

dichotomous: Nominal measurement when only two possible fixed responses exist such as yes or no

FIGURE 10-4	Examples of Nominal Level Measurement

Gender:	Male = 1
	Female = 2
Race:	African American = 1
	Asian = 2
	Caucasian = 3
	Hispanic = 4
	Native American = 5
	Other = 6
Type of dementia:	Alzheimer's disease = 1
	Lewy body dementia = 2
	Vascular dementia = 3
	Frontotemporal dementia = 4
	Unknown = 5

| FIGURE 10-5 | Examples of Ordinal Level Measurement |

To what extent are you satisfied with the quality of care you received?

Extremely dissatisfied	Very dissatisfied	Somewhat satisfied	Very satisfied	Extremely satisfied
1	2	3	4	5

Put the following in order of importance to you. Assign 1 to the most important and 5 to the least important.

_____ Time with family
_____ Satisfaction with work
_____ Income
_____ Health
_____ Personal appearance

is the term used when there are only two possible fixed responses, such as true or false and yes or no.

Ordinal measurement represents the second lowest level of measurement. A continuum of numeric values is used with small numbers representing lower levels on the continuum and larger numbers representing higher values. However, although the values are ordered or ranked, the intervals are not meant to be equal. For example, in a marathon the distance and time among those who finish in first, second, and third are not equal; however, there is value to the number assigned. Many questionnaires and scales use ordinal measurements. **Figure 10-5** provides examples of ordinal measures.

Interval measurement is a third level of measurement and uses a continuum of numeric values, also known as *continuous data*. At this level, the values have meaning and the intervals are equal. On interval scales, the zero point is arbitrary and not absolute. The zero is not an indication of the true absence of something. The best example of this is the Celsius scale. When measuring temperature in Celsius, 0 does not mean the absence of temperature. In fact, it is quite cold. Other examples of interval scores include intelligence measures, personality measures, and manual muscle testing.

KEY TERM

continuous data: Interval- or ratio-level data that use a continuum of numeric values with equal intervals

Continuous data are also collected using ratio measurement, which is the highest level of measurement and uses a continuum of numeric values with equal intervals and a zero point that is absolute. Age, weight, height, and income are good examples of this type of measurement. VAS also provides ratio measurement along with many other biochemical and physiological measures.

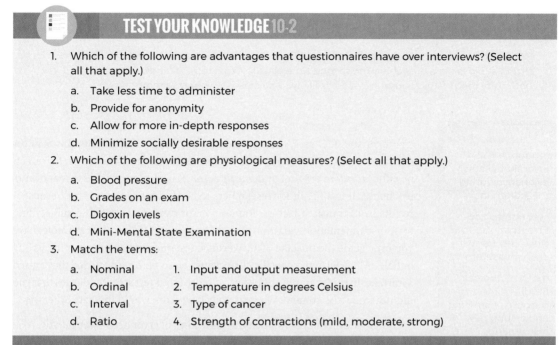

10.3 Validity and Reliability

At the end of this section, you will be able to:

‹ Identify types of random and systematic measurement errors
‹ Define validity and reliability
‹ Name strategies that researchers use to establish reliability and validity of various measures
‹ Recognize questions used to appraise quantitative data collection methods

Measurement Error

Although it may seem that creating surveys and instruments is easy, researchers actually spend a significant amount of time designing them. They do this to reduce *measurement error* so that they know the measurements provide a true reflection of the sample characteristics. In any measurement, the goal is for the observed measurement to be as close to the true measurement as possible. The equation $O = T + E$ illustrates this concept. O stands for the observed score. This is the actual number or value that is obtained from the instrument regarding the characteristic. T stands for the true score, the actual amount of the

KEY TERM

measurement error: The difference between the true score and the observed score

CRITICAL THINKING EXERCISE 10-2

What if you were to take an exam two times? The first time would be in a comfortable room sitting at a desk in a nice chair. The second time you are expected to stand with a clipboard in a hot, stuffy room. Which observed score is likely to be closer to your true score? Why?

characteristic. If $O = T$, there would be a perfect instrument, but this is never the case because error (E) is always present during measurements. Error can be either *random error* or *systematic error*. Random error is error that occurs by chance. It is difficult for researchers to control for random error because it results from transient factors. Random error can be attributed to subject factors, instrumentation variations, or environmental factors. For example, have you ever made the mistake of answering a test question by filling in the wrong bubble? Although you knew the correct answer, something occurred that caused a mistake. In this example, the observed score (your test score) indicates that you did not know the content, whereas your true score would indicate otherwise.

Systematic error occurs when the same kind of error occurs repeatedly. Also known as consistent error, it can result from subject, instrumentation, and environmental factors. For example, a researcher measures body temperatures after an intervention. The researcher assumes that the electronic thermometer is measuring accurately; however, the device has not recently been calibrated. Body temperatures are being reported a half degree lower than the actual temperatures. Because every temperature measured is affected, this is systematic error.

If there is error in all measurement, how do researchers know when instruments are useful? Instruments can be tested using a variety of strategies to identify error. Researchers conduct *methodological* studies to test instruments. The nursing literature, as well as literature from other disciplines, contains such reports. Another term, *psychometrics*, is also associated with instrument testing. Psychometrics refers to the development of measures for psychological attributes.

Validity

When selecting an instrument, researchers must first ask themselves if it is valid. *Validity* refers to the degree an instrument measures what it is supposed to measure. A valid instrument reflects the characteristics or concept that is being measured. For example, a researcher might want to measure the amount of fear patients have prior to surgery. The researcher would need to carefully select an instrument that measures fear, and not anxiety, which is a similar but different concept. There are three kinds of validity: *content validity*, *criterion-related validity*, and *construct validity* (**Table 10-2**).

TABLE 10-2	Validity: Does the Instrument Accurately Measure What It Is Supposed to Measure?

Type	Test	Description
Content validity: Is the content representative of the content domain under study?	Face validity	Colleagues or subjects examine an instrument and are asked whether it appears to measure the concept.
	Content validity testing	Experts on the topic are asked to judge each item on an instrument by assigning a rating to determine its fit with the concept being measured.
Criterion-related validity: To what degree are the "observed score" and the "true score" related?	Concurrent validity	New instrument is administered at the same time as an instrument known to be valid. Scores of the two instruments are compared. Strong positive correlations indicate good validity.
	Predictive	New instrument is given at two different times and scores are correlated. Strong positive correlations indicate good validity.
Construct validity: To what extent does the instrument measure the theoretical construct or trait?	Hypothesis testing	Hypotheses derived from theories are tested with the new instrument.
	Convergent	New instrument is administered at the same time as an instrument known to be valid. Scores of the two instruments are compared. Strong, positive correlations indicate good validity.
	Divergent	New instrument is administered at the same time as an instrument measuring the opposite of the concept. Scores of the two instruments are compared. Strong negative correlations indicate good validity.
	Multitrait-multimethod	New instrument, established instrument of same concept, and established instrument of opposite concept are given at the same time. Strong positive and negative correlations indicate good validity.
	Known groups	New instrument is administered to individuals known to be high or low on the characteristic being measured.
	Factor analysis	Statistical approach to identify items that group together.

Content validity is established when researchers know that the instrument measures the concept intended to be measured. This requires that researchers clearly define the concept being studied to ensure that the selected instrument fits.

Researchers test for content validity in two ways: *face validity* and *content validity testing*. Both methods involve letting others examine the instruments. When researchers try to obtain face validity, they ask colleagues or subjects to examine an instrument and indicate whether the instrument appears to measure the concept. Face validity is less desirable than content validity because face validity uses an intuitive approach. To implement content validity testing, researchers give an instrument to a panel consisting of experts on the concept. The experts judge the instrument by rating each item for the degree to which it reflects the concept being measured. After researchers receive feedback from the panel, they make adjustments to the instrument. Items that receive high ratings are kept, and items with low ratings are altered or eliminated. For example, when Beyer, Denyes, and Villarruel (1992) developed a pediatric photographic pain scale, they asked children, rather than adults, to rank pictures of a child experiencing pain. Children placed the pictures in order from no pain to most pain. Researchers found consensus among children regarding some photographs and eliminated others when children disagreed about the amount of pain being expressed.

Criterion-related validity is concerned with the degree to which the observed score and the true score are related. Researchers test for criterion-related validity in two ways: *concurrent validity* and *predictive validity*. Concurrent validity is tested when researchers simultaneously administer two different instruments measuring the same concept. Usually, the new instrument being developed is compared to an instrument already shown to be valid. Researchers use correlations to compare scores from the two instruments. High correlations indicate agreement between the instruments, whereas low correlations indicate that the instruments are measuring different concepts. Predictive validity refers to whether a current score is correlated with a score obtained in the future. For example, suppose that a class of sophomore nursing students completed an instrument measuring critical thinking today, and they will complete the instrument again 1 month from now. If the instrument has good criterion-related validity, their scores will be correlated.

Construct validity focuses on theory. Constructs are theoretical concepts that are tested empirically. When researchers test for construct validity, they ask how well the instrument measures a theoretical concept. Because establishing construct validity requires empirical testing, more sophisticated strategies implemented over a longer period of time are needed. There are a number of ways to determine construct validity: *hypothesis testing*, *convergent testing*, *divergent testing*, *multitrait-multimethod testing*, *known group testing*, and *factor analysis*.

For hypothesis testing, researchers use theories to make predictions about the concept being measured. Data are gathered, and a determination is made as to whether the findings support the hypothesis. In the study by Beyer et al. (1992), the authors hypothesized that pain scores would be highest on the day of the surgical procedure and then gradually decrease. They found that scores were highest on the operative day and gradually decreased over the course of the hospital stay. The construct validity of the Oucher, a children's pain scale, was supported because data were consistent with predicted pain patterns.

When researchers use two or more instruments to measure the same theoretical component, they are testing for convergent validity. Convergent validity focuses on how the observed scores compare to one another. For example, Beyer et al. (1992) compared the Oucher to a VAS pain scale. Pain ratings were highly correlated, thus establishing convergent validity. Divergent validity testing involves comparing scores from two or more instruments that measure different theoretical constructs. In this strategy, it is not unusual for researchers to compare opposites; for example, depression and happiness. In this situation, negative correlations support construct validity. When convergent testing and divergent testing are combined, researchers are using a strategy known as multitrait-multimethod. This approach is especially helpful to reduce systematic error.

Another way to test for construct validity is to use the known group approach. Instruments are administered to individuals known to be high or low on the characteristic being measured. Researchers expect that there will be significantly different scores between the high group and the low group. Beyer et al. (1992) tested known groups by comparing pain scores for children who had experienced extensive surgical procedures with pain scores for children who had minor surgical procedures. Children who had spinal fusions reported significantly higher pain scores using the Oucher than did children who had a cardiac catheterization.

Most concepts have more than one dimension. These dimensions are known as factors. Researchers use factor analysis, a statistical approach, to identify questions that group around different factors. Thus, items that group together as one factor have high correlations. These items may or may not highly correlate with items around a different factor. Questions that do not fit are altered or eliminated. Because factor analyses require complex, simultaneous computations of correlations, computers are needed.

Reliability

Instruments are considered to be reliable when researchers obtain consistent measurements over time. *Reliability* must be considered in relation to

KEY TERMS

convergent testing: A test for construct validity in which new instruments are administered at the same time as an instrument known to be valid; scores of the two instruments are compared, and strong, positive correlations indicate good validity

divergent testing: Test for construct validity in which new instruments are administered at the same time as an instrument measuring the opposite of the concept; scores of the two instruments are compared, and strong negative correlations indicate good validity

multitrait-multimethod testing: Test for construct validity in which a new instrument, established instrument of the same concept, and established instrument of the opposite concept are given at the same time; strong positive and negative correlations indicate good validity

KEY TERMS

known group testing: A test for construct validity in which new instruments are administered to individuals known to be high or low on the characteristic being measured

factor analysis: A test for construct validity that is a statistical approach to identify items that group together

reliability: Obtaining consistent measurements over time

correlation coefficient: An estimate, ranging from 0.00 to +1.00, that indicates the reliability of an instrument; a statistic used to describe the relationship between two variables

stability: An attribute of reliability when instruments render the same scores with repeated measures under the same circumstances

equivalence: An attribute of reliability in which there is agreement between alternate forms of an instrument or alternate raters

validity. An instrument can be reliable but not valid. If you weighed yourself 10 times in a row on your bathroom scale this morning, you would expect the scale to show the same weight each time. You would conclude that the scale is reliable. If you are anxious about your weight, you cannot conclude that the scale measured your level of anxiety. Whereas the scale is a valid instrument to measure your weight, it is not a valid instrument to measure your anxiety even though the scale was shown to be reliable. Estimates of reliability are usually presented in the form of a *correlation coefficient*. Although correlations range from −1.00 to +1.00, reliability coefficients are typically reported as values between 0.00 and +1.00 because that is the nature of relationships that are tested. Reliability coefficients of 0.80 and above are acceptable for well-established instruments, whereas reliability coefficients of 0.70 and above are acceptable for newly developed instruments (Griffin-Sobel, 2003).

When testing instruments for reliability, researchers are interested in three attributes: *stability*, *equivalence*, and *internal consistency*. Instruments are stable when the same scores are obtained with repeated measures under the same circumstances (as in the bathroom scale example). An instrument is said to be equivalent when there is agreement between alternate forms or alternate raters. Internal consistency, also known as homogeneity, exists when all items on a questionnaire measure the same concept. Seven ways are commonly used to test instruments for reliability. They are *test-retest reliability*, *parallel* or *alternate form*, *interrater reliability*, *split-half reliability*, *item to total correlation*, *Kuder-Richardson coefficient*, and *Cronbach's alpha* (**Table 10-3**).

Test-retest reliability determines stability by administering the instrument to the same subjects under the same conditions at two different times. Scores are used to calculate a Pearson *r*, a type of correlation coefficient. Parallel or alternate form testing is used to test for both stability and equivalence. Researchers create parallel forms by altering the wording or layout of items. Because the forms are similar, researchers expect high positive correlations. For example, Beyer et al. (1992) compared a pocket-sized Oucher with a poster-sized Oucher and obtained similar pain ratings.

Interrater reliability also tests for equivalence. This method is used when instruments record observations. A common way to determine interrater reliability is to have two observers score the same event. Ratings are compared, and if the ratings are similar, the instrument is considered to have strong reliability. Another way to establish interrater reliability is to have one individual make multiple observations over time.

TABLE 10-3	Reliability: Does the Instrument Yield the Same Results on Repeated Measurements?

Type	What Is Determined?	Description
Test-retest	Stability	New instrument is given at two different times under the same conditions. Scores are correlated. Strong positive correlations indicate good reliability.
Parallel or alternate	Stability Equivalence	New instrument is given in two different versions. Scores are correlated. Strong positive correlations indicate good reliability.
Interrater reliability	Equivalence	Two observers measure the same event. Scores are correlated. Strong positive correlations indicate good reliability.
Split-half	Internal consistency	The items are divided to form two instruments. Both instruments are given and the halves are compared using the Spearman-Brown formula.
Item to total	Internal consistency	Each item is correlated to the total score. Reliable items have strong correlations with the total score.
Kuder-Richardson coefficient	Internal consistency	Used with dichotomous items. A computer is used to simultaneously compare all items.
Cronbach's alpha	Internal consistency	Used with interval or ratio items. A computer is used to simultaneously compare all items.

KEY TERMS

internal consistency: An attribute of reliability when all items on an instrument measure the same concept

test-retest reliability: A test for instrument reliability when new instruments are given at two different times under the same conditions; scores are correlated, and strong positive correlations indicate good reliability

parallel form: A test for instrument reliability in which two different versions of new instruments are given. Scores are correlated, and strong positive correlations indicate good reliability; also known as alternate form

alternate form: A test for instrument reliability in which two different versions of new instruments are given. Scores are correlated, and strong positive correlations indicate good reliability; also known as parallel form

KEY TERMS

interrater reliability:
A test for instrument
reliability when
two observers
measure the same
event. Scores are
correlated, and
strong positive
correlations indicate
good reliability

split-half reliability:
A test for instru-
ment reliability in
which the items
are divided to form
two instruments.
Both instruments
are given and the
halves are com-
pared using the
Spearman-Brown
formula

**item to total
correlation:** A test
for instrument
reliability in which
each item is
correlated to the
total score; reliable
items have strong
correlations with
the total score

**Kuder-Richardson
coefficient:** A test
for instrument
reliability for use
with dichotomous
items; all items are
simultaneously
compared using a
computer

Cronbach's alpha:
A test for instrument
reliability used with
interval or ratio
items; all items are
simultaneously
compared using a
computer

Sometimes, researchers divide the items on a questionnaire in half to make two versions, a technique known as split-half reliability. Researchers use the Spearman-Brown formula to compare the two halves. Split-half testing is used to establish internal consistency. Item to total calculations are also used to test for internal consistency. Each item on the instrument is compared to the total score obtained. Strong items have high correlations with the total score. Items with low correlations to the total score are examined, and decisions are made to change or eliminate them. When the level of measurement is dichotomous, researchers determine internal consistency using the Kuder-Richardson coefficient (K-20). This correlation compares all items at the same time. Cronbach's alpha is the most common method used by nursing researchers to assess internal consistency. This method can be used when data are interval level or higher. Like the Kuder-Richardson, all items are compared simultaneously to obtain a single correlation (Trochim, 2000). Computer software is required to perform these sophisticated tests.

As nurses appraise the methods section of any research article, it is important to consider the issues of validity and reliability (Roberts & Priest, 2006) before making practice decisions. The report should contain information about the validity and reliability of each instrument used. References for the original development of the instruments should be provided. Occasionally researchers include instruments in articles that allow readers to observe how the questions align with the concepts that were being measured.

Appraising Data Collection in Quantitative Studies

When reading the methods section of any research article, nurses should determine that each instrument is described and the reliability and validity are reported. The level of measurement should be noted for each variable measured. Nurses should also appraise whether instruments represent the concepts and variables being operationalized. Interventions should be detailed so that nurses know what was done in the research. If a pilot was done prior to the study, its instruments, interventions, and findings should be presented. If subjects are grouped, the author should describe how grouping was accomplished.

Many quantitative studies fall short of significant findings if there are holes in the methods section. If the instruments do not adequately measure the concepts or variables, or if they lack validity and reliability, the study may be flawed (Ioannidis, 2005). **Box 10-1** lists questions that nurses should consider when appraising the methods section.

<table>
<tr><td>**BOX 10-1**</td><td>Assessing the Quality of Quantitative Data Collection Methods</td></tr>
</table>

What are the variables being measured?

Does the data collection method fit with the study variables?

What is the intervention?

Is there sufficient detail given about the intervention and the control group?

Was the setting described?

What steps were taken to minimize measurement error?

What instruments are used? Were validity and reliability discussed for each instrument?

Was the level of measurement considered?

Were there any difficulties with enrollment, attrition, or missing data?

TEST YOUR KNOWLEDGE 10-3

True/False

1. Validity is concerned with an instrument obtaining accurate and repeatable measures.
2. Content validity is established by having a panel of experts review the instruments.
3. Face validity is the strongest method to establish validity.
4. Equivalence, internal consistency, and stability are tested to ensure instrument reliability.
5. An instrument with a reported Cronbach's alpha of .65 has good reliability.

How did you do? 1. F; 2. T; 3. F; 4. T; 5. F

10.4 Collecting Qualitative Data

At the end of this section, you will be able to:

‹ Identify the researcher as the most important data collection instrument
‹ Describe various methods used to collect qualitative data
‹ Discuss the advantages and disadvantages of qualitative data collection methods
‹ Recognize questions used to appraise qualitative data collection methods

Collecting Words

In recent years, the use of qualitative methods has become more common in health services research, resulting in an increase in publication of these studies in healthcare journals (Sandelowski, 2004). Qualitative researchers collect data that are in-depth and descriptive in order to understand the phenomena being studied. The methods allow participants to express their thoughts and describe their actions and intentions in their own words. The researcher is the most important data collection instrument (Miller, 2010). Researchers gather qualitative data through questionnaires, *interviews*, *focus groups*, *case studies*, *direct observations*, and *storytelling*. **Table 10-4** lists data collection strategies associated with the four major qualitative methods.

Questionnaires

Questionnaires are frequently used to collect qualitative data from individuals or groups of participants. The questionnaire is typically a list of written questions that can be self-administered. It can also be administered using the Internet or can be read to the participant by the data collector. Questionnaires can use open-ended questions, closed-ended questions, or both. Open-ended questions are used to elicit statements without providing a fixed answer. An example of an open-ended question is, "Tell about your experience as a caregiver for a person with Parkinson's disease." Closed-ended questions offer fixed choices that must be selected. For example, a closed-ended question may ask participants to

TABLE 10-4	Qualitative Research Methods and Instruments
Method	**Instrument/Tool**
Phenomenology	In-depth interviews Diaries Artwork
Grounded theory	Observations Open-ended question interviews with individuals or small groups
Ethnography	Participant and direct observations Open-ended question interviews Diagrams Documents Photographs
Historical	Open-ended question interviews Interviews Documents Photographs Artifacts

respond "yes" or "no" to a list of questions. Thoughtful consideration should be given to wording questions in a clear and concise manner. A sufficient number of questions must be included so that accurate descriptions can be obtained. The font size should be large enough for easy reading.

The advantages of questionnaires are that they are usually easy to administer, can provide a wealth of data, and are relatively inexpensive. They can provide anonymity when desired; however, researchers cannot ensure that intended participants actually answered the questions. The sample may be limited to literate participants when individuals are expected to self-administer the questionnaire.

Interviews

The one-on-one nature of interviews makes them more personal than self-administered questionnaires are, and researchers are able to probe more deeply with follow-up questions. Interviews can be conducted in person or over the telephone. Structured interviews emphasize obtaining answers based on carefully predetermined questions. For some qualitative methods, an in-depth interview guide is used that does not follow this structured form. Rather, a general or "grand tour" question is asked, and a dialogue between the researcher and the participant unfolds, leading to more detailed information. Interviews are frequently tape recorded so they can be transcribed word for word at a later date. Researchers must take care to minimize distractions and interruptions to allow participants to focus on the topic. Although interviews provide the opportunity to clarify questions and answers, they are more expensive and take more time to conduct than questionnaires do. Because anonymity is impossible to achieve, participants may be inclined to answer in socially desirable ways. Face-to-face interviews provide an opportunity for researchers to assess nonverbal communication and the context in which the interview occurs. Self-reported data, whether obtained from questionnaires or interviews, provide a rich source of information. Additionally, response rates are generally high for participants who are willing to express their opinions.

Focus Groups

Focus groups are small groups composed of usually fewer than 12 participants (Beyea & Nicoll, 2000). Participants are brought together to explore attitudes and thoughts about a particular subject. Through group interaction, insights are often gained that may not have emerged through individual interviews. When focus groups are used, researchers must identify and define the objectives of the focus group. A facilitator guides the group process by stating ground rules, objectives, and questions. This role is essential to keep participants comfortable and the group process flowing and on track. Facilitators must be skilled at involving all participants and ensuring that the conversation is not monopolized by one or two individuals. It is recommended that the researcher not be the facilitator of the group but rather an observer who can listen, take notes, and ask specific follow-up questions.

Focus group participants must represent the intended population identified by the researcher. An adequate number of participants should be represented because participants are not randomly selected. They should be notified in advance regarding the date, time, and location of the focus group. Focus group sessions are usually audiotaped and involve a note taker. Approximately 60 to 90 minutes are given to ask no more than 10 structured questions. Following the session, the data are transcribed and analyzed to look for trends and patterns.

There are both advantages and disadvantages to using focus groups. This data collection method is an economical way to bring participants together to gather information. Often participants selected for focus groups are pleased to offer their answers, opinions, and insights about the objectives identified for the group. However, participants must feel secure about the topic. For example, a researcher investigating the attitudes of nurses about employment practices may be wise to put nursing managers in separate focus groups from staff nurses. Like other qualitative methods, the transcription and analysis may be costly and time consuming (Curtis & Redmon, 2007).

Case Studies

Case studies are often used to gain an understanding of the circumstances around a rare or sentinel health event. A group of individuals involved in the situation is brought together to analyze and draw conclusions about the event. Researchers use this method to examine participants' behaviors and decision making. Although this method may be used less in research, it is an important method in quality improvement programs in almost every healthcare setting. For example, healthcare providers may convene when a major error is made such as amputating the wrong limb. Circumstances of the situation are examined and strategies to ensure that this type of error is avoided are identified.

Observation

Observations are another type of qualitative data collection method and must be consistent with the aims of the study (Casey, 2006). Researchers capture information in the natural and often unstructured setting either by being present or by recording on videotape to view at a later time. *Unstructured observations* use an inductive approach. Phenomena of interest are allowed to emerge over time as observations are being made. Researchers may be both observers and participants. Participants are aware of the researchers' roles and the research taking place, but researchers are also participants to gain insiders' perspectives about the phenomena (Casey, 2006).

Researchers usually make observations in settings where research projects take place. Observations can be expensive and time consuming. When more than one individual is involved in making observations, the observers should confer occasionally to make sure that data are being collected in the same manner. The presence of researchers may alter behaviors that are observed. Therefore, researchers may need to spend additional time in the setting so that participants feel more comfortable and the behaviors that are observed are more likely to be typical (Casey, 2006).

Storytelling

Sometimes qualitative researchers collect data though the use of storytelling. Using interviews, participants and researchers share their stories about the research topic. To establish trust, storytelling begins with the researcher revealing a story that is personal in nature. Participants are encouraged to follow with their stories, which are recorded and later transcribed verbatim. This works well when studying topics of a sensitive nature (Hayman, Wilkes, Jackson, & Halcomb, 2011), as well as with ethnography and narrative qualitative methods. Storytelling is particularly useful when participants are from a culture that engages in the tradition of oral history (Lee, Fawcett, & DeMarco, 2016; Palacios et al., 2015). This technique is also successful for gaining perspectives from elders and individuals diagnosed with dementia (Mendes, 2016).

There are three types of storytelling (Lee et al., 2016). One type involves personal stories that describe a significant event in one's life. For example, a researcher may ask women to tell the story about how they were diagnosed with breast cancer. The second type focuses on significant, historical events that help to document the event to better understand the past. For example, marathon runners might recount their experiences of seeing other runners and spectators being injured during the Boston Marathon bombing. The third type of storytelling engages participants for the purpose of changing the attitudes or perceptions of the storytellers. For example, smokers may be asked to tell their stories about how and why they began to smoke. Doing this may help them glean new insights about their attitudes and change their smoking behaviors. Storytelling can be effective because there is a balance of power between the researchers and the participants (Blythe, Wilkes, Jackson, & Halcomb, 2013; Hayman et al., 2011). When the data are analyzed, researchers focus not only on the stories, but also on how the stories were told. While storytelling typically is oral in nature, stories can be expressed through other mediums such as writing, dance, song, or digital media (Palacios et al., 2015).

Preparing to Go into the Field

After consent has been obtained from participants and researchers go into the field to collect data, they should be prepared with additional materials and anticipate needs that may arise. Researchers should go prepared with additional consent forms in case additional participants are identified, participant information sheets that explain the study, stamped self-addressed return envelopes, and additional interview guides. Because field notes are essential in qualitative research methods, it is helpful to have notebooks with extra pens and pencils available. If interviews are being conducted, extra tape recorders, additional batteries, and audiotapes need to be available as backups. Likewise, if video is being used for observations, extra video cameras, additional batteries, and extra videotapes should be available. When mobile devices are utilized, it is imperative to be sure wireless access is available if required. The device should be fully charged, and/or charging capability should be available. Additionally, when using devices, it is imperative that a secure network be used so that others cannot access the information that is being entered. When compensation is given to participants, researchers should be prepared with monetary and nonmonetary rewards (Ripley, Macrina, Markowitz, & Gennings, 2010).

Appraising Data Collection in Qualitative Studies

As nurses read and interpret evidence from qualitative studies, it is essential that they determine whether data collection methods are appropriate. **Box 10-2** outlines critical questions that can be used to appraise data collection methods of qualitative research. Data collection methods should be congruent with the research question. For example, when appraising an ethnographic study, the reader must ask whether a broad question is clearly stated. This question may become more focused as time is spent in the field and the researcher identifies emerging themes. Do emerging questions make sense to participants and therefore accurately reflect what participants are saying? Does the particular group or do individuals in the study sample represent the experiences into which the researcher hopes to gain insight? The sample of the study should also be assessed. The setting should be adequately described so that readers can determine whether the findings relate to other settings. Readers need to ask if a systematic method or procedure for data collection was described so that others could replicate the study and if enough data were collected to reach saturation. Williams (2015) recommended that readers ask, "Does the researcher describe steps in data collection and analysis in sufficient detail for you to judge if he or she actually followed the method selected?" (p. 32).

FYI

As nurses read and interpret evidence from qualitative studies, it is essential that they determine whether data collection methods are appropriate. Data collection methods should be congruent with the research question.

BOX 10-2   Appraising Data Collection Methods in Qualitative Studies

Where was the setting of the study?

What was the rationale for choosing the setting?

Who were the participants and what were their roles and characteristics?

Why were they chosen?

What data collection methods were used?

What role did the researcher adopt within the setting?

Who collected the data and were they qualified for their roles?

How were data collectors trained? Was the training adequate?

Was the process of the fieldwork adequately reported?

How did the event unfold?

Was data collection continued until saturation was achieved?

Were the researchers' assumptions or biases acknowledged?

CRITICAL THINKING EXERCISE 10-3

Recall the last time you performed a physical assessment on a client. What type of data were you able to gather through interview? Through observation? What open-ended questions did you use? What closed-ended questions did you use?

TEST YOUR KNOWLEDGE 10-4

1. Which of the following statements is true regarding the collection of qualitative data?
   a. Questionnaires are an economical way to collect anonymous data.
   b. Researchers can probe for more data when using questionnaires than when using interviews.
   c. Focus groups can be led by anyone interested in the subject.
   d. Researchers should never interact with individuals they are observing.
2. Which of the following should nurses consider when appraising qualitative data collection methods? (Select all that apply.)
   a. The cost of the study
   b. The setting of the study
   c. The ages of the data collectors
   d. The role of the researcher

How did you do? 1. a; 2. b, d

10.5 Keeping It Ethical

At the end of this section, you will be able to:

‹ Discuss the importance of protecting human subjects during data collection

Protecting human subjects is essential throughout the data collection process. In healthcare research, subjects or participants are considered to be more vulnerable because of alterations in health status. Dilemmas can arise when advocating for the rights of individuals conflicts with the need to promote nursing science. It is not uncommon for nurses to find themselves caring for individuals involved in research studies; therefore, it is helpful for nurses to understand some basic safeguards.

Prior to data collection, informed consent must be obtained. One of the fundamental responsibilities of researchers is to make sure each person understands the nature of the research project and the implications of participating. Potential research participants should not be given too much hope that the intervention will benefit them because this could influence their decisions to participate. Individuals, or the proxy decision makers, must be able to freely decide whether to participate. They must be assured that they can withdraw from the study at any time without fear of reprisal. If nurses determine that potential subjects are not fully informed or lack understanding, they have an obligation to notify primary investigators. If proxy decision makers are involved in informed consent, nurses should determine that decisions are in the best interest of participants (Dunn et al., 2013).

Sometimes research studies raise sensitive issues among nurses who feel protective of their patients. Nurses may be reluctant to identify and recruit subjects or may collect only partial data. For example, Moody and McMillan (2002) reported that hospice nurses shielded their patients from a study even though the study was supported by the hospice administrative staff. Only 60 patient–caregiver dyads were enrolled despite there being 475 eligible patients. It was noted that many nurses believed that patients who were in the final stage of life should not be disturbed.

RCTs also create dilemmas for nurses because subjects are randomized into treatment and control groups. Nurses

FYI

One of the fundamental responsibilities of researchers is to make sure each person understands the nature of the research project and the implications of participating. Potential research participants should not be given too much hope that the intervention will benefit them because this could influence their decisions to participate.

must accept that randomization occurs to better understand the differences between groups, particularly when it is not known if treatments are beneficial. In blinded studies, nurses should not speculate with subjects or their families about the intervention. When nurses are informed of RCTs, they are more likely to assist researchers in recruiting, enrolling, and retaining participants (Roll et al., 2013).

The Internet is an accepted source of data and method used to collect data; therefore, it is important for nurses to be aware of some ethical considerations, namely, privacy and confidentiality. Because Internet communications leave a trail of archived records, privacy and confidentiality might be threatened. There is growing debate about whether information on the Internet is private or public. If the site is considered to be public, researchers may use information without obtaining informed consent (Coons, 2014). Whenever collecting data from the Internet, consideration should be given to questions such as: "1) What is private?, 2) What is identifiable?, 3) How can IRBs and researchers protect subjects' online privacy and confidentiality interests?, and 4) Can they minimize risks when using sensitive online data?" (Coons, 2014, p. 77). There is mounting concern that data collected via the Internet could be sold to others, posing threats to individuals who are willing to meet via the Internet and share health-related experiences. Additionally, data that currently are not linked to individuals may be identifiable in the future. When online methods are used, individuals should access the Internet via a secure site and use usernames and passwords. Security issues must be monitored continuously throughout the data collection process, and researchers also need to update and upgrade security measures frequently (Im & Chee, 2006). It is essential that researchers protect any personal data or IP addresses and comply with the Health Insurance Portability and Accountability Act (HIPAA).

Regardless of how data are collected, researchers must implement strategies to keep data secure. Attention to data collection methods is imperative to prevent error. Researchers should not feel pressured to falsify or fabricate data because there are statistical methods to address missing data. Security measures must be in place to ensure that only authorized individuals have access to data. For example, data should be kept in secured computer files that require passwords to access. Codes, rather than names of subjects, must be used on data collection instruments such as questionnaires and laboratory reports to ensure anonymity. Raw data should be stored in locked cabinets, and audiotapes should be destroyed after they are transcribed.

TEST YOUR KNOWLEDGE 10-5

True/False

1. When collecting data via the Internet, the rights of human subjects can be ignored because the Web is a public domain.

2. Nurses should not speculate about the treatments subjects receive in a blinded RCT.

3. Data collection instruments should have codes rather than subject names to ensure anonymity.

How did you do? 1. F; 2. T; 3. T

Apply What You Have Learned

The work by your EBP committee is progressing. Now, the focus shifts to how researchers collected data about hand hygiene compliance. For the articles inserted into your grid, enter information in the outcomes and time columns. What do you notice about how researchers measure hand hygiene? Read the articles by Whitby and McLaws (2007) and Dyson et al. (2013) to explore challenges of measuring hand hygiene compliance.

RAPID REVIEW

» Data collection takes a significant amount of time and resources when conducting research. Pilot studies can help identify unexpected problems.

» Quantitative data collection methods involve measurements that gather numbers.

» Questionnaires, observation, scales, and physiological measures are data collection methods used in quantitative studies.

» There are four levels of measurement: nominal, ordinal, interval, and ratio. Statistical tests used in data analysis are selected based on the level of measurement.

» All measurement contains error. There are two types of error: random and systematic.

» Validity refers to whether an instrument measures what it should be measuring. There are three kinds of validity: content validity, criterion-related validity, and construct validity.

» Reliability refers to the accuracy and consistency of an instrument. Reliable instruments have stability, equivalence, and internal consistency.

» A correlation coefficient of 0.70 or greater indicates that an instrument has good reliability. Cronbach's alpha is one correlation coefficient that is commonly reported for interval and ratio data.

» The purpose of qualitative data collection is to collect words.

» The researcher is the most important data collection instrument in qualitative data collection. Researchers use questionnaires, interviews, focus groups, case studies, observation, and storytelling to collect qualitative data.

» Protecting human subjects is an important aspect of all research studies and one in which nurses play a key role.

REFERENCES

Anastasi, J., Capili, B., Kim, G., & Chung, A. (2005). Clinical trial recruitment and retention of a vulnerable population: HIV patients with chronic diarrhea. *Gastroenterology Nursing, 28*, 463–468.

Beyea, S., & Nicoll, L. (2000). Collecting, analyzing, and interpreting focus group data. *AORN Journal, 71*, 22–30.

Beyer, J. E., Denyes, M. J., & Villarruel, A. M. (1992). The creation, validation, and continuing development of the Oucher: A measure of pain intensity in children. *Journal of Pediatric Nursing, 7*, 335–346.

Blythe, S., Wilkes, L., Jackson, D., & Halcomb, E. (2013). The challenges of being an insider in storytelling research. *Nurse Researcher, 21*(1), 8–13.

Casey, D. (2006). Choosing an appropriate method of data collection. *Nurse Researcher, 13*, 75–92.

Coons, S. (2014). Internet research issues for IRBs: Context is important in determining privacy of information. *Research Practitioner, 15*(4), 76–79.

Curtis, E., & Redmon, R. (2007). Focus groups in nursing research. *Nurse Researcher, 14*, 25–37.

Drayton, K. (2013). How mobile technology can improve healthcare. *Nursing Times, 109*, 1–3.

Dunn, L., Fisher, S., Hantke, M., Appelbaum, P., Dohan, D., Young, J., & Roberts, L. (2013). "Thinking about it for somebody else": Alzheimer's disease research and proxy decision makers' translation of ethical principles into practice. *American Journal of Geriatric Psychiatry, 21*, 337–345. doi:10.1016/j.jagp.2012.11.014

Dyson, J., Lawton, R., Jackson, C., & Cheater, F. (2013). Development of a theory-based instrument to identify barriers and louvers to best hand hygiene practice among healthcare practitioners. *Implementation Science, 8*(111), 1–9.

Granger, B., Zhao, Y., Rogers, J., Miller, C., Gilliss, C., & Champagne, M. (2013). The language of data: Tools to translate evidence for nurses in clinical practice. *Journal of Nurses Professional Development, 29*, 294–300.

Griffin-Sobel, J. (2003). Evaluating an instrument for research. *Gastroenterology Nursing, 26*, 135–136.

Haeok, L., Fawcett, J., & DeMarco, R. (2015). Storytelling/narrative theory to address health communication with minority populations. *Applied Nursing Research, 30*, 58–60.

Havens, G. A. (2001). A practical approach to the process of measurement in nursing. *Clinical Nurse Specialist, 15*, 146–152.

Hayman, B., Wilkes, L., Jackson, D., & Halcomb, E. (2011). Story-sharing as a method of data collection in qualitative research. *Journal of Clinical Nursing, 21*, 285–287.

Hunter, L. (2012). Challenging the reported disadvantages of e-questionnaires and addressing methodological issues of online data collection. *Nurse Researcher, 20*, 11–20.

Im, E., & Chee, W. (2006). An online forum as a qualitative research method. *Nursing Research, 55*, 267–273.

Ioannidis, J. P. A. (2005). Why most published research findings are false. *PLOS Medicine, 8*, 696–701. Retrieved from http://dx.doi.org/10.1371/journal.pmed.0020124

Marwit, S., & Meuser, T. (2002). Development and initial validation of an inventory to assess grief in caregivers of persons with Alzheimer's disease. *Gerontologist, 42*, 751–765.

Meadows, K. A. (2003). So you want to do research? 5: Questionnaire design. *British Journal of Community Nursing, 12*, 562–570.

Mendes, A. (2016). The value of storytelling for people living with dementia. *Nursing & Residential Care, 18*(12), 667–669.

Merchant, J., & Mateo, M. (1993). Accurate data: The basis of decision. *Gastroenterology Nursing, 16*, 163–169.

Meuser, T., & Marwit, S. (2001). A comprehensive, stage-sensitive model of grief in dementia caregiving. *Gerontologist, 41*, 658–700.

Miller, W. (2010). Qualitative research findings as evidence: Utility in nursing practice. *Clinical Nurse Specialist, 24*, 191–194.

Moody, L., & McMillan, S. (2002). Maintaining data integrity in randomized clinical trials. *Nursing Research, 51*, 129–133.

Myers, G., & Meccariello, M. (2006). From pet rock to rock-solid: Implementing unit based research. *Nursing Management, 37*, 24–29.

Palacios, J. F., Salem, B., Hodge, F. S., Albarrán, C. R., Anaebere, A., & Hayes-Bautista, T. M. (2015). Storytelling: A qualitative tool to promote health among vulnerable populations. *Journal of Transcultural Nursing, 26*(4), 346–353.

Ripley, E., Macrina, F., Markowitz, M., & Gennings, C. (2010). Who's doing the math? Are we really compensating research participants? *Journal of Empirical Research on Human Research Ethics, 5*, 57–65. doi:10.1525/jer.2010.5.3.57

Roberts, P., & Priest, H. (2006). Reliability and validity in research. *Nursing Standard, 20*, 41–45.

Roll, K., Stegenga, V., Hendricks-Ferguson, Y., Barnes, B., Cherven, S., Docherty, S., & Haase, J. (2013). Engaging nurses in research for a randomized clinical trial of a behavioral health intervention. *Nursing Research and Practice*. Retrieved from http://dx.doi.org/10.1155/2013/183984

Sandelowski, M. (2004). Using qualitative research. *Qualitative Health Research, 14,* 1366–1386.

Sinkowitz-Cochran, R. (2013). Survey design: To ask or not to ask? That is the question. *Clinical Infectious Diseases, 56*(8), 1159–1164.

Trochim, W. (2000). *The research methods knowledge base* (2nd ed.). Cincinnati, OH: Atomic Dog Publishing.

Whitby, M., & McLaws, M. (2007). Methodological difficulties in hand hygiene research. *Journal of Hospital Infection, 67,* 194–195.

Williams, B. (2015). How to evaluate qualitative research. *American Nurse Today, 10*(11), 31–38.

Wolf, Z. R. (2003). Teaching the code book. *Nurse Educator, 38,* 132–135.

At the end of this chapter, you will be able to:

- Identify the basic concepts associated with sampling
- Differentiate between probability and nonprobability samples
- Describe various sampling methods
- Identify quantitative and qualitative research sampling strategies
- Discuss factors that should be considered when determining sample size
- Describe strategies that enhance the recruitment and retention of subjects
- Identify factors related to sampling that must be considered when appraising studies for evidence-based practice
- Describe ethical considerations related to sampling

accessible population
anonymity
assent
attrition rate
cluster sampling
coercion
confidentiality
convenience sampling
data saturation
effect size
elements
exclusion criteria
heterogeneous
homogeneity

inclusion criteria
informed consent
network sampling
nonprobability sampling
population
power analysis
probability sampling
purposive sampling
quota sampling
randomization
representativeness
sample
sampling bias
sampling error

sampling frame
sampling interval
sampling plan
significance level
simple random sampling
snowball sampling
stratified random sampling
subjects
systematic random sampling
target population
theoretical sampling
vulnerable population

CHAPTER 11

Using Samples to Provide Evidence

Ann H. White

11.1 Fundamentals of Sampling

At the end of this section, you will be able to:

‹ Identify the basic concepts associated with sampling

Nurses make decisions every day and are using the best evidence from research as one method to guide these decisions (Hopp, 2012). The ultimate goal of evidence-based practice (EBP) is high-quality health care with beneficial outcomes (Hall & Roussel, 2014). Collecting evidence to change clinical practice by identifying relevant nursing research on clinical topics is critical. After research studies are identified, nurses must appraise whether the research is valid and relevant to clinical practice. One consideration when appraising evidence is to determine whether the sample and the sampling method were appropriately selected for the study.

Learning the Terms

When designing a research study, researchers must define the population as specified in the research question. A *population* is the entire group of elements that meet study criteria (Fawcett & Garity, 2009). *Elements*, also called population units, are the basic unit of the population and may be people, events, experiences, or behaviors (Fawcett & Garity, 2009). When elements are people, they are referred to as *subjects*. After determining the population of interest, researchers must create a *sampling plan* that includes the size of the sample, who will be eligible to be in the study, how individuals will be selected, and how they will be recruited (Bloom & Trice, 2011). It is not economical, feasible, or time efficient to include all possible subjects in a study. An alternative is to identify a select group of subjects that is representative of all eligible subjects. These individuals constitute the *sample*.

To obtain the sample needed for the study, researchers must identify the *target population*, which is defined as all elements that meet the study criteria. For example, if a researcher is conducting a study on individuals ages 13–17 who have type 1 diabetes, then every single adolescent who has type 1 diabetes and who is 13–17 years of age would be included in the target population. The researcher may choose to narrow the scope of the study by defining the target population as a more specific group of subjects. For example, the target population could be defined as adolescents 13–17 years of age with type 1 diabetes whose care is managed by a local diabetic clinic. The researcher determines the target population based on the purpose of the study, the design, and the type of data collection being planned (Fawcett & Garity, 2009).

After the target population is defined, researchers identify the *accessible population*, which is the group of elements to which the researcher has reasonable access. Typically, the accessible population is a smaller group than the target population; however, in some cases it may be the same group. In the previous example of adolescent diabetics who received care in one local clinic, the sample target population and accessible population may be the same. Regardless, researchers select subjects from the accessible population (see **Figure 11-1**).

Learning these terms means using them correctly when appraising research studies. Frequently, individuals use the words *population* and *sample* interchangeably, which is incorrect. The term *sample* is used appropriately when one

FIGURE 11-1 Relationship of Sample to Population

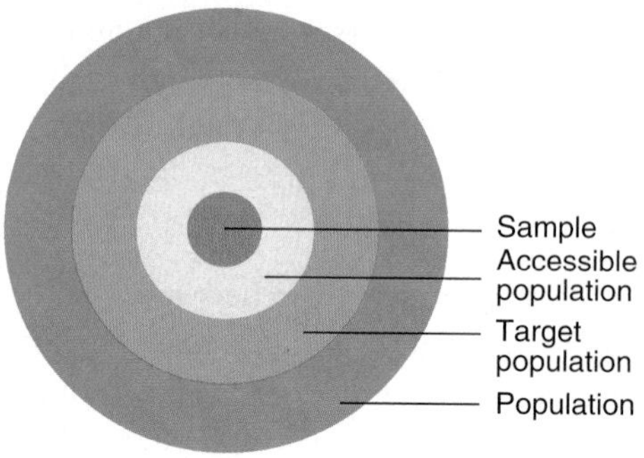

- Sample
- Accessible population
- Target population
- Population

CRITICAL THINKING EXERCISE 11-1

The next time you use the term *sample* or *population,* pause and consider whether you have used the term correctly. Were you referring to the individuals who participated in a study or were you referring to the group of individuals to whom the findings would be generalized? Listen to how others use these terms. Are they using them correctly?

discusses the elements of a study. The term *population* is used appropriately when one is generalizing findings to all possible elements (Bloom & Trice, 2011).

The Hallmark of a Sample: Representativeness

Researchers place much importance on *representativeness*. This means obtaining representative samples so that results of studies can be generalized to target populations (Albert, O'Connor, & Buelow, 2012). Generalizability, also referred to as external validity, is the applicability of study findings to target populations. There is greater concern for generalizability in quantitative research studies than in qualitative studies. Generalizabilty of study findings is a critical factor in EBP. As nurses identify and read research studies to determine best practice, they must determine whether results of the studies are applicable to patients in their organizations. Confidence in generalizability can be increased if samples accurately represent the target population. This means that the elements of a sample must possess characteristics similar to the elements composing the target population (see **Figure 11-2**). Melnyk and Cole (2011) identified a four-step method to ensure that samples are representative of target populations (see **Box 11-1**). By following this process, the potential for obtaining a representative sample is high. When the population, target population, accessible population, and sample are similar, the sample can be said to be representative.

Inclusion criteria are used to determine subjects to be included in the sample. Researchers identify characteristics that each element must possess to be included in the sample. Inclusion criteria are guided by the research question and careful identification of the target and accessible populations. For example, in the study of adolescent diabetics, the researcher would first identify the essential characteristics or inclusion criteria for the target population. These characteristics could include age, a diagnosis of type 1 diabetes, receiving care at a local diabetic clinic, and ability to speak English. Researchers often report inclusion criteria to clearly identify the subjects of the study.

FYI

In order to collect evidence that changes clinical practice, nurses must identify and appraise research that is relevant to clinical practice. Key to this appraisal is determining that the sample and the sampling method are appropriate for the study and generalizable. Confidence in generalizability can be increased if samples accurately represent the target population.

KEY TERMS

representativeness: The degree to which elements of the sample are like elements in the population

inclusion criteria: Characteristics that each element must possess to be included in the sample

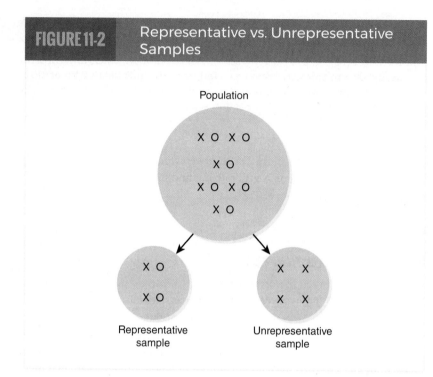

FIGURE 11-2	**Representative vs. Unrepresentative Samples**

Representative vs. Unrepresentative Samples

BOX 11-1   Four Steps to Ensure Representative Samples

1. Define and clearly articulate the target population for the study by listing all of the essential characteristics of the target population or eligibility criteria for inclusion in the study.
2. Identify the population the researcher has access to for the study, taking care to verify that the accessible population closely resembles the target population by using the same eligibility criteria.
3. Develop a method to approach the accessible population. Some researchers refer to this as a sampling frame. The sampling frame is a practical method used to gain access to the population that is readily available to the researcher.
4. Select subjects from the accessible population to include in the sample.

Modified from Melnyk, B. M., & Cole, R. (2011). Generating evidence through quantitative research. In B. Melnyk & E. Fineout-Overholt (Eds.), *Evidence-based practice in nursing and healthcare* (2nd ed., pp. 397–434). Philadelphia, PA: Lippincott Williams & Wilkins.

KEY TERM

exclusion criteria: Characteristics of elements that will not be included in the sample

Researchers may also designate *exclusion criteria*, which are characteristics of elements that will not be included in a sample. The use of exclusion criteria may decrease the risks of certain characteristics influencing the results of a study (Bloom & Trice, 2011). For example, the researcher wants to study coping in adolescents with type 1 diabetes. Individuals having another chronic disease such as asthma may be excluded from the study. The researcher may believe that having another chronic disease is an extraneous variable that could affect coping. If researchers choose to set exclusion criteria, the criteria must be clearly delineated, and researchers must have valid explanations to support the reasons for the exclusions.

Inclusion and exclusion criteria are also important to appraise when considering evidence. When criteria are explicit, nurses can determine whether results are applicable to the clinical practice topic being considered. Clearly defined inclusion and exclusion criteria tend to improve studies because the precision of sample selection is enhanced. This precision leads to stronger evidence when looking at research relevant to clinical practice (Bloom & Trice, 2011).

When samples are not representative of target populations, the potential for sampling errors and bias is increased. *Sampling error* occurs when subjects in a study do not adequately represent the population. In most instances, sampling error is a result of small sample size that could not adequately represent all of the elements of the target population. *Sampling bias* occurs when the sample includes elements that over- or underrepresent characteristics when compared to elements in the target population. This is a threat to the external validity of the study or how the study can be generalized and reported to reflect the target population.

KEY TERMS

sampling error: Error resulting when elements in the sample do not adequately represent the population

sampling bias: A threat to external validity when a sample includes elements that over- or underrepresent characteristics when compared to elements in the target population

TEST YOUR KNOWLEDGE 11-1

Match the following:

1. Population
2. Target population
3. Accessible population
4. Sample
5. Inclusion criteria
6. Exclusion criteria
7. Representativeness
8. Element

a. The elements included in a study

b. All elements that meet a well-defined set of criteria

c. Degree to which the sample reflects the population

d. Characteristics that eliminate elements from a study

e. A population that meets sampling criteria

f. Basic unit of the population

g. Population from which a researcher can sample

h. Characteristics of elements in a study

How did you do? 1. b; 2. e; 3. g; 4. a; 5. h; 6. d; 7. c; 8. f

11.2 Sampling Methods

At the end of this section, you will be able to:

‹ Differentiate between probability and nonprobability samples
‹ Describe various sampling methods
‹ Identify quantitative and qualitative research sampling strategies

Once inclusion criteria have been determined, researchers identify a method to select subjects for the sample. Researchers can use several sampling methods to select subjects. These methods are divided into two categories: probability and nonprobability sampling.

Probability Sampling Methods

When researchers use *probability sampling*, every element in the accessible population has an equal chance of being selected for inclusion in the study. Three conditions must be met in probability sampling. First, an accessible population must be identifiable. Next, the researcher must create a *sampling frame*; that is, a list of all possible elements in the accessible population. Finally, random selection must be used to choose elements from the sampling frame. The use of *randomization* is important because it reduces the threat of selection bias. The probability that the characteristics of elements in the sample will be similar to elements of the population is increased (Graff, 2014; Stevens, 2011). There are four probability sampling methods: simple random sampling, stratified random sampling, cluster sampling, and systematic random sampling.

Each of the four probability sampling methods has advantages and disadvantages. Researchers should select a method based on the purpose of the research, the research question, and the research design. **Table 11-1** provides an overview of the assumptions, potential bias, and representativeness of probability sampling methods.

Simple Random Sampling

Simple random sampling involves randomly selecting elements from the accessible population and is considered by some authorities to be the most effective method to obtain a representative sample. If the accessible population is small, simple random sampling may be as easy as drawing names. For example, if the accessible population is 25 nursing students and the researcher needs 10 students for the study, the name of each student could be placed in a container. The first name is drawn and recorded as a potential participant. The name is

KEY TERMS

probability sampling: Sampling method in which elements in the accessible population have an equal chance of being selected for inclusion in the study

sampling frame: A list of all possible elements in the accessible population

randomization: The selection, assignment, or arrangement of elements by chance

simple random sampling: Randomly selecting elements from the accessible population

TABLE 11-1	Overview of Probability Sampling Methods

Type of Sampling	Assumptions	Possibility of Bias	Representativeness	Other Comments
Simple random sampling	Each subject has the same chance to be selected Strategy used to select subjects upholds randomization	Low risk of bias if randomization of subjects is upheld	With each subject having the same chance for selection, high probability the sample will represent the population as long as sample size is sufficient	Time consuming for researcher if the study has a large sample size
Stratified random sampling	Strata must be mutually exclusive so a subject can be assigned to only one stratum Random sampling used to select subject from each stratum	Low risk of bias if randomization of subjects is upheld	If assumptions are upheld, high probability the sample will represent the population if the number of subjects in each stratum is sufficient	Time consuming for researcher if the study has a large sample size
Cluster sampling	Simple random sampling used to first select groups or clusters and then select subjects within each cluster	Potential for bias greater if the initial clusters selected under- or overrepresent groups within the population	Greater potential for the sample to not represent the population depending on how the initial clusters are selected	Less time consuming than the first two because the initial clusters focus the sites for subject selection
Systematic sampling	Begin sampling with a random start. Start counting each *k*th subject on the list by first identifying the start location. Or, close eyes and point to a number on the list to start the counting	Some bias may be introduced if randomization of start location is not maintained	If bias occurs, not as representative of population as other three sampling methods	Simpler to complete than the other three forms of probability sampling

Data from Gray, J., Grove, S., & Sutherland, S. (2016). *Burns and Grove's the practice of nursing research: Appraisal, synthesis, and generation of evidence* (8th ed.). St. Louis, MO: Saunders; Polit, D., & Beck, C. T. (2014). *Essentials of nursing research: Appraising evidence for nursing practice*. Philadelphia, PA: Lippincott Williams & Wilkins.

FYI

Researchers can use several sampling methods to select subjects. The methods can be divided into two categories: probability and nonprobability sampling. Researchers should select a method based on the purpose of the research, the research question, and the research design.

returned to the container and this process continues until 10 student names have been selected. Should one of the selected students decline to participate in the study, another name would be selected in the same manner.

When the accessible population is large, it may be easier for researchers to use a random numbers table. Such a table contains columns of digits (see **Table 11-2**). Each element in the sampling frame is assigned a number. The researcher points to a number on the random numbers table to begin the selection process. The researcher then proceeds through the table either horizontally, vertically, or diagonally. Numbers are selected until the desired sample size is achieved. Elements corresponding to the numbers selected form the sample. For example, in a study to determine student interest in creating a smoke-free campus, the accessible population is 5,500 undergraduate and graduate students. The researcher secures a list of all students enrolled in the university and assigns each name on the list a number. It has been determined

TABLE 11-2	Table of Random Numbers		
5	2	25	52
57	63	12	72
29	31	84	20
27	80	48	11
59	1	26	6
8	19	28	86
83	53	64	22
14	45	35	37
7	23	21	46
22	4	15	57
17	61	82	85
44	34	31	10
60	24	58	55
16	54	13	71
56	62	65	33
81	9	87	47

that a sample of 200 students is necessary to achieve representativeness. After selecting the start point, the researcher selects additional elements by proceeding vertically through the columns until 200 subjects are selected. Computer programs are also available that select a random sample, and these programs are frequently used when the researcher is using a large sample.

Stratified Random Sampling

Stratified random sampling involves selecting elements from a population that has been divided into groups or strata. Researchers identify characteristics that they want to stratify. These determinations are frequently based on what is already known about the phenomenon being studied. For example, findings show that boys and girls respond differently to pain. Therefore, a researcher may want to stratify subjects on the variable of gender to ensure that they have enough boys and girls to make comparisons.

Strata must be mutually exclusive. This means that each element can be put into one and only one stratum (Gray, Grove, & Sutherland, 2016). For example, if the sample is stratified according to gender, subjects can be categorized only as a boy or a girl. These strata are mutually exclusive because subjects cannot fit into both categories. After strata are established, researchers assign each element from the accessible population to a stratum. Participants are then randomly selected from each stratum. For example, the researcher may want to study nursing student attitudes toward treatment of pain. Because there are significantly fewer male than female nursing students, the researcher needs to account for gender disparity in the study. If less than 10% of the accessible population is male, the researcher uses stratified random sampling so that 10% of the sample is male. After strata are determined, subjects are randomly selected from each stratum.

One advantage to stratified random sampling is that sampling error can be reduced because elements are selected by strata that are known to represent the population. Representative samples increase the likelihood that findings can be generalized to the population. Stratifying can also decrease data collection time and costs of collecting data (Gray et al., 2016). However, care must be taken when using this method. Each stratum must have a sufficient number of elements. In the preceding example, if 50 males are needed to constitute 10% of the sample, there must be at least 50 males in the accessible population.

Cluster Sampling

Cluster sampling is also known as multistaging sampling. Cluster sampling is an effective and efficient method to collect data from large populations. A manageable sample is obtained by randomly selecting elements from larger to smaller clusters or subsets of a population. First, researchers identify all elements that could be included in a study. Then they determine logical subsets of the populations using random selection techniques. The participants are then randomly selected within those groups. For example, a researcher wants to study baccalaureate nursing education in the United States. Using cluster sampling, the researcher first randomly selects 10 states that will be included in the study. Then all baccalaureate nursing programs in each of the 10 states are identified. The researcher then randomly selects three schools from each state and obtains the names of baccalaureate students enrolled in each of the programs selected. Sampling is concluded by randomly selecting 30% of the names on each list.

Although cluster sampling is an effective method to sample large populations, there are limitations. In the preceding example, suppose the researcher decided to select 50 students from each program rather than selecting 30%. This could result in oversampling of students from small programs and undersampling of students from large programs. Selecting a percentage of students provides a more representative sample.

Systematic Random Sampling

A fourth type of probability sampling is *systematic random sampling*. In this method, researchers select subjects by creating a numbered list of elements and then selecting every *k*th element. Sometimes every odd- or even-numbered element may be chosen. To determine the *sampling interval*, researchers must know two things: the desired size of the sample and the size of the sampling frame. The formula for determining sample interval is as follows (Gray et al., 2016):

$$k = \frac{\text{Size of sampling frame}}{\text{Size of sample}}$$

For example, a researcher desires to study infant feeding patterns and has access to a well-baby clinic. At this clinic, 300 infants are registered as patients. The researcher needs 20 subjects for the study. Using systematic sampling, the researcher would obtain a list of names of all infants seen in the clinic and assign each name a number. The sampling interval would be calculated by dividing 300 by 20, which equals 15. After randomly selecting a starting point on the list, every 15th (*k*th) name would be invited to participate in the study.

Sampling bias may be introduced with this method. This method should not be used if there is a pattern inherent in the list of elements. For example, if every 10th name on the list is a baby with formula intolerance, these infants would either be over- or undersampled, resulting in a biased sample.

CRITICAL THINKING EXERCISE 11-2

Suppose you are on a task force at your university. The task force needs to survey students about attitudes toward adopting a smoke-free campus. What are the advantages and disadvantages to using each of the probability sampling methods?

Nonprobability Sampling Methods

A second category of sampling methods is *nonprobability sampling*. These methods do not require random selection of elements and therefore are less likely to be representative of the target population. Researchers use nonprobability sampling methods when a sampling frame cannot be determined. Because randomization is not used, the threat of selection bias is increased; therefore, samples selected using nonprobability are likely to be less representative than are samples selected using probability methods. The researcher should make every effort to create a representative sample and clearly describe the method of sampling for the reader (Houser, 2011; Melnyk & Cole, 2011). There are four nonprobability sampling methods: convenience, quota, purposive, and theoretical. **Table 11-3** provides an overview of nonprobability sampling methods.

Convenience Sampling

In *convenience sampling*, also known as accidental sampling, researchers select elements for inclusion in the sample because they are easy to access. For example, a researcher desires to conduct a study of patients with type 2 diabetes presenting for treatment at an emergency department. Because the researcher cannot predict which diabetic patients will use the emergency department over the course of the study, it is impossible for the researcher to create a sampling frame and randomly select subjects. Therefore, the researcher elects to use a convenience sample that includes all patients with type 2 diabetes who seek care at the emergency department.

Although sampling bias is a concern with this method, strategies can be used to control for bias. Comparing demographic data from individuals in the sample to population demographics can help researchers determine whether the sample is representative. Researchers should present a thorough description of the convenience sample in the study results and compare it to the target population. A careful explanation of why and how the sample was selected allows nurses to determine the potential for sampling bias and whether study findings should be used as evidence for clinical practice.

KEY TERMS

nonprobability sampling: Sampling methods that do not require random selection of elements

convenience sampling: Nonprobability sampling method in which elements are selected because they are easy to access

TABLE 11-3	Overview of Nonprobability Sampling			

Type of Sampling	Assumptions	Possibility of Bias	Representativeness	Other Comments
Convenience sampling	1. Inclusion criteria identified prior to selection of subjects 2. All subjects are invited to participate	Highest probability of bias	Because sample is selected for ease of data collection, may not be representative of the target population	Seen in many nursing studies because of ease of data collection
Quota sampling	1. Strata must be mutually exclusive so a subject can be assigned to only one stratum 2. Convenience sampling used to select subject from each stratum	May have some bias resulting from convenience sampling after strata are identified	Because sample within each stratum is selected using convenience sampling method, may not represent the population	Similar to stratified random sampling except convenience sampling is used to obtain the sample in each stratum
Purposive sampling	1. Researcher has sufficient knowledge of topic to select sample of experts 2. Researcher should identify criteria to include in selection of subjects 3. Commonly used in qualitative research	May have minimal bias if identification of participants adheres to selection criteria and sample in study is homogenous	Because sample is selected by researcher, cannot generalize to population; generalizing the results is not an expected outcome of qualitative research	Focus of this research is to learn more about and understand the phenomenon being studied
Theoretical sampling	1. Data collection and data analysis occur simultaneously 2. Commonly used in grounded theory research	Not applicable with this type of sampling	Cannot generalize to population; generalizing the results is not an expected outcome of grounded theory research	Used in grounded theory

Data from Gray, J., Grove, S., & Sutherland, S. (2016). *Burns and Grove's the practice of nursing research: Appraisal, synthesis, and generation of evidence* (8th ed.). St. Louis, MO: Saunders; Polit, D., & Beck, C. T. (2014). *Essentials of nursing research: Appraising evidence for nursing practice.* Philadelphia, PA: Lippincott Williams & Wilkins.

Quota Sampling

When researchers sample from strata without randomly selecting elements, they are using quota sampling. Like stratified random sampling, researchers select strata based on what is already known about the phenomenon being studied. The desired number, or quota, needed to fill each stratum should be proportionate to the population to obtain a representative sample.

The difference between *quota sampling* and stratified random sampling is the use of random selection. In quota sampling, elements are conveniently selected from each strata rather than being randomly selected. For example, in a study about how age is related to success in nursing programs, a researcher could stratify according to age by creating three age groups: 18–22, 23–30, and older than 30. Suppose 80% of nursing students are ages 18–22, 15% are ages 23–30, and 5% are older than age 30. If the researcher needs a sample size of 100, the sampling would continue until 80 students between the ages of 18 and 22 years, 15 students between the ages of 23 and 30 years, and 5 students older than age 30 had been recruited. By establishing proportional quotas that mirror the nursing student population, the researcher is more likely to obtain a representative sample.

Convenience and quota sampling are predominantly used in quantitative research studies. They are frequently used because it is often difficult in nursing research to determine a sampling frame in advance of a study. They also are less time consuming and less costly than probability sampling methods. The ability to generalize results to the target population depends heavily on the appropriateness of the sampling method used.

Purposive Sampling

Purposive sampling, which is a nonprobability sampling method, is used in qualitative studies. Sampling methods used in qualitative research must be appropriate to allow researchers to gain insight into the experience or event being studied. There is less focus on the results of the study being generalized to the target population, and more emphasis is placed on the interpretation and understanding of the event or experience, including relevant contextual factors being studied (Leeman & Sandelowski, 2012). Researchers use purposive sampling in qualitative research to select a distinct group of individuals who either have lived the experience or have expertise in the event or experience being studied. In qualitative studies, individuals in the sample are referred to as participants. For example, researchers investigating the lived experience of women younger than the age of 25 years who have survived a liver transplant would use purposive sampling. Because the focus of the study is so specific, the researcher can hand select women who meet the inclusion criteria. Researchers must carefully document the process used to select subjects.

KEY TERMS

snowball sampling:
Recruitment of
participants based
on word of mouth
or referrals from
other participants

network sampling:
Recruitment of
participants based
on word of mouth
or referrals from
other participants;
snowball sampling

**theoretical
sampling:**
Nonprobability
sampling method
used in grounded
theory to collect
data from an
initial group of
participants

When obtaining a purposive sample, researchers often use what is known as *snowball sampling*, or *network sampling*. When using this approach, an initial participant who meets the study criteria is identified. This participant then identifies other individuals who meet the criteria for inclusion in the study. To protect confidentiality, researchers must ascertain from the referring participant that it is permissible to contact suggested potential participants. When using snowball sampling, researchers assume that individuals will identify others who are similar to themselves. Snowball sampling is a useful method to identify participants who would otherwise be difficult for the researchers to find. Suppose a researcher is investigating the lived experience of young women with eating disorders. By first identifying a small group of women who meet the criteria and then asking them to identify other young women that they know, researchers can find a larger number of potential participants.

Theoretical Sampling

Another sampling method, used specifically in grounded theory, is *theoretical sampling*. When using this sampling method, researchers collect data from an initial group of participants. After conducting some preliminary analyses of data, researchers identify additional participants for inclusion in the sample (Fawcett & Garity, 2009).

TEST YOUR KNOWLEDGE 11-2

1. A researcher desires to study the effect of a memory game on older adults' abilities to recall a short-term task list. The researcher randomly selects 20 elders from a list of residents at a local nursing home. The sampling method used is
   a. convenience sampling.
   b. quota sampling.
   c. simple random sampling.
   d. purposive sampling.

2. Which of the following sampling methods involves randomization? (Select all that apply.)
   a. Systematic sampling
   b. Snowball sampling
   c. Stratified random sampling
   d. Cluster sampling

3. To use random sampling, a researcher must know the
   a. sampling frame.
   b. characteristics of the population.
   c. exclusion criteria.
   d. sampling interval.

How did you do? 1. c; 2. a, c, d; 3. a

11.3 Sample Size: Does It Matter?

At the end of this section, you will be able to:

< Discuss factors that should be considered when determining sample size
< Describe strategies that enhance the recruitment and retention of subjects
< Identify factors related to sampling that must be considered when appraising studies for evidence-based practice

Determining Sample Size

After the sampling method is identified, researchers must decide how large a sample is needed. Various factors determine sample sizes for quantitative and qualitative studies. In either type of design, the sample size must be sufficient to adequately support the research purpose and design of the study. *Homogeneity* of the population is one factor that needs to be considered when determining sample size in quantitative studies. *Homogeneity* refers to the degree to which elements are homogenous or similar (Bloom & Trice, 2011). If a population has a number of common characteristics, the sample size does not need to be as large as a more *heterogeneous*, or diverse, population (see **Figure 11-3**).

Another factor to consider when determining sample size is the purpose of the study and what is being studied. If the focus of the study is narrow, the sample may not need to be as large as a sample for a very broadly focused study. A study investigating eating habits of fifth graders is very broad and would require a large sample. A study on eating habits of fifth graders who have diabetes is narrower in focus; thus, the number of subjects needed for the study may be smaller.

FIGURE 11-3	Homogeneous vs. Heterogeneous Samples

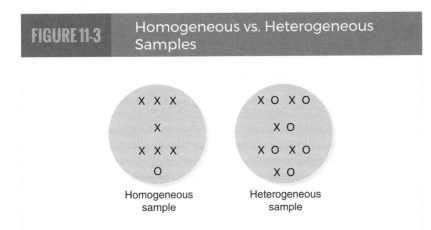

Homogeneous sample   Heterogeneous sample

KEY TERMS

attrition rate:
Dropout rate; loss of subjects before a study is completed; threat of mortality

power analysis: A statistical method to determine the acceptable sample size that will best detect the true effect of the independent variable

significance level:
The alpha level established before the beginning of a study

effect size: An estimate of how large a difference will be observed between the groups

Another factor that researchers need to consider when conducting quantitative studies is *attrition rate,* also known as dropout rate. Typically, there will be subjects who agree to participate in a study and, for whatever reason, do not complete the study. Attrition is a threat to internal validity, and the researcher should attempt to create a study design that minimizes loss of subjects. One method to address attrition is to increase the number of subjects in the sample so that even with losing subjects, the researcher will have a sufficient sample size for the research study (Albert et al., 2012).

The design of the study also influences decisions about sample size. The number of variables being investigated is an important factor. Typically, the greater the number of variables being tested in a study, the larger the sample size needed to detect changes in the variables. The sensitivity of instruments used to collect data also affects the sample size. A very precise instrument typically requires fewer subjects than does a less precise instrument (Bloom & Trice, 2011). In addition, decisions about sample size are influenced by practical matters such as cost, convenience, and feasibility.

There is one accepted rule for determining sample size when using quantitative research designs (Bloom & Trice, 2011). The rule of 30 is used by many quantitative researchers (Gray et al., 2016). This rule states that in order to have a sufficient sample size to adequately represent the target population, there needs to be a minimum of 30 subjects in each group being studied. For example, in an experiment using a control group and an intervention group, a sample size of 60 would be indicated. The rule of 30 should be considered the minimal number of subjects in each group.

A more powerful and accurate method to determine sample size for quantitative studies is to conduct a *power analysis*. A power analysis is a statistical method used to determine the acceptable sample size to detect the true effect or difference in the outcome variable (Houser, 2011). When nurses read that a power analysis was conducted and used correctly, they can have greater assurance that the sample size was appropriate for the study and be confident applying the findings to the target population (Polit & Beck, 2014).

Two factors must be established to conduct a power analysis: significance level and effect size. The *significance level* is the alpha level established prior to the beginning of the investigation. A vast majority of nursing researchers use $p = .05$ as the significance level. The *effect size* is an estimate of how large a difference will be observed between the groups (Hayat, 2013). When researchers expect that the effect size is large, fewer subjects are needed to detect differences between the groups. If the effect of an intervention is small, a larger sample is needed to statistically demonstrate that the intervention was effective. A review of relevant literature on the research topic can assist the researchers in identifying the effect size (Albert et al., 2012).

There are also factors that determine sample sizes in qualitative studies. These factors include the scope of the study, the phenomenon being investigated, the quality of data collected, and the study design. The size of the sample is sufficient when qualitative researchers achieve *data saturation*. Saturation means that collecting data from additional participants adds no new information to what has already been collected (Fawcett & Garity, 2009). Researchers should provide information about sample selection so that nurses can make determinations about the adequacy of the sample. Because the focus is on the data collected, the richness of data, and the researchers' conclusions, qualitative studies tend to have smaller samples than quantitative studies do.

Recruitment and Retention of Subjects

Effective recruitment and retention of subjects are imperative to the credibility of research studies. Failure to attend to recruitment and retention details can critically affect the size of samples. Initial contacts made by researchers may determine whether subjects will participate and remain in the study. Because researchers may have only one opportunity to encourage participation, information should be professional, informative, and culturally sensitive for the accessible population. Flyers, letters, and advertisements are all methods used to recruit subjects.

Decisions about recruitment strategies are based on cost, predicted success, and appropriateness for the accessible population. Recruitment materials should include a brief description of the study purpose, inclusion criteria, and information explaining how to enroll in the study. It is helpful to indicate in recruitment materials if incentives are being offered for participation. Researchers should determine reasons that subjects elect not to participate in studies. Being cognizant of who is not participating in a study should be included in the discussion of the results because selection bias affects generalizability of the results. Even with mailed, anonymous questionnaires, researchers may discover, by trending demographic data, similarities among subjects who did not respond. Researchers should be aware that certain age groups, socioeconomic groups, or ethnic groups may be underrepresented.

It is important to retain subjects after they have been recruited to participate in a study. Strategies to reduce threats of mortality can be effective in reducing subject attrition. Reasons why subjects withdraw from studies should be monitored, and conditions causing subjects to withdraw should be modified if possible.

Considerations for EBP

It is imperative that nurses use the best possible evidence to make decisions about clinical practice. When considering research studies for EBP, nurses must critically appraise whether samples represent target populations. Nurses should expect detailed accounts of sampling methods, sample sizes, and recruitment and retention strategies. When critically appraising studies, nurses should look for discussion about power analyses in quantitative studies and data saturation in qualitative studies. By carefully examining attributes of samples and sampling methods, nurses can make decisions about the applicability of findings to clinical practice (Hopp, 2012).

CRITICAL THINKING EXERCISE 11-3

Suppose you are in charge of designing recruitment materials for a study examining Hispanic mothers' attitudes toward breastfeeding. What factors would need to be considered when designing these materials?

TEST YOUR KNOWLEDGE 11-3

True/False

1. Attrition has little effect on the generalizability of study findings.
2. The best way to determine sample size for a quantitative study is through power analysis.
3. A study involving three groups needs a minimum of 30 subjects.
4. A group with elements having similar attributes would be considered heterogeneous.
5. Characteristics of the accessible population should be considered when creating recruitment materials.

How did you do? 1. F; 2. T; 3. F; 4. F; 5. T

11.4 Keeping It Ethical

At the end of this section, you will be able to:

< Describe ethical considerations related to sampling

Individuals who participate in research have fundamental rights that must be protected. The American Nurses Association (ANA) code of ethics and human rights guidelines direct researchers to protect the rights of each and every subject (ANA, 2001). The ANA code addresses five human rights that mandate protection when conducting research. These rights include the right to anonymity and/or confidentiality, the right to self-determination, the right to privacy, the right to fair treatment, and the right to protection from discomfort and harm.

Researchers have a responsibility to protect all subjects, especially those who are considered to be in a *vulnerable population*. Children, pregnant women, the unborn, frail elderly, prisoners, and individuals with some level of mental incapacity are considered to be members of vulnerable populations. In some situations, factors such as ethnicity, gender, socioeconomic status, education, and language may create potential vulnerability for certain subjects (Polit & Beck, 2014).

To ensure subject protection, researchers maintain *anonymity* and *confidentiality*. Anonymity means keeping the names of the subjects separated from the data so that no one, not even the researcher, knows their identities. In some studies, it is not possible for subjects to remain anonymous. In these situations, confidentiality must be protected. Confidentiality refers to protecting subjects' identities. One way identities are protected is to keep a master list with the names of subjects and the codes assigned to the data collected. The list is locked away from other data and destroyed after all data are collected. The principal researcher or designee should be the only person who has the list of names and code numbers. Another way to ensure confidentiality is by reporting results as group data, not as individual data. Actions such as these are in accordance with the ANA code of ethics and human rights guidelines (ANA, 2001), as well as the Health Insurance Portability and Accountability Act (HIPAA) guidelines.

Another major responsibility of researchers is maintaining subjects' rights to self-determination by obtaining *informed consent*. Prior to beginning a research study, institutional review board (IRB) approval must be obtained. This board consists of individuals who review research proposals to ensure that research is conducted in an ethical manner and that the rights of subjects are not violated. The IRB pays particular attention to the process of informed consent and ensures that mandatory content is included in consent forms. See **Box 11-2** for a list of essential components of consent forms.

Subjects must be informed that they may choose to participate or not participate in the study and that they may withdraw at any time without harm or consequences. There must be a clear and concise explanation of the study and what subjects will be asked to do in the study. There should also be a discussion of the potential benefits and risks of participation in the study. If there are monetary benefits, there must be a description of the amount of money participants will receive and what is required to receive that monetary amount.

KEY TERMS

vulnerable population: A special group of people needing protection because of members' limited ability to provide informed consent or because of their risk for coercion

anonymity: Keeping the names of subjects separate from data so that no one, not even the researcher, knows subjects' identities; concealing the identity of subjects, even from the researcher

confidentiality: The protection of subjects' identities from everyone except the researcher

informed consent: An ethical practice requiring researchers to obtain voluntary participation by subjects after subjects have been informed of possible risks and benefits

CRITICAL THINKING EXERCISE 11-4

Check out the Health Insurance Portability and Accountability Act (HIPAA) regulations at http://www.hhs.gov/ocr/privacy/hipaa/understanding/index.html. How do these guidelines provide direction to researchers about protecting confidentiality of subjects?

BOX 11-2	Mandatory Components of Consent Forms

Title of study
Invitation to participate in the research study
Participation is voluntary
Basis for subject selection
Purpose of study
Explanation of procedures
Benefits and risks
Alternatives to participation
Financial obligations/compensation
Confidentiality assurance
HIPAA disclosure
Subject withdrawal without penalty or consequences
Offer to answer questions
Consent statement
Identification of researchers

Modified from U.S. Department of Health and Human Services. (2009). Code of Federal Regulations. Title 45: Public welfare. Part 46: Protection of human subjects. Retrieved from http://www.hhs.gov/ohrp/humansubjects/guidance/45cfr46.html

FYI

When inviting subjects to participate in studies, researchers must obtain informed consent, with particular regard for vulnerable populations. With children, nurses should obtain assent. Nurses should also maintain anonymity and confidentiality as well as avoid coercion when sampling.

If there are risks to subjects, those risks must be clearly detailed and include any physical, emotional, spiritual, economic, social, or legal risks.

There are other factors to consider when obtaining informed consent. Informed consents should be written in simple language. If subjects cannot read, forms should be read to potential subjects. For subjects who speak English as a second language, consent forms should be read by an interpreter or written in the subjects' native language. Subjects should have sufficient time to carefully think about whether or not to participate. Both subjects and researchers must sign consent forms after researchers assure subjects that participation is voluntary. Consent forms should not be kept with data; this protects subjects' confidentiality. A copy of the signed form should also be given to subjects.

There can be some unique circumstances for obtaining informed consent. For example, if there is minimal risk associated with participation in the study, the IRB may not require the signing of consent forms. Rather, it may be required that a statement indicating that completion and submission of the survey imply that the subject is giving informed consent. With vulnerable populations, the researcher needs to have clearly stated guidelines as to how the informed consent will be obtained (Polit & Beck, 2014).

One reason that considerable attention is given to the process of obtaining informed consent is that it is unethical for subjects to feel coerced into participating in research. *Coercion* is the threat of harm or the offer of an excessive reward with the intent to force an individual to participate in a research study. Healthcare providers must be extremely careful when conducting clinical research to ensure that patients do not feel coerced into participating in studies. Patients may feel particularly vulnerable if they decline participation because they may fear that treatment may be withheld (Polit & Beck, 2014). Coercion can also be a factor in studies involving nursing education. Faculty who conduct research involving nursing students must be careful that students do not feel coerced into participating and must recognize the power faculty has over students when assigning grades.

Children, because they are minors, cannot give consent to participate in research; however, researchers are obligated to obtain *assent* when possible. Children may have difficulty understanding what a study involves, and they may agree to participate to please adults. Typically, children 7 years of age and older must give oral assent, while children 12 years and older must sign an assent form. Regardless of the age, parents or legal guardians must sign consent forms.

Despite the importance placed on adherence to IRB guidelines and informed consent, there usually is little discussion about the process used to ensure that subjects' rights were not violated. In research articles, authors typically state that IRB approval was obtained and that the rights of subjects were protected. When such a statement is made, nurses can assume that ethical principles were upheld.

Sampling methods and how subjects are selected and protected through the IRB process are critical components in nursing research. The nurse evaluating nursing research for best evidence to influence clinical practice must understand the implications of the entire research process.

KEY TERMS

coercion: The threat of harm or the offer of an excessive reward with the intent to force an individual to participate in a research study

assent: Permission given by children to participate in research

---

TEST YOUR KNOWLEDGE 11-4

Indicate whether the following actions are ethical or unethical.

1. Allowing a subject who does not speak English to sign a consent form without providing an interpreter.
2. Allowing a nursing administrator to see group data from surveys conducted in the organization.
3. Keeping a folder for every subject that contains a signed consent form and raw data.
4. Providing subjects with money to reimburse their travel expenses to the data collection site.
5. Promising health care for life to individuals if they choose to participate in a study.

How did you do? 1. Unethical; 2. Ethical; 3. Unethical; 4. Ethical; 5. Unethical

Apply What You Have Learned

As your EBP committee has progressed in its assignment to identify strategies to improve hand hygiene compliance, you have been challenged to apply research principles for the purpose of establishing best practices. The next step is to review your articles, paying particular attention to details about the sample. Fill in the column for population on your grid by including details such as sample characteristics, sampling method, and size. Consult the examples already done.

RAPID REVIEW

» Sampling methods are determined by the research purpose and the research design.

» There are two major types of sampling: probability and nonprobability.

» Probability sampling and selected nonprobability sampling are used in quantitative research. Fundamental to probability sampling, but not nonprobability sampling, is random selection of subjects.

» Probability sampling methods include simple random sampling, stratified random sampling, cluster sampling, and systematic random sampling.

» Nonprobability sampling methods include convenience sampling, quota sampling, purposive sampling, and theoretical sampling.

» In quantitative research, the goal of sampling is to select a representative sample by identifying subjects that reflect the same characteristics as the population.

» The more representative the sample, the more confidence there is generalizing to the population.

» Nonprobability sampling is used in qualitative research.

» Sample size is determined by homogeneity of the population, purpose of the study, attrition rate, design, number of variables being investigated, and the sensitivity of instruments used.

» Power analysis is used to calculate the minimal number of subjects required in a quantitative study.

» Sample size for qualitative research continues until saturation is achieved.

» When making decisions about EBP, critical appraisal of the sampling method and sample size is desirable.

» Researchers must attend to many factors to ensure that the rights of subjects are protected. Researchers must ensure that informed consent is obtained and that individuals choose freely, without coercion, to participate in studies.

» Vulnerable populations must be especially protected by researchers.

REFERENCES

Albert, N., O'Connor, P., & Buelow, J. (2012). How many subjects do I need in my research sample? *Clinical Nurse Specialist, 26*(2), 302–304.

American Nurses Association. (2001). *Code of ethics for nurses with interpretative statements*. Washington, DC: Author.

Bloom, K. C., & Trice, L. B. (2011). Sampling. In C. Boswell & S. Cannon (Eds.), *Introduction to nursing research: Incorporating evidence-based practice* (2nd ed., pp. 145–163). Sudbury, MA: Jones & Bartlett Learning.

Fawcett, J., & Garity, J. (2009). *Evaluating research for evidence-based nursing practice*. Philadelphia, PA: F. A. Davis.

Graff, J. C. (2014). Mixed methods research. In H. Hall & L. Roussel (Eds.), *Evidence-based practice: An integrative approach to research, administration, and practice* (pp. 45–64). Burlington, MA: Jones & Bartlett Learning.

Gray, J., Grove, S., & Sutherland, S. (2016). *Burns and Grove's the practice of nursing research: Appraisal, synthesis, and generation of evidence* (8th ed.). St. Louis, MO: Saunders.

Hall, H., & Roussel, L. (2014). Interdisciplinary collaboration and the integration of evidence-based practice. In H. Hall & L. Roussel (Eds.), *Evidence-based practice: An integrative approach to research, administration, and practice* (pp. xxi–xxvi). Burlington, MA: Jones & Bartlett Learning.

Hayat, M. (2013). Understanding sample size determination in nursing research. *Western Journal of Nursing Research, 35*(7), 943–956.

Hopp, L. (2012). Professional nursing and evidence-based practice. In L. Hopp & L. Rittenmeyer (Eds.), *Introduction to evidence-based practice: A practical guide for nursing* (pp. 2–11). Philadelphia, PA: F. A. Davis.

Houser, J. (2011). *Nursing research: Reading, using and creating evidence*. Sudbury, MA: Jones & Bartlett Learning.

Leeman, J., & Sandelowski, M. (2012). Practice-based evidence and qualitative inquiry. *Journal of Nursing Scholarship, 44*(2), 171–179.

Melnyk, B. M., & Cole, R. (2011). Generating evidence through quantitative research. In B. Melnyk & E. Fineout-Overholt (Eds.), *Evidence-based practice in nursing and healthcare* (2nd ed., pp. 397–434). Philadelphia, PA: Lippincott Williams & Wilkins.

Polit, D., & Beck, C. T. (2014). *Essentials of nursing research: Appraising evidence for nursing practice*. Philadelphia, PA: Lippincott Williams & Wilkins.

Stevens, K. (2011). Critically appraising knowledge for clinical decision making. In B. Melnyk & E. Fineout-Overholt (Eds.), *Evidence-based practice in nursing and healthcare* (2nd ed., pp. 73–80). Philadelphia, PA: Lippincott Williams & Wilkins.

U.S. Department of Health and Human Services. (2009). Code of Federal Regulations. Title 45: Public welfare. Part 46: Protection of human subjects. Retrieved from http://www.hhs.gov/ohrp/humansubjects/guidance/45cfr46.html

CHAPTER OBJECTIVES

At the end of this chapter, you will be able to:

< List the 5 Ss
< Discuss the types and purposes of other sources of evidence
< List interdisciplinary databases that can provide evidence for practice
< Use the 5 Ss to locate evidence in a logical fashion
< Discuss one ethical dilemma when using other sources of evidence

KEY TERMS

case studies
concept analyses
integrative review
meta-analysis
meta-synthesis
nonpropositional
    knowledge

practice guidelines
propositional knowledge
studies
summaries
synopses
syntheses
systematic review

systems
traditional literature
    review

CHAPTER 12

Other Sources of Evidence

Cynthia L. Russell

12.1 The Pyramid of the 5 Ss

At the end of this section, you will be able to:

‹ List the 5 Ss
‹ Discuss the types and purposes of other sources of evidence

Nursing is both an art and a science. We learn and practice nursing by using both propositional knowledge and nonpropositional knowledge. *Propositional knowledge* is the science of nursing, or knowledge that is "formal, explicit, derived from research and scholarship and concerned with generalisability" (Rycroft-Malone et al., 2004, p. 83). For example, the knowledge we gain from research studies is propositional knowledge. *Nonpropositional knowledge* is the art of nursing, or knowledge that is "informal, implicit and derived primarily through practice" (Rycroft-Malone et al., 2004, p. 83). When we learn to prepare adhesive tape before dressing a wound, we are gaining nonpropositional knowledge. Both of these ways of knowing must come from many sources, be critically evaluated by experts, and be integrated into the evidence that guides nursing practice.

An organizing framework to explain the importance and contribution of various levels of information to evidence-based healthcare delivery has been developed (Haynes, 2006). The framework is organized in a pyramid with five levels, including *studies*, *syntheses*, *synopses*, *summaries*, and *systems* (see **Figure 12-1**). These levels are known as the 5 Ss (Haynes, 2006). Research studies form the base of the pyramid. The use

propositional knowledge: The science of nursing or knowledge that is obtained from research and scholarship

nonpropositional knowledge: The art of nursing or knowledge that is obtained through practice

studies: A level in the pyramid of the 5 Ss that contains quantitative and qualitative studies, case studies, and concept analyses

syntheses: A level in the pyramid of the 5 Ss containing evidence to present a whole depiction of a phenomenon

synopses: A level in the pyramid of the 5 Ss containing brief descriptions of evidence

summaries: A level in the pyramid of the 5 Ss containing detailed descriptions of evidence

systems: A level in the pyramid of the 5 Ss involving electronic medical records integrated with practice guidelines

FIGURE 12-1 The Pyramid of the 5 Ss

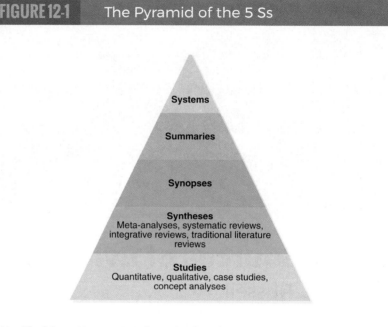

Modified from Haynes, R. B. (2006). Of studies, syntheses, synopses, summaries, and systems: The "5 S" evolution of information services for evidence-based health care decisions [Editorial]. *ACP Journal, 145*(3), A8.

of research studies (i.e.: RCTs, correlational, qualitative) as sources of evidence has been presented previously. Additional types of evidence that form this bottom layer of the pyramid include *case studies* and *concept analyses*. Haynes identifies other layers of the information pyramid moving upward. These levels are syntheses or systematic reviews, synopses or brief evidence-based journal abstracts, summaries such as evidence-based textbooks, and finally systems such as computerized decision support systems.

The First S: Studies

The case study report contributes to nursing's body of knowledge; it can expand and generalize theory, represent a typical case, and provide great detail about a phenomenon for which little information is known (Yin, 2013). A case study enhances our understanding of clinical care and clinical decision making, specifically the process of care for a particular case (Aitken & Marshall, 2007).

Yin (2013) notes that a case study "is an empirical inquiry that investigates a contemporary phenomenon within its real-life context, especially when the boundaries between the phenomenon and context are not clearly evident" (p. 13). Sandelowski (2011) provides an expanded definition, stating that "case studies are singular combinations of diverse arrays of methodological approaches directed toward maintaining empirical intimacy with the one or more temporally and spatially defined objects researchers construct and target for study" (p. 153). What does this mean? In nursing, case studies are frequently used to report the story of one patient, including details such as diagnosis, nursing care, and influential environmental factors. Articles about quality improvement projects are also considered case studies. The case study report provides enough detail so that the reader feels informed about that particular situation.

The case study approach, which originated from sociology, informs nurses about phenomena through the information that it provides. Case studies can be exploratory, but they are typically descriptive or explanatory and answer research questions that ask "how" or "why" (Yin, 2013). The selection of a case or cases for study is based on the cases' representativeness of a particular situation. Cases may also be selected for their potential to describe or explain a theory.

Case studies involve direct observation of the situation and are best used as a research approach when studying events that are currently happening and when the researcher has little or no control over these events. Yin (2013) notes that "the case study's unique strength is its ability to deal with a full variety of evidence—documents, artifacts, interviews, and observations" (p. 8). A case study typically includes an introduction that focuses on the area of clinical practice and provides a review of the literature about the current knowledge in the area (Aitken & Marshall, 2007). The introduction can also present a description about a unique case and include information such as history, care, and outcomes. Aitken and Marshall note "the discussion should provide a critique of the care in the context of the known literature, including commentary on care that was not effective and exploration of possible reasons for this" (p. 132). Implications for practice and recommendations for future research should be included.

Just like for research studies, the merit of the case study must be evaluated to determine its contribution to the evidence. **Box 12-1** lists criteria for evaluating a case study. Although the findings from case studies are not regarded as highly as findings from research studies are, in some instances case study findings can provide insight and understanding when little evidence is available, thus contributing to the body of knowledge in a specific clinical area. For example, when a novel innovation is implemented, a case study may be the only published information about the innovation.

Other sources of evidence in the first S of the pyramid are concept analyses. Rogers and Knafl (2000) defined concepts as being "formed by the identification of characteristics common to a class of objects or phenomena and the abstraction and clustering of these characteristics, along with some means of expression (most often a word)" (p. 78). For example, pain is an important concept in patient

KEY TERMS

case studies: A description of a single or novel event; a unique methodology used in qualitative research that may also be considered a design or strategy for data collection

concept analyses: Scholarly papers that explore the attributes and characteristics of a concept

BOX 12-1	Criteria for Evaluating a Case Study

Does the introduction focus on a specific area of practice?

Is the purpose of the case study appropriate?

Does the background literature clearly indicate a literature gap that this case study fills?

Are multiple sources of evidence from the literature included?

If appropriate, is a theoretical framework presented for the case study?

Is the case history presented clearly?

Is the process of clinical care clearly described?

Are outcomes identified?

Are all appropriate history, process, and outcome elements included?

Does the discussion address the case in the context of what is known, offering rationale for successful and unsuccessful outcomes?

Are appropriate implications for practice provided?

Are specific suggestions for future research delineated?

Is the case study presented clearly?

Is the case study presented logically?

CRITICAL THINKING EXERCISE 12-1

Consider the last time that you read a case study. How did the study enhance your understanding of the situation? How did the case study strengthen your theory about an issue? How did it clarify clinical processes and outcomes for you?

care. One way to define pain is an uncomfortable feeling, but this definition is problematic because it is too broad and other concepts, such as itching, could be defined the same way. Therefore, concepts must be described, understood, and communicated so they can be used for building theory (Risjord, 2009).

Concept analyses provide for the exploration of the attributes and characteristics of a concept (Walker & Avant, 2010). Specific steps for concept analyses have been described (Walker & Avant, 2010). Understanding these steps can assist nurses in evaluating concept analyses for application to theories and evidence-based practice (EBP). The author of the concept analysis should begin by clearly stating the aims of the analysis. The contribution of the concept analysis to research and practice should be clearly described. Assumptions made about the concept may also be presented and may assist in understanding

FYI

The pyramid of the 5 Ss is an organizing framework explaining the importance and contribution of various levels of information to evidence-based healthcare delivery. The 5 Ss are: studies, syntheses, synopses, summaries, and systems.

CRITICAL THINKING EXERCISE 12-2

Read a concept analysis article on a concept that is of interest to you. How does the report increase your understanding of the concept? Describe how the concept analysis report helped you clarify the "edges" of the concept.

the perspective of the author's analysis. Possible uses of the concept should be presented, including definitions and descriptions found in all types of literature. Related and interchangeable concepts may also be described. This further assists in clarifying the concept being studied. After this, the author can state specific characteristics of the concept, known as defining attributes. Antecedents, or conditions that must precede the concept, are also presented. For example, a person must have functioning neurons to feel pain. Next, the consequences, or outcomes, of the concept should be discussed.

The most interesting part of the concept analysis is the presentation of various cases. In the pain example, one case describes pain, another may describe itching, and yet another may describe pleasure. These cases represent, almost represent, and do not represent the concept. Critiquing the rigor with which the author has approached the concept analysis report is of utmost importance in determining the contribution of the report to evidence. When the author has carefully and thoughtfully followed the concept analysis steps, the results and implications for practice and research can contribute to the development of evidence.

Although qualitative findings are considered lower-level evidence, they do provide the patient perspective for EBP. *Meta-synthesis* is the analysis of a group of qualitative studies. Finfgeld (2003) noted the goal is "to produce a new and integrative interpretation of findings that is more substantive than those resulting from individual investigations" (p. 894). Meta-synthesis involves breaking down findings, examining them, discovering essential features, and finally transforming the essential features into a new, integrated whole.

The Second S: Syntheses

Syntheses integrate various pieces of evidence to present a whole depiction of a phenomenon. A *systematic review* is a common type of synthesis found in nursing. It is a rigorously conducted process of obtaining and reviewing the literature to answer pre-established theoretical or practice questions. The word *systematic* is the key to understanding the nature and intent of a systematic review. According to the *Encarta* dictionary, *systematic* means "done methodically or carried out in a methodological and organized manner."

FYI

Within the 5 Ss are several types of evidence, including case studies, concept analyses, meta-syntheses, systematic reviews, traditional literature reviews, integrative reviews, meta-analyses, practice guidelines, and abstracts.

KEY TERMS

meta-synthesis: A systematic review that contains only qualitative studies; a scholarly paper that combines results from qualitative studies

systematic review: A rigorous and systematic synthesis of research findings about a clinical problem

The Cochrane Library (2017) stated, "A systematic review attempts to identify, appraise and synthesize all the empirical evidence that meets prespecified eligibility criteria to answer a given research question." A systematic review of the literature includes both a systematic approach to obtaining the literature and a systematic approach to conducting the review of the literature after it is obtained. "Researchers conducting systematic reviews use explicit methods aimed at minimizing bias, in order to produce more reliable findings that can be used to inform decision making" (Cochrane Library, 2017).

Understanding the critical steps to these processes assists in evaluating the quality of a systematic review. The Cochrane Library offers specific guidelines for conducting systematic reviews. There are three types of Cochrane systematic reviews: (1) intervention reviews to assess the benefits and harms of interventions used in health care and health policy, (2) diagnostic test accuracy reviews to assess how well a diagnostic test performs in diagnosing and detecting a particular disease, and (3) methodology reviews to address issues relevant to how systematic reviews and clinical trials are conducted and reported. The *Cochrane Handbook for Systematic Reviews of Interventions* and the *Cochrane Handbook for Diagnostic Test Accuracy Reviews* offer specific guidance for these reviews.

Before beginning the systematic review process, the author of the review clarifies the problem and the questions to be answered (Cochrane Library, 2017; Cooper, 1998). Questions that can be answered by a systematic review include: What is the state of the theoretical knowledge in this area? What are the methodological gaps in the current studies? What is the impact of interventions on patient outcomes from these studies? What should be the focus of the next research study? and How are two bodies of literature related or unrelated? Because the systematic review can assist in answering many types of questions, the author must define what variables and/or concepts are important to the problem or question. Furthermore, the author may also identify the relationships between variables if these relationships are important to the problem being investigated.

The author must decide what kinds of studies to include in the systematic review. Therefore, inclusion and exclusion criteria must be established based on the problem and question to be answered. For example, if the question relates to a particular age group, then research reports that include only that particular age group would be included in the systematic review. If studies with a particular design are the target—for example, a randomized controlled trial—then only reports with this design would be included. The inclusion and exclusion criteria must logically flow from the problem and questions.

After the problem and question to be answered by the systematic review are clarified and the inclusion and exclusion criteria are identified, the author obtains relevant literature (Cooper, 1998). This begins the data collection phase of the systematic review. Through an exhaustive process, both published and unpublished literature is sought for the review. Because most published studies have significant findings, including unpublished literature helps to decrease bias. Computerized databases are searched, including *Cumulative Index to Nursing and Allied Health Literature* (CINAHL), MEDLINE, Psyc INFO, Health-STAR, the Cochrane Library, Google Scholar, and Dissertation Abstracts Online. Keywords are used to query the databases. Additional computerized databases may also be used, depending on the selected topic. For example, if the author were conducting a systematic review on a topic related to geriatric nursing, the Age Line Database would be included.

The author of the review should consult with expert health science information specialists during the search. These specialists can locate more studies than less experienced researchers can (Conn, Valentine, Cooper, & Rantz, 2003; Cook, Guyatt, & Ryan, 1993). The author must also search for additional published literature through the ancestry approach. This strategy is completed when the reference lists of articles are carefully reviewed for any additional articles that are pertinent to the review. Hand searches of journals in which other eligible articles have been found should also be completed. Locating all pertinent research reports is critical to enhancing external validity of the systematic review. External validity is the ability to generalize the findings from a study, in this case a systematic review, to another situation (e.g., clinical practice).

The next phase of the systematic review involves evaluation of the literature (Cooper, 1998). Each piece of literature can be conceptualized as a subject, much like a subject in primary research. Each piece of literature is evaluated for its contribution to the problem and posed questions. A typical approach for data evaluation involves a data collection tool similar to the grid within this text's digital resources that you are developing in the Apply What You Have Learned exercise. A table such as this is often created, where each evaluation criterion is listed and data that are extracted from each report are placed into the format. Depending on the question to be answered by the systematic review, data evaluation may include gathering author, year, study purpose, research question/hypothesis, variables studied, sample size, sample age, setting, research design, research instruments used to measure each variable, instrument psychometrics, procedures used for data collection, and study results.

The next phase of the systematic review process is data (Cooper, 1998). This stage is defined as "reducing the separate data collection points collected by the inquirer into a unified statement about the research problem" (Cooper, 1998, p. 104). The goal of the systematic review determines the data analysis approach used. On one hand, reviews of concepts, definitions, and methods are best summarized qualitatively. On the other hand, if the body of reports

KEY TERMS

traditional literature review: Article based on common or uncommon elements of works with little concern for research methods, designs, or settings; narrative literature review

integrative review: A scholarly paper that synthesizes published studies to answer questions about phenomena of interest

meta-analysis: A scholarly paper that combines results of studies, both published and unpublished, into a measurable format and statistically estimates the effects of proposed interventions

is still relatively small and quantitative results are reported, then descriptive statistics can be applied to the group of studies.

The final step of the systematic review is interpretation of the data and dissemination of the results (Cooper, 1998). The stated results should flow logically from the data presented in the systematic review. The problem and research questions should be answered from the data. Systematic reviews are written using a format similar to that used in primary research reports, including the introduction, methods, results, and discussion. Most often a table of the data collected from each study is included in the systematic review article.

There are two additional types of syntheses that are less rigorous than systematic reviews. These include the *traditional literature review* and the *integrative review*. A traditional literature review differs from a systematic review because when a literature review is conducted, the author typically does not go to the extreme lengths of obtaining all possible literature on a topic. When conducting a traditional literature review, the author may include only literature that supports a particular point, excluding reports that have conflicting findings. Nurses are very familiar with the traditional literature review because this is the type of paper they wrote for many of their nursing courses.

Integrative reviews are more rigorous than traditional literature reviews, but they are less rigorous compared to systematic reviews. Authors of integrative reviews seek only published reports, whereas systematic reviewers use a more rigorous method of obtaining both published and unpublished reports. Authors follow very methodical approaches for both types of reviews. Because the scope of integrative reviews is narrower, the findings are less likely to have external validity than are the findings from a systematic review.

When the body of reports is large and homogenous, a *meta-analysis* can be conducted. Meta-analysis is a statistical procedure that involves quantitatively pooling data from a group of independent studies that have studied the same or similar clinical problems using the same or similar research methods (Cooper, Hedges, & Valentine, 2009). A pooled estimate of effect, called effect size (ES), and a confidence interval (CI) are calculated. Effect size estimates the strength of the relationship between two variables, and a confidence interval shows the

CRITICAL THINKING EXERCISE 12-3

Locate a systematic review of the literature that addresses a topic pertinent to your patients. Evaluate the rigor of the study using the information presented in Box 12-1. How will you use the results of the systematic review to enhance the evidence that you use to provide the best care possible?

reliability of the estimate, in this case, effect size (Cooper et al., 2009). Due to the sophisticated analysis, a meta-analysis is considered to be a very high level of evidence.

Network meta-analysis, also known as multiple treatments meta-analysis or mixed treatment comparison meta-analysis, is a method used to assess the comparative effectiveness of experimental treatment among similar patient populations that have not been compared directly in a randomized clinical trial. Unlike traditional meta-analyses, which summarize the results of trials that have evaluated the same treatment/placebo combination, network meta-analyses compare the results from two or more studies that have one treatment in common (Bafeta, Trinquart, Seror, & Ravaud, 2013; Cipriani, Higgins, Geddes, & Salanti, 2013; Lumley, 2002). Unlike the systematic review, the author obtains both published and unpublished evidence. Authors may even contact researchers for their data to perform the analysis. Meta-analyses are critical because information may be used to guide clinical practice decision making and direct the development of future research strategies (Moore, 2012).

The Preferred Reporting Items for Systematic Reviews and Meta-Analyses (PRISMA) guidelines were created to help authors improve the reporting of systematic reviews and meta-analyses (Moher, Liberati, Tetzlaff, & Altman, 2009). PRISMA consists of a 27-item checklist and a flow diagram. For each checklist item, this document contains an example of good reporting, a rationale for its inclusion, and supporting evidence, including references, whenever possible.

In nursing and other practice disciplines, an important kind of synthesis is *practice guidelines*. They are "systematically developed statements to assist practitioner and patient decisions about appropriate health care for specific clinical circumstances" (Institute of Medicine [IOM], 1990, p. 8). These guidelines are systematically created by a group of experienced experts and key affected persons who read, critique, and prioritize the pertinent evidence. Practice guidelines have been introduced into practice for several reasons. These consensus recommendations are developed for use in practice to improve patient and system outcomes. These tools seek to reduce variations in practice, resulting in more consistent care delivery by those who use the guidelines. Guidelines also enhance efficient use of resources, which frequently results in reducing the cost of care delivery. Guidelines should have the following characteristics (IOM, 2011):

> » "be based on a systematic review of the existing evidence;
> » be developed by a knowledgeable, multidisciplinary panel of experts and representatives from key affected groups;

KEY TERM

practice guidelines: Systematically developed statements to assist healthcare providers with making appropriate decisions about health care for specific clinical circumstances

> **CRITICAL THINKING EXERCISE 12-4**
>
> Locate a nursing clinical guideline and explore the process that was used to develop the guideline. How do you think the guideline changes practice patterns?

» consider important patient subgroups and patient preferences, as appropriate;

» be based on an explicit and transparent process that minimizes distortions, biases, and conflicts of interest;

» provide a clear explanation of the logical relationships between alternative care options and health outcomes, and provide ratings of both the quality of evidence and the strength of the recommendations; and

» be reconsidered and revised as appropriate when important new evidence warrants modifications of recommendations." (p. 3)

Nursing practice guidelines can be found at the Registered Nurses' Association of Ontario Nursing Best Practice Guidelines Program (http://www.rnao .org), the National Guideline Clearinghouse (http://www.guideline.gov), and the Royal College of Nursing (http://www.rcn.org.uk). Clinical practice guidelines may also be written and made available to educate and enhance decision making for the public. The guidelines can be very helpful to the layperson who is faced with making choices about health care.

Understanding the process of clinical practice guideline development can assist nurses in evaluating the merit of clinical practice guidelines. Depending on the area of practice, the team of experts may be multidisciplinary in nature. Guidelines are typically focused on patient problems that involve many disciplines working toward similar patient goals. Practice guidelines may be created locally, nationally, or internationally. Often they are developed by professional organizations or federal agencies. Examples include the Gerontological Nursing Interventions Research Center (http://www.nursing .uiowa.edu/excellence/evidence-based-practice-guidelines), the Association of Women's Health, Obstetric and Neonatal Nurses (http://www.awhonn.org /awhonn/), the American Pain Society (http://americanpainsociety.org/), and the Oncology Nursing Society (http://www.ons.org). Systematic reviews of the literature are frequently used to assist a group of experts with integrating the larger body of literature pertinent to the practice guideline development. If current systematic reviews of the literature are not available, the experts must use the rigorous systematic review process for assimilating the body of literature to create practice guidelines.

As new evidence is generated from primary research reports, systematic reviews of the literature and practice guidelines must be revised and updated. The Agency for Healthcare Research and Quality (AHRQ, 2014) has developed a series of questions that can be used to guide systematic review updates. As the number of guidelines has increased, guideline syntheses are

> systematic comparisons of selected guidelines that address similar topic areas. Key elements of each synthesis include a discussion of areas of agreement and difference, the major recommendations, the corresponding strength of evidence and recommendation rating schemes, and a comparison of guideline methodologies. Also included are the benefits/harms of implementing the guideline recommendations and any associated contraindications. (AHRQ, 2017)

The Third S: Synopses

A synopsis is a brief description of evidence, typically presented in a paragraph. Abstracts obtained through CINAHL and MEDLINE are essentially synopses. A variety of evidence-based journals have emerged that provide synopses of valid and clinically useful studies (DiCenso et al., 2005; Melnyk & Fineout-Overholt, 2015; Straus, Glasziou, Richardson, & Haynes, 2011). Although most of these require subscriptions, many websites allow guests access to some full-text articles.

The Fourth S: Summaries

Integrative summaries are addressed in the fourth level of the pyramid of the 5 Ss (Haynes, 2006). For example, the "Evidence Summaries" and "Recommended Practices" are available at Johanna Briggs Institute (JBI) and fit in this level. Evidence is presented in a succinct, easy-to-read format in two to three pages. This format allows nurses to review evidence about best practices quickly, which can be an advantage when caring for patients. Other source of summaries can be found at BMJ Clinical Evidence (http://www.clinicalevidence.com/ceweb/index.jsp), the AHRQ's National Guideline Clearinghouse (http://www.guideline.gov), and Physicians' Information and Education Resource (American College of Physicians, 2017; Haynes, 2006).

The Fifth S: Systems

If you deliver nursing care in a healthcare organization that has an integrated computerized decision support system, such as Epic, you have the system in place to implement evidence-based care (Haynes, 2006; Epic, 2017). This system model uses an electronic medical record that has integrated practice guidelines that provide alerts to healthcare providers. This makes it easier for healthcare providers to follow guidelines, because it can be challenging to keep up with the volume of new and revised guidelines (Epic, 2017). Many healthcare organizations have or are implementing this technology. As technology advances, the ability to link other types of evidence to electronic medical records will improve.

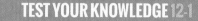

12.2 Using the Pyramid of the 5 Ss for Evidence-Based Practice

At the end of this section, you will be able to:

< List interdisciplinary databases that can provide evidence for practice
< Use the 5 Ss to locate evidence in a logical fashion

FYI

Because the purpose of EBP is to answer clinical questions, and the goal is to efficiently find information, nurses should begin the search for information at the top of the pyramid and work down the various levels. The best option is having a system already in place that brings the information to the medical record.

FYI

Fortunately, few ethical dilemmas arise when considering use of evidence. When nurses find evidence that can be applied to practice, they must consider changes carefully because lives are at stake; however, it is unethical *not* to adopt practice guidelines when the evidence is clear.

Because the purpose of EBP is to answer clinical questions, and the goal is to efficiently find information, nurses should begin the search for information at the top of the pyramid and work down the various levels. The best option is having a system already in place that brings the information to the nurse. However, because such systems are not very common, the next best source of evidence is integrative summaries. If you are unable to locate summaries of the evidence, you should attempt to locate synopses of the evidence in *Evidence-Based Nursing* (http://ebn.bmjjournals.com) or another selected evidence-based journal. If you are unable to find what you need there, you should look for systematic and other types of reviews of the literature. The Cochrane Library (http://www.cochrane.org) is a good place to begin. When none of these are available, you must rely on individual studies, case studies, and concept analyses. **Box 12-2** presents a multidisciplinary list of online resources that can assist in accessing all levels of evidence.

BOX 12-2   Databases to Search for Evidence

Agency for Healthcare Research and Quality (AHRQ)

http://www.ahrq.gov

AHRQ works with 12 Evidence-Based Practice Centers that develop evidence reports and technology assessments on topics relevant to clinical, social science/behavioral, economic, and other healthcare organization and delivery topics. Professional societies, health plans, insurers, employers, and patient groups can nominate topics. AHRQ sponsors a National Guideline Clearinghouse at http://www.guideline .gov.

American College of Physicians DynaMed Plus

https://www.acponline.org/clinical-information/clinical-resources-products/dynamed-plus

DynaMed Plus provides evidence-based guidance to improve clinical care. Topics include diseases, screening and prevention, complementary/alternative medicine, ethical/legal issues, procedures, quality measures, and drug resources.

BMJ Clinical Evidence

http://www.clinicalevidence.com/ceweb/index.jsp

BMJ Clinical Evidence presents summaries that address common or important clinical conditions seen in primary and hospital care and benefits and harms of preventive and therapeutic interventions. A rigorous process of developing the summaries is described. Drug safety alerts and links to national guidelines are included.

DynaMed

http://www.dynamed.com/home/

DynaMed provides clinically organized summaries of nearly 1,800 evidence-based topics for use at the point of care via the Internet.

Evidence-Based Medicine

http://ebm.bmj.com/

Evidence-Based Medicine presents abstracts of international medical journals with commentary on its clinical application to primary medicine.

Evidence-Based Nursing

http://ebn.bmj.com/

Evidence-Based Nursing presents abstracts of selected research with an expert commentary on its clinical application.

(continued)

| **BOX 12-2** | Databases to Search for Evidence (continued) |

Health Services/Technology Assessment Texts

http://www.ncbi.nlm.nih.gov/books/NBK16710/

The Health Services/Technology Assessment Texts is a free, Web-based resource of full-text documents including guidelines that provide health information and support healthcare decision making for healthcare providers, health service researchers, policymakers, payers, consumers, and the information professionals who serve these groups.

Joanna Briggs Institute

http://www.joannabriggs.org/

The Joanna Briggs Institute is an International Research and Development Unit of Royal Adelaide Hospital and an Affiliated Institute of the University of Adelaide that supports the development and dissemination of international systematic reviews and summaries of best practices to consumers, healthcare professionals, and all levels of the healthcare systems, governments, and service provider units.

Physiotherapy Evidence Database

http://www.pedro.org.au/

PEDro is the Physiotherapy Evidence Database, which was developed to provide rapid access to bibliographic details and abstracts of randomized controlled trials, systematic reviews, and evidence-based clinical practice guidelines in physiotherapy.

Primary Care Clinical Practice Guidelines

http://medicine.ucsf.edu/education/resed/ebm/practice_guidelines.html

This site, compiled by the UCSF School of Medicine, includes links to guidelines from professional organizations.

SUM Search

http://sumsearch.org/

SUM Search provides references to answer clinical questions about diagnosis, etiology, prognosis, and therapy (plus physical findings, adverse treatment effects, and screening/prevention) by searching sources such as Merck Manual, MEDLINE, National Guideline Clearinghouse from AHRQ, Database of Abstracts of Reviews of Effects, and Pub Med.

The Cochrane Library

http://www.thecochranelibrary.com

The Cochrane Library provides systematic reviews related to clinical topics. The complete reviews are available by subscription, either on CD-ROM or via the Internet. Abstracts of the reviews are available on the website.

| BOX 12-2 | Databases to Search for Evidence (continued) |

The Guide to Community Preventive Services

http://www.thecommunityguide.org

The Guide to Community Preventive Services is a multidisciplinary, independent, nonfederal group that develops evidence-based practice guidelines for community preventive services.

UpToDate

http://www.uptodate.com/

UpToDate provides evidence-based clinical information to a variety of clinicians on the Internet.

U.S. Preventive Services Task Force (USPSTF)

https://www.uspreventiveservicestaskforce.org/

The U.S. Preventive Services Task Force systematically reviews the evidence of effectiveness of a wide range of clinical preventive services, including screening tests, counseling, immunizations, and chemoprophylaxis.

CRITICAL THINKING EXERCISE 12-5

Consider each of the types of evidence and how to locate each type. How will you integrate the use of these other sources of evidence into your practice?

TEST YOUR KNOWLEDGE 12-2

1. Put the following sources of evidence in order, beginning at the top of the pyramid of the 5 Ss.

    a. Synopses

    b. Systems

    c. Studies

    d. Summaries

    e. Syntheses

How did you do? 1. b, d, a, e, c

12.3 Keeping It Ethical

At the end of this section, you will be able to:

< Discuss one ethical dilemma when using other sources of evidence

Fortunately, few ethical dilemmas arise when considering use of evidence. Care must be taken to label evidence correctly and to be true to the process of review. Shortcuts should not be taken when searching for evidence, and attention to detail is critical. On occasion, an author might mislabel the type of review conducted because there are many commonalities. Authors sometimes generalize beyond the scope of the evidence or ignore limitations of studies (Gambrill, 2011). It is therefore important for nurses to critically read and be familiar with the various types of review to determine the usefulness of the findings. Gambrill noted that discretion must be used when choosing how to describe new ideas (e.g., accurately or in a distorted form) and that original (rather than secondary) sources must be read.

It is normal to become excited when finding evidence that can be applied to practice. Such enthusiasm makes providing nursing care stimulating. On one hand, practice changes must be considered carefully because lives are at stake. On the other hand, it is unethical not to adopt practice guidelines when the evidence is clear. Our nursing efforts must focus on providing the best care to achieve optimum patient outcomes, with the least variation in practice, in a resource-conscientious manner while integrating the evidence with patient preferences. Using other sources of evidence upon which to base your nursing practice enhances your abilities to achieve these goals.

TEST YOUR KNOWLEDGE 12-3

True/False

1. Nurses are ethically obligated to follow practice guidelines when evidence is clear.
2. Authors who publish their work in professional journals never draw conclusions beyond their findings.

How did you do? 1. T; 2. F

Apply What You Have Learned

Your committee has found three additional articles. They are not reports about research studies, yet they contain some very pertinent information about hand hygiene compliance.

The first piece of evidence is from the Joanna Briggs Institute. It is a summary of the evidence with a best practice recommendation. This evidence falls in the fourth level of the 5 Ss, making it a high level of evidence.

> Nguyen, P. (2016). Hand hygiene: Alcohol-based solutions. The Joanna Briggs Institute. Retrieved January 12, 2017, from http://ovidsp.tx.ovid.com.ezproxy.valpo.edu/sp-3.23.1b /ovidweb.cgi3.10.0b/ovidweb.cgi?&S=NJCIFPGFJODDKDEKNCNKIAOBGLKBAA00&Link +Set=S.sh.21%7c1%7csl_190

To obtain this, you will need to access JBI through your library's subscription. Once at the website, you can mark the title option and then enter the title "Hand Hygiene: Alcohol-Based Solutions" as shown here:

(continued)

Apply What You Have Learned *(continued)*

Once you have searched for the item, it will appear. To obtain the summary, click on the link "JBI Database PDF." The summary will open in a full-text mode.

The second item is a systematic review. Like the summary, this is considered a high level of evidence because it provides a critical analysis of multiple sources of evidence. This resource can be obtained by searching in PubMed, CINAHL, or Nursing and Allied Health Database. Use information in the citation to find this article quickly.

Kingston, L., O'Connell, N. H., & Dunne, C. P. (2016). Hand hygiene-related clinical trials reported since 2010: A systematic review. *The Journal of Hospital Infection, 92*, 309–320.

The third source of evidence obtained by the EBP committee comes from *The New York Times*. In this article, the author has also combined information from multiple sources, but this item is intended for lay people. Therefore, it is ranked low on the hierarchy of evidence; however, this does not mean that it cannot contribute to the body of evidence. This article is posted on the Web, and you can obtain it by entering the http website listed in the citation. Or, you can enter the phrase "you've been washing your hands wrong" into a search engine such as Google or Bing. Here is the citation:

Bromwich, J. E. (2016, April 20). You've been washing your hands wrong. *The New York Times*. Retrieved from https://www.nytimes.com/2016/04/21/health/washing-hands .html?_r=0

Read these articles and complete the grid for each of them. Be aware that because these are not studies, you may not have information to put in each of the columns. When this is the case, simply indicate "not applicable."

⚡ RAPID REVIEW

» Propositional knowledge is the science of nursing, and nonpropositional knowledge is the art of nursing.

» The pyramid of the 5 Ss is an organizing framework that explains the importance of various levels of evidence. It uses the 5 Ss: studies, syntheses, synopses, summaries, and systems.

» Syntheses include case studies, concept analyses, meta-synthesis systematic reviews, traditional literature reviews, integrative reviews, and meta-analyses.

» Case studies provide great detail about phenomena for which little is known.

» Concept analyses are an example of a synthesis. Nurses use them to clarify understanding about concepts that are important in patient care.

» Meta-syntheses combine the results of multiple qualitative studies about the same topic.

» Although all reviews require searching for evidence, the amount and kind of evidence included vary among the types of reviews.

» Practice guidelines are developed by experts who systematically review the literature and develop recommendations about patient care.

» Nurses can use synopses, summaries, and systems to efficiently obtain evidence for practice.

» To avoid ethical dilemmas, nurses must critically read and be familiar with the various types of review to determine the usefulness of the findings.

REFERENCES

Agency for Healthcare Research and Quality. (2014). Updating systematic reviews. Retrieved from https://www.ahrq.gov/research/findings/evidence-based-reports/sysreviews.html

Agency for Healthcare Research and Quality. (2017). National Guideline Clearinghouse: Guideline syntheses. Retrieved from http://www.guideline.gov/syntheses/index.aspx

Aitken, L. M., & Marshall, A. P. (2007). Writing a case study: Ensuring a meaningful contribution to the literature. *Australian Critical Care, 20*(4), 132–136. doi:10.1016/j.aucc.2007.08.002

American College of Physicians. (2017). Dynamed-plus: A benefit for ACP members. Retrieved from https://www.acponline.org/clinical-information/clinical-resources-products/dynamed-plus

Bafeta, A., Trinquart, L., Seror, R., & Ravaud, P. (2013). Analysis of the systematic reviews process in reports of network meta-analyses: Methodological systematic review. *British Medical Journal, 347*, f3675. doi:10.1136/bmj.f3675

Biron, A. D., Loiselle, C. G., & Lavoie-Tremblay, M. (2009). Work interruptions and their contribution to medication errors: An evidence review. *Worldviews on Evidence-Based Nursing, 6,* 70–86.

Cipriani, A., Higgins, J., Geddes, J. R., & Salanti, G. (2013). Conceptual and technical challenges in network meta-analysis. *Annals of Internal Medicine, 159*(2), 130–137. doi:10.7326/0003–4819–159–2–201307160–00008

Cochrane Library. (2017). About Cochrane systematic reviews and protocols. Retrieved from http://www.cochranelibrary.com/about/about-cochrane-systematic-reviews.html

Conn, V. S., Valentine, J. C., Cooper, H. M., & Rantz, M. J. (2003). Grey literature in meta-analyses. *Nursing Research, 52,* 256–261.

Cook, D. J., Guyatt, G. H., & Ryan, G. (1993). Should unpublished data be included in meta-analyses? *Journal of the American Medical Association, 269,* 749–753.

Cooper, H. M. (1998). *Synthesizing research: A guide for literature reviews* (3rd ed., Vol. 2). Thousand Oaks, CA: Sage.

Cooper, H., Hedges, L. V., & Valentine, J. C. (2009). *The handbook of research synthesis and meta-analysis* (2nd ed.). New York, NY: Russell Sage Foundation.

DiCenso, A., Ciliska, D., Marks, S., McKibbon, A., Cullum, N., & Thompson, C. (2005). Evidence-based nursing. In S. E. Straus, W. S. Richardson, P. Glasziou, & R. B. Haynes (Eds.), *Evidence-based medicine: How to practice and teach EBM* (3rd ed.; electronic media). Edinburgh, Scotland: Churchill Livingstone.

Epic. (2017). *Making it easy to follow clinical guidelines.* Retrieved from http://www.epic.com/epic/post/2744

Finfgeld, D. L. (2003). Meta-synthesis: The state of the art—so far. *Qualitative Health Research, 13*(7), 893–904. doi:10.1177/1049732303253462

Gambrill, E. (2011). Evidence-based practice and the ethics of discretion. *Journal of Social Work, 11*(1), 26–48. doi:10.1177/1468017310381306

Haynes, R. B. (2006). Of studies, syntheses, synopses, summaries, and systems: The "5 S" evolution of information services for evidence-based health care decisions [Editorial]. *ACP Journal, 145*(3), A8.

Institute of Medicine. (2011). *Clinical practice guidelines we can trust.* Washington, DC: National Academies Press.

Lumley, T. (2002). Network meta-analysis for indirect treatment comparisons. *Statistics in Medicine, 21*(16), 2313–2324. doi:10.1002/sim.1201

Melnyk, B. M., & Fineout-Overholt, E. (2015). *Evidence-based practice in nursing and healthcare: A guide to best practice* (3rd ed.). Philadelphia, PA: Wolters Kluwer/Lippincott Williams & Wilkins.

Moher, D., Liberati, A., Tetzlaff, J., & Altman, D. G., for the PRISMA Group. (2009). Preferred reporting items for systematic reviews and meta-analyses: The PRISMA statement. *British Medical Journal Open Access, 339,* b2535.

Moore, Z. (2012). Meta-analysis in context. *Journal of Clinical Nursing, 21*(19–20), 2798–2807. doi:10.1111/j.1365–2702.2012.04122.x

Risjord, M. (2009). Rethinking concept analysis. *Journal of Advanced Nursing, 65*(3), 684–691. doi:10.1111/j.1365-2648.2008.04903.x

Rogers, B. L., & Knafl, K. A. (2000). *Concept development in nursing: Foundations, techniques, and applications* (2nd ed.). Philadelphia, PA: Saunders.

Rycroft-Malone, J., Seers, K., Titchen, A., Harvey, G., Kitson, A., & McCormack, B. (2004). What counts as evidence in evidence-based practice? *Journal of Advanced Nursing, 47*(1), 81–90.

Sandelowski, M. (2011). "Casing" the research case study. *Research in Nursing and Health, 34*(2), 153–159. doi:10.1002/nur.20421

Straus, S. E., Glasziou, P., Richardson, W. S., & Haynes, R. B. (2011). *Evidence-based medicine: How to practice and teach EBM* (4th ed.). Edinburgh, Scotland: Churchill Livingstone.

Walker, L., & Avant, K. (2010). *Strategies for theory construction in nursing* (5th ed). Upper Saddle River, NJ: Pearson Prentice Hall.

Yin, R. K. (2013). *Case study research: Design and methods.* Thousand Oaks, CA: Sage.

Decision

UNIT 4

Decisions about practice should always be based on a careful appraisal of the evidence.

At the end of this chapter, you will be able to:

< Define statistics
< Differentiate between descriptive and inferential statistics
< Identify how frequencies can be graphically depicted
< Describe measures of central tendency and their uses
< Name patterns of data distribution correctly
< Describe measures of variability and their use
< Discuss the purpose of inferential statistical tests
< Explain how statistical testing is related to chance
< Distinguish between type I and type II errors
< Describe alpha levels commonly used in nursing research
< Match common notations with associated statistical tests

< Identify common statistical tests as parametric or nonparametric
< Describe tests used to determine statistically significant differences between groups
< Discuss tests used to determine statistically significant differences among variables
< Assign commonly used statistical tests to examples based on type of research question and level of measurement
< Interpret data reported in statistical tables
< Differentiate between statistical significance and clinical significance
< Appraise data analysis sections of an article
< Discuss ethical considerations when conducting statistical analyses

alpha level
amodal
analysis of variance
bimodal
bivariate analysis
Chi square
coefficient of variation
confidence intervals
correlated *t* test
correlation coefficients
degrees of freedom
descriptive statistics
direction
heterogeneous
homogenous
independent *t* test
inferential statistics
kurtosis
magnitude

mean
measures of central tendency
measures of variability
median
modality
mode
multiple regression
multivariate analysis
negatively skewed
nonparametric
nonsignificant
normal distribution
parametric
Pearson's *r*
percentage distributions
percentile
population parameters
position of the median
positively skewed

probability
range
Rule of 68–95–99.7
sample statistics
sampling distribution
sampling error
semiquartile range
skewed
standard deviation
statistically significant
statistics
Statistics
t statistic
tailedness
type I error
type II error
unimodal
univariate analysis
z scores

CHAPTER 13

What Do the Quantitative Data Mean?

Rosalind M. Peters, Nola A. Schmidt, and Moira Fearncombe

13.1 Using Statistics to Describe the Sample

At the end of this section, you will be able to:

‹ Define statistics
‹ Differentiate between descriptive and inferential statistics

Originally the term *statistics* referred to information about the government because the word is derived from the Latin *statisticum*, meaning "of the state." It was given its numerical meaning in 1749 when Gottfried Achenwall, a German political scientist, used the term to designate the analysis of *data* about the state (Harper, 2013). Currently, there are two meanings of the term *statistics*. *Statistics*, with a capital S, is used to describe the branch of mathematics that collects, analyzes, interprets, and presents numerical data in terms of samples and populations, while *statistics*, with a lowercase s, is used to describe the numerical outcomes and the probabilities derived from calculations on raw data.

When reporting the results of their study, researchers often present two types of statistics: descriptive and inferential. *Descriptive statistics* deal with the collection and presentation of data used to explain characteristics of variables found in a sample. As its name implies, descriptive statistics describe, summarize, and synthesize collected data. Calculations and information presented with descriptive statistics must be accurate. *Inferential statistics* involve analysis of data as the basis for predictions related to the phenomenon of interest. Inferential statistics are used to make inferences or draw conclusions about a population based on a sample. They are used to develop *population parameters* from the *sample statistics*. For example, a researcher conducted a study on the efficiency of vitamin C in preventing the common cold. Descriptive statistics would be used to report that 60% of subjects in the experimental group had fewer colds than did subjects receiving the placebo. The researcher would then use inferential statistics to determine whether the difference in the number of colds between the two groups was statistically significant. If it was, then it could be inferred that taking vitamin C would be advantageous. Descriptive statistics are used to provide information regarding univariate or bivariate analyses.

Univariate analysis is conducted to present organized information about only one variable at a time and includes information regarding frequency distributions, measures of central tendency, shape of the distribution, and measures of variability, sometimes known as dispersion. *Bivariate analysis* is performed to describe the relationship between two variables that can be expressed in contingency tables or with other statistical tests. *Multivariate analysis* is done when the researcher wants to examine the relationship among three or more variables.

The results of descriptive analysis are frequently presented in table format, and scientific notations are often used. Therefore, it may be helpful to review common notations used in tables as shown in **Table 13-1**.

TABLE 13-1	Statistical Symbols for Descriptive Statistics

Symbol/Abbreviation	Definition
f	Frequency
M	Mean
Mdn	Median
n	Number in subsample
N	Total number in a sample
%	Percentage
SD	Standard deviation
z	A standard score

1. To describe the frequency of the single variable myocardial infarction in adults ages 30–49, which of the following could be used? (Select all that apply.)

    a. Descriptive statistics
    b. Inferential statistics
    c. Univariate analysis
    d. Bivariate analysis

How did you do? 1. a, c

KEY TERMS

bivariate analysis: The use of statistics to describe the relationship between two variables

multivariate analysis: The use of statistics to describe the relationships among three or more variables

13.2 Using Frequencies to Describe Samples

At the end of this section, you will be able to:

‹ Identify how frequencies can be graphically depicted

Information about the frequency, or how often, a variable is found to occur may be presented as either ungrouped or grouped data. Ungrouped data are primarily used to present nominal and ordinal data where the raw data represents some characteristic of the variable. In contrast, with interval- and ratio-level data, the raw data are collapsed (grouped) into smaller classifications to make the data easier to interpret. **Table 13-2** provides an example of how categorical data about a sample may be presented in ungrouped format.

FYI

There are two types of statistics: descriptive and inferential. Descriptive statistics describe, summarize, and synthesize collected data, while inferential statistics involve analysis of data as the basis for predictions related to the phenomenon of interest.

Ungrouped data are rarely presented when reporting on continuous variables such as age, scores on scales, time, or physiological variables (e.g., temperature, blood pressure, cell counts). For example, if readers of an article were presented with a set of ages for 20 different participants in the study, it would be difficult to make sense of this raw data (see **Table 13-3**). However, if the numbers were arranged in a frequency distribution and graphed, they would make much more sense to the readers. Before a graph can be constructed, the researcher must create a frequency distribution table. First, the raw data are sorted, usually in ascending order. Next, the number of times each value occurs is tallied, and the frequency of each event is recorded in the table. Table 13-3 shows how the raw data can be organized to more clearly present the information. The table

TABLE 13-2	Example of Categorical Data Presented in Ungrouped Format

Variable	n(%)
Gender	
Men	14 (41)
Women	20 (59)
Race/Ethnicity	
White/Caucasian	190 (76.0)
Black/African American	32 (12.8)
Hispanic/Latino	12 (4.8)
Native American/Eskimo	3 (1.2)
Asian/Pacific Islander	2 (0.8)
No answer	11 (4.4)
Self-Care Behaviors	
Current smoker	7 (18)
Alcohol > 1 drink/day	0 (0)
Exercise	
No regular exercise	9 (27)
1–2 days/week	10 (29)
3–4 days/week	8 (24)
≥ 5 days/week	5 (15)

n = number in group; % = percent

shows how raw data are tallied and the resulting frequencies and percentages are recorded. The left-hand side of the table shows the frequency with which individual age data occur. Because all possible data points are presented, it is still somewhat difficult to comprehend this presentation of the ungrouped data. The right-hand side of the table shows a grouped frequency and percentage distribution with the ages grouped in 2-year increments. It should be obvious that the grouped data are more meaningful than either the raw or ungrouped data.

Although there are few fixed rules regarding how and when to group data, it is imperative that there be no overlap of categories. Each group must have well-defined lower and upper limits so that the groups are mutually exclusive, yet the groups must include all data collected. For example, if the groupings in Table 13-3 had been 18–20 and 20–22, people who are 20 years old would have been counted in both groups, and the statistics would have been compromised. Group size also should be consistent. If the groups had been 18–20 (a 3-year span), 21–25 (a 4-year span), and older than 25 (a 3-year span), then inaccurate analysis of data would occur. Although grouping data might make

TABLE 13-3	Example of Frequency and Percentage Distributions of Ages

Raw Data
18 18 18 19 19 19 20 21 21 21 21 21 22 22 22 23 23 25 27 28

	Ungrouped Data				Grouped Data		
Age	**Tally**	**Frequency**	**Percentage**	**Age**	**Tally**	**Frequency**	**Percentage**
18	|||	3	15	18–19	₩₩		6	30
19	|||	3	15	20–21	₩₩		6	30
20			1	5	22–23	₩₩	5	25
21	₩₩	5	25	24–25			1	5
22	|||	3	15	> 25	||	2	10
23	||	2	10	**Total**		20	100
25			1	5				
27			1	5				
28			1	5				
Total		20	200				

it easier to understand, it also results in some loss of information. The grouped data presented in Table 13-3 indicate that 30% of the subjects were between 20 and 21 years of age; however, there is no way of knowing that most subjects (five of the six) were 21, and only one subject was 20 years of age.

In addition to frequency distributions, *percentage distributions* are often used to present descriptive statistics. A percentage distribution is calculated by dividing the frequency of an event by the total number of events. For example, in Table 13-3 the three 18-year-old subjects in the study represent 15% of the total number of subjects reported. Providing information about percentages is another way to group data to make results more comprehensible and allow for easier comparisons with other studies.

After data are tallied and a frequency distribution is determined, data may be converted to graphic form. Graphs provide a visual representation of data and often make it easier to discern trends. The most common types of graphs are line charts, bar graphs, pie charts, histograms, and scattergrams (or scatterplots). **Figure 13-1** depicts two different ways to present the age data from Table 13-3.

KEY TERM

percentage distributions: Descriptive statistics used to group data to make results more comprehensible; calculated by dividing the frequency of an event by the total number of events

FIGURE 13-1	Frequency Polygon and Histogram of Age Data

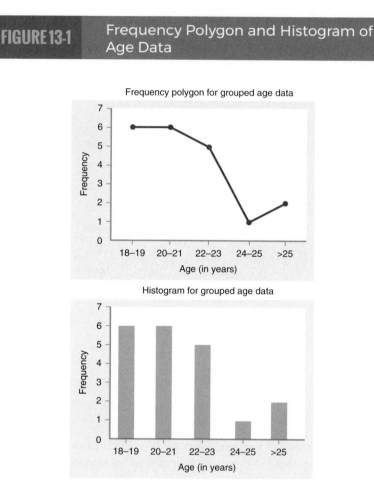

TEST YOUR KNOWLEDGE 13-2

True/False

1. Frequency distributions are an effective way to present inferential statistics.

2. Categories in grouped data must be mutually exclusive.

3. Percentages are often used to describe characteristics of samples.

4. The total number of subjects in a sample is represented by the symbol *n*.

How did you do? 1. F; 2. T; 3. T; 4. F

13.3 Measures of Central Tendency

At the end of this section, you will be able to:

‹ Describe measures of central tendency and their uses

Measures of central tendency offer another way to describe raw data. These measures provide information about the "typical" case to be found in the data. The *mean, median,* and *mode* are the three terms most commonly used to describe the tendency of data to cluster around the middle of the data set (i.e., "averages" for the data). The mean and median are used to describe continuous-level data, while the mode is used to describe both continuous- and nominal-level data. Because the mean and median may be calculated values, they can be rounded to the nearest number; however, the mode is never rounded because it is an actual data point.

Mode

The *mode* is the easiest measure of central tendency to determine because it is the most frequently occurring value in a data set. It is the highest tally when counting and is the highest frequency in a distribution table. *Modality* refers to the number of modes found in a data distribution. Data can be *amodal* (without a mode), *unimodal* (with one mode), or *bimodal* (with two modes). There is no specific term to indicate when data have more than two modes. The mode does not mean that a data value occurs more than once in a frequency distribution because the mode is an actual data point. The mode is not affected by the existence of any extreme values in the data. **Table 13-4** demonstrates how the

TABLE 13-4	Mode	
Data Points	**Type of Mode**	**Location of Mode**
{0, 1, 2, 3}	amodal	N/A
{0, 1, 2, 2}	unimodal	2
{1, 1, 2, 2}	bimodal	1 and 2
{1, 1, 1, 2, 2}	unimodal	1
{1, 1, 1, 2, 596}	unimodal	1

TABLE 13-5	Mode of Age Data for 20 Subjects

Ungrouped Data			Grouped Data		
Age	**Tally**	**Frequency**	**Age**	**Tally**	**Percentage**
18	|||	3	18–19	##|	6
19	|||	3	20–21	##|	6
20	|	1	22–23	##	5
21	##	5	24–25	|	1
22	|||	3	> 25	||	2
23	||	2	**Total**		20
25	|	1			
27	|	1			
28	|	1			
Total		20			

change in just one data point affects the modality of the data. In the age data presented in Table 13-3, note that the ungrouped data are unimodal with the mode being 21. However, when the data are grouped, they become bimodal with modes at 18–19 years as well as 20–21 years of age (**Table 13-5**). It is easy to see the modes on the frequency polygon and histogram in Figure 13-1 because the modes have the highest peaks and tallest bars. The mode is considered to be an unstable measure of central tendency because it tends to vary widely from one sample to the next. Given its instability, the mode is rarely presented as the sole measure of central tendency.

Median

The *median* is the center of the data set. Just as the median of the road divides the highway into two halves, the median of a data set divides data in half. If there are an odd number of data points, the median is the middle value or the score where exactly 50% of the data lie above the median and 50% of the data lie below it. If there is an even number of values in the data set, the median is the average of the two middle-most values and as such may be a number not actually found in the data set. The median actually refers to the average position in the data, and it is minimally affected by the existence of an outlier.

The *position of the median* is calculated by using the formula $(n + 1)/2$, where n is the number of data values in the set. It is important to remember that this formula gives only the position, and not the actual value, of the median. For example, in a study describing the number of hours that five ($n = 5$) sedentary subjects spent watching television last week, the following data were collected: {4, 6, 3, 38, 6} hours. To determine the median, the researcher would perform a number of easy steps.

1. Sort the data: 3 4 6 6 38
2. Determine the median's location. The median is at the $(5 + 1)/2$, or third, position from either end.
3. Count over three places to find that the median is 6. In this example, 6 is also the mode because it is the most frequently occurring value.

If the data set is changed to {3, 4, 6, 6}, then the position of the median would be 2.5, or halfway between the second and third sorted data points. In this example, the median is 5, and 6 is the mode. If the data set is changed again to include {3, 4, 6, 100}, the position of the median still will be 2.5, or halfway between the second and third sorted data points, and the median remains 5. This example demonstrates that the outlier value of 100 did not affect the median value. For this reason, the median is generally used to describe average when there is an extreme value in the data.

When data are grouped, the median is determined using cumulative frequencies. In **Table 13-6** age data are reported for 20 subjects. The median is located at $(20 + 1)/2$, the 10.5th position, and it is the average of the 10th and 11th data values. In the ungrouped data, the median is 21 years old, while the grouped median is 20–21 years.

Mean

When people refer to an average, what they are really referring to is the *mean*. The mean is calculated by adding all of the data values and then dividing by the total number of values. The mean is the most commonly used measure of central tendency. It is greatly affected by the existence of outliers because every value in the data set is included in the calculation. The larger the sample size, the less an outlier will affect the mean. For example, using the previous data example about number of hours spent watching television, subjects reported watching 4, 6, 3, 38, and 6 hours of television per week. Using these data, the mean is calculated to be 11.4 hours ($57 / 5 = 11.4$). However, 11.4 hours does not present a clear picture of the amount of television watched by most subjects because the one extreme value of 38 hours skews the data. Because the mean is the measure of central tendency used in many tests of statistical significance, it is imperative for researchers to evaluate data for outliers before performing statistical analyses.

KEY TERM

mean: The mathematical average calculated by adding all values and then dividing by the total number of values

TABLE 13-6	Median of Age Data for 20 Subjects

	Ungrouped Data				Grouped Data		
Age	**Tally**	**Frequency**	**Cumulative Frequency**	**Age**	**Tally**	**Frequency**	**Cumulative Frequency**
18	|	3	3	18–19	⊪|	6	6
19	|||	3	6	20–21	⊪|	6	12
20	|	1	7	22–23	⊪	5	17
21	⊪	5	12	24–25	|	1	18
22	|||	3	15	> 25	||	2	20
23	||	2	17	**Total**		20	
25	|	1	18				
27	|	1	19				
28	|	1	20				
Total		20					

When reading articles in which averages are used, nurses must carefully examine the conclusions drawn. For example, suppose a nursing unit employs five staff nurses and a nursing manager. Annual salaries of these employees are $66,500, $66,500, $67,000, $68,000, and $69,000. The nursing manager earns $133,000. During contract negotiations, nurses indicate that they need a raise. One individual claims the "average" salary is $67,000 per year (median), while another says the "average" salary is $66,500 (the mode). When confronted by the administration, the nurse manager responds by saying the "average" salary is actually $78,333.33 (mean). So, who is correct? In fact, they are all correct. They are just using different meanings of *average*. This example demonstrates how easy it is to manipulate statistics and why careful attention must be given to the interpretation of data being presented.

When appraising evidence, it is helpful to remember that the mean is the best measure of central tendency if there are no extreme values, and the median is best if there are extreme values. Because they are calculated, the mean and median are not necessarily actual data values, whereas the mode must be an exact data point. The mean and median are unique values (again, because they are calculated), but the mode might be unique or might not exist at all, or there might be multiple modes. The mean is greatly affected by extreme values, the median is marginally affected, and the mode is not affected. The

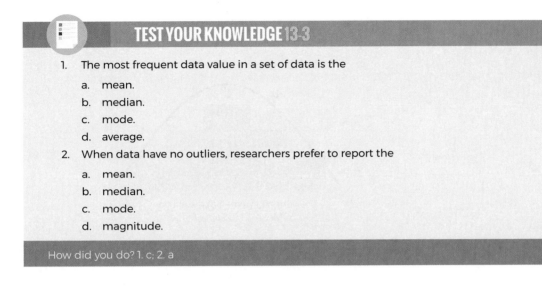

1. The most frequent data value in a set of data is the
   a. mean.
   b. median.
   c. mode.
   d. average.
2. When data have no outliers, researchers prefer to report the
   a. mean.
   b. median.
   c. mode.
   d. magnitude.

How did you do? 1. c; 2. a

mean and median use continuous-level data values for their calculations, while the mode can use either continuous- or nominal-data values. The mean is the most stable in that if repeated samples were drawn from the same population, the mean would vary less than either the median or the mode would from sample to sample.

Because it is the most stable, the mean is most often used when computing other statistics. The median is used when the center of a data set is desired, and the mode is used to determine the most frequent case.

13.4 Distribution Patterns

At the end of this section, you will be able to:

‹ Name patterns of data distribution correctly

Normal Distributions: Symmetrical Shapes

Measures of central tendencies are used to define distribution patterns. When the distribution of the data is symmetrical (that is, when the two halves of the distribution are folded over, they would be superimposed on each other and therefore be unimodal), then the mean, median, and mode are equal. In this situation, the data are considered to be normally distributed. A *normal distribution* has a distinctive bell-shaped curve and is symmetric about the mean. In **Figure 13-2**, note that the decreasing bars, or area under the curve, indicate that the data cluster at the center and taper away from the mean.

KEY TERM

normal distribution: Data representation with a distinctive bell-shaped curve, symmetric about the mean

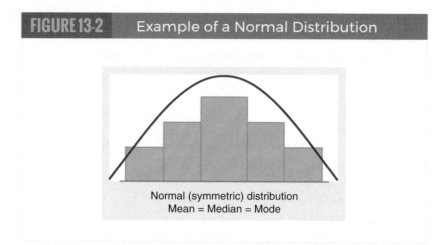

FIGURE 13-2 Example of a Normal Distribution

Normal (symmetric) distribution
Mean = Median = Mode

A number of human traits, such as intelligence and height, are considered to be normally distributed in the population.

When Data Are Not Normally Distributed

Often data do not fit a normal distribution and are considered to be asymmetric or *skewed*. In asymmetric distributions, the peak of the data is not at the center of the distribution, and one tail is longer than the other. Skewed distributions are usually discussed in terms of their direction. If the longer tail is pointing to the left, the data are considered to be *negatively skewed* (**Figure 13-3**). In this situation, the mean is less than the median and mode. For example, a group of students take a test for which all but one student studied. The one student, who did not study, scores very low. This low score, because it is an outlier, affects the mean because the scores of students who studied are high. This outlier contributes to a negatively skewed distribution. The low score pulls down the mean and pulls with it the tail of the distribution to the left. If the mean is greater than the median and mode, then the data are *positively skewed*, pulling the tail to the right. For example, an instructor gives a difficult test. Only one or two students scored high on the test. The rest of the students' scores were low. Most students' scores are lower than the mean because the outliers affect the mean. The distribution of these scores is positively skewed. The extremely high scores pull up the mean and pull the tail in a positive direction toward the right (**Figure 13-4**).

Attention should be given to how the data are spread, or dispersed, around the mean. Just as schoolchildren or military personnel wear uniforms to be like each other, uniform data have very little spread and look like each other.

KEY TERMS

skewed: An asymmetrical distribution of data

negatively skewed: A distribution when the mean is less than the median and the mode; the longer tail is pointing to the left

positively skewed: Distribution when the mean is greater than the median and the mode; the longer tail is pointing to the right

FIGURE 13-3   Example of a Negatively Skewed Distribution

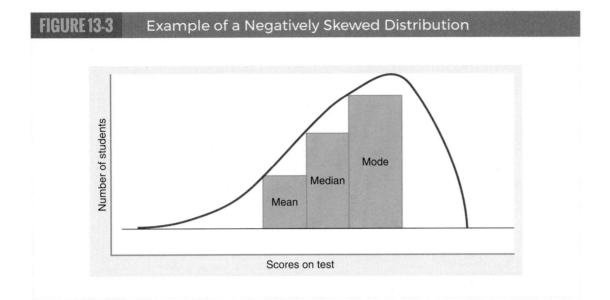

FIGURE 13-4   Example of a Positively Skewed Distribution

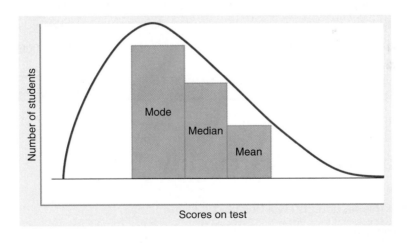

When there is greater variation in data, a wider spread results. In graphic representations of data (see **Figure 13-5**), highly uniform data have a high peak and highly variable data have a low peak. *Kurtosis* is the term used to describe the peakedness or flatness of a data set.

KEY TERM

kurtosis: The peakedness or flatness of a distribution of data

| FIGURE 13-5 | Example of Kurtosis |

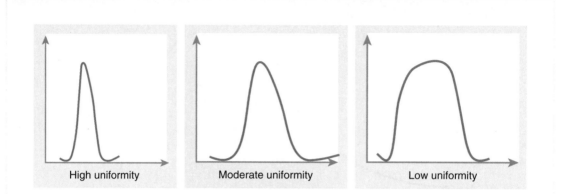

High uniformity   Moderate uniformity   Low uniformity

TEST YOUR KNOWLEDGE 13-4

True/False

1. If the tail of a distribution is skewed to the left, the data are negatively skewed.
2. In a normal distribution, the mean, median, and mode are the same value.
3. If data are highly uniform, a low peak will be observed in a graphic representation of the data.

How did you do? 1. T; 2. T; 3. F

13.5 Measures of Variability

At the end of this section, you will be able to:

‹ Describe measures of variability and their use

Measures of variability provide information regarding how different the data are within a set. These can also be known as measures of dispersion because they provide information about how data are dispersed around the mean. If the data are very similar, there is little variability, and the data are considered to be *homogenous*. If there is wide variation, the data are considered to be *heterogeneous*. Common measures of variation include range, semiquartile

TABLE 13-7	Example of Ranges of Income	
	Control	**Experimental**
	$30,000	$15,000
	$38,000	$23,000
	$42,000	$42,000
	$57,000	$57,000
	$73,000	$103,000
Range	$43,000	$88,000

range, percentile, and standard deviation. z scores and variance are used to compare the variability among data using different units of measure.

Range

A statistical *range* is the difference between the maximum and minimum values in a data set. Because the range is very sample specific, it is considered to be an unstable measure of variability. **Table 13-7** shows the income reported for subjects in the experimental and control groups of a study designed to evaluate health literacy. The mean for both data sets is $48,000, and the medians are each $42,000. However, the data are quite different because the data for the experimental group are more heterogeneous than for the control group. The experimental group's income varies from a minimum of $15,000 to a maximum of $103,000, with a range of $88,000. The control group's income has a minimum of $30,000 and a maximum of $73,000. Although salaries are still quite variable, they are more uniform than the experimental group's salaries because their range is $43,000. In data comparisons, the smaller the range, the more uniform the data; the greater the range, the more variable the data.

Semiquartile Range

Just as the median divides data into two halves, other values divide these halves in half, meaning into quarters. The *semiquartile range* is the range of the middle 50% of the data. **Figure 13-6** illustrates the semiquartile range of the age data from a previous example. The semiquartile range lies between the lower (first) and upper (third) quartile of ages. The first quartile value is the median of the lower half of the data set; one fourth of the data

FIGURE 13-6	Semiquartile Range of Age Data

18 18 18 19 19 | 19 20 21 21 21 | 21 21 22 22 22 | 23 23 25 27 28

$Q_1 = 19$ Median = 21 $Q_3 = 22.5$

lies below the first quartile and three fourths of the data lie above it. The third quartile value is the median of the upper half of the data; three fourths of the data lie below the third quartile and one fourth of the data lies above it. The semiquartile range is the difference between the third and first quartile values and describes the middle half of a data distribution. In Figure 13-6, note that 50% of the data lie between 19 and 22.5, and the range is 3.5.

Percentile

A *percentile* is a measure of rank. Each percentile represents the percentage of cases that a given value exceeds. The median is the 50th percentile, the first quartile is the 25th percentile, and the third quartile is the 75th percentile score in a given data set. For example, if a newborn baby boy's weight is in the 39th percentile, he weighs more than 39% of babies tested weigh but less than 61% of the other babies.

Standard Deviation

The most commonly reported measure of variability is the *standard deviation*, which is based on deviations from the mean of the data. Whereas the mean is the expectation value (the expected "average" of the data set), the standard deviation is the measure of the average deviations of a value from the mean in a given data set. Because it is a measure of deviation from the mean, a standard deviation should always be reported whenever a mean is reported. Standard deviation is based on the normal curve and is used to determine the number of data values that fall within a specific interval in a normal distribution. Understanding the standard deviation allows you to interpret an individual score in comparison with all other scores in the data set. Recall the salary example presented earlier. The data were variable because of the extreme ranges of

KEY TERMS

percentile: A measure of rank representing the percentage of cases that a given value exceeds

standard deviation: A measure of variability used to determine the number of data values falling within a specific interval in a normal distribution

CRITICAL THINKING EXERCISE 13-1

Consider how your ACT or SAT scores were reported. What was your raw score? What was your percentile? What do these data indicate about your performance on these tests?

TABLE 13-8	Standard Deviations of Income	
	Control	**Experimental**
	$30,000	$15,000
	$38,000	$23,000
	$42,000	$42,000
	$57,000	$57,000
	$73,000	$103,000
SD	$17,073.37	$34,842.50

salary values. Calculating a standard deviation provides different information about variability. It is now apparent that the average deviation from the mean for the experimental group is $34,842.50, which is more than double that of the control group's $17,073.37 deviation (see **Table 13-8**).

Comparing Variability When Units of Measure Are Different

Because standard deviations are based on the mean of the data set, information collected using different measurement scales cannot be directly compared. For example, the mean of a sample's age is reported in years, whereas the mean of a sample's weight is reported in pounds. To make comparisons among unlike data requires that all the data means be converted to standardized units called standardized or *z scores*. *z* scores are then used to describe the distance a score is away from the mean per standard deviation. A *z* score of 1.25 means that a data value is 1.25 standard deviations above the mean. A *z* score of –2.53 means that a data value is 2.53 standard deviations below the mean. Using the *z* score allows researchers to compare results of age and weight.

The *coefficient of variation* is a percentage used to compare standard deviations when the units of measure are different or when the means of the distributions being compared are far apart. The coefficient of variation is computed by dividing the standard deviation by the mean and recording the result as a percentage. For example, if you were to compare age and income of a sample of nurses, you could not use range or standard deviations to discuss the variables' comparative spread because they are measured with different units. If the mean salary for nurses is $66,000, with a standard deviation of $6,000 and the mean age is 32 years, with a standard deviation of 4 years, the coefficient of variation for the salary is 9.1%, and the coefficient of variation for age is 12.5%.

KEY TERMS

z scores: Standardized units used to compare data gathered using different measurement scales

coefficient of variation: A percentage used to compare standard deviations when the units of measure are different or when the means of the distributions being compared are far apart

CRITICAL THINKING EXERCISE 13-2

Do you have a professor who uses means and standard deviations, known as norm referencing, for grading exams? What are the advantages to using this approach as opposed to straight scales for grading? What are some disadvantages? Why would it be false to assume that having more questions on exams would be advantageous to students when norm referencing is used?

Using the coefficient of variation shows that age is more variable than salaries among this group of nurses.

Tailedness: The Rule of 68–95–99.7

The concept of *tailedness* is important to understand when reading statistical reports. Recall that a normal distribution is one in which the mean, median, and mode are all equal and the data are symmetrical. In discussing tailedness, the graph of a normal distribution is depicted as a bell-shaped curve, centered about the mean (x), with three standard deviations marked to the right (positive) and also to the left (negative) (see **Figure 13-7**). Normal distributions are not shown beyond three standard deviations in either direction because approximately 99.7% of the data will lie within this range. Approximately 68% of all data in a normal curve lie within one standard deviation of the mean, and 95% of the data lie within two standard deviations of the mean. Thus, the *Rule of 68–95–99.7* tells us that for every sample, 99.7% of the data will fall within three standard deviations of the mean. In **Figure 13-8**, note the symmetry about the mean for the standard deviations as they are divided in half for each distribution percentage. For example, one standard deviation contains

KEY TERMS

tailedness: The degree to which a tail in a distribution is pulled to the left or to the right

Rule of 68-95-99.7: Rule stating that for every sample 68% of the data will fall within one standard deviation of the mean; 95% will fall within two standard deviations; 99.7% of the data will fall within three standard deviations

FIGURE 13-7	Normal Distribution with Standard Deviations

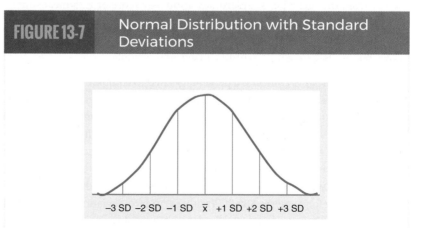

–3 SD –2 SD –1 SD $\bar{x}$ +1 SD +2 SD +3 SD

FIGURE 13-8 Standard Deviations and Percentage Distribution

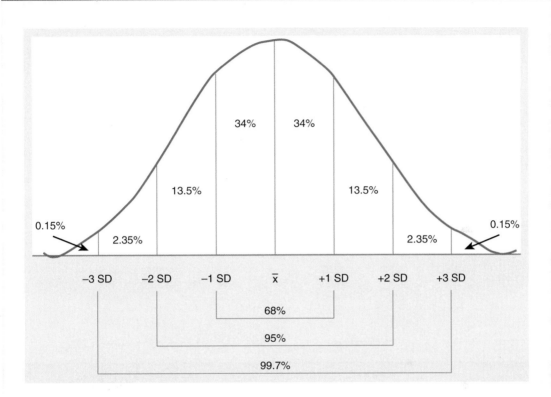

34% of the scores above and 34% of the scores below the mean to total 68%; two standard deviations contain 34% plus 13.5% above and below the mean to equal 95% of the scores. On a standard deviation graph, the mean has a z score of zero. Other z-score percentages may be determined by using a table showing the area under the curve data.

Figure 13-9 shows that normal distributions may also be used to approximate percentile ranks. Actual percentile values must always be determined by using a normal distribution table to look up a given z score.

The age data from previous examples do not approximate a normal distribution because the mean, median, and mode are not equal. If, however, we used data that were standardized with a mean of 23 and a standard deviation of 1.5 years, the normal curve for these data would look like the graph in **Figure 13-10**. Sixty-eight percent of these people would be between 21.5 and 24.5 years of age, and someone 26 years old would be in the 95th percentile.

FIGURE 13-9 Percentile Rank Based on Normal Distribution

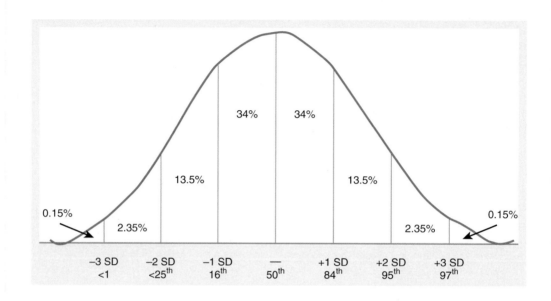

−3 SD	−2 SD	−1 SD	—	+1 SD	+2 SD	+3 SD
<1	<25th	16th	50th	84th	95th	97th

FIGURE 13-10 Standard Deviations of Age Data

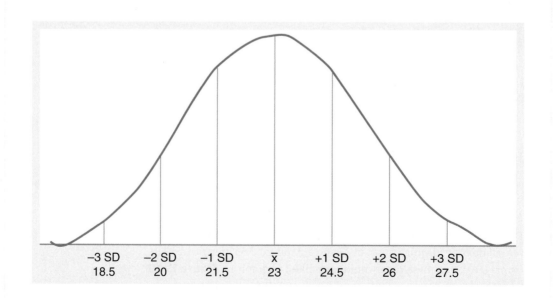

−3 SD	−2 SD	−1 SD	$\bar{x}$	+1 SD	+2 SD	+3 SD
18.5	20	21.5	23	24.5	26	27.5

Half of the people would be 23 years or older, while half would be younger than 23 years.

Correlation Coefficients

Bivariate analyses are performed to calculate *correlation coefficients*, which are used to describe the relationship between two variables. Correlation coefficients provide information regarding the degree to which variables are related. Correlations are evaluated in terms of magnitude direction and sometimes significance. Scatterplots of data can provide hints about direction and magnitude of the correlation (**Figure 13-11**). *Direction* refers to the way the two variables covary. A positive correlation occurs when an increase in one variable is associated with an increase in another or when a decrease in one variable is associated with a decrease in the other. For example, if a researcher found that as weight increased so did systolic blood pressure, or if weight decreased so did systolic blood pressure, a "positive" relationship between weight and blood pressure exists. A negative correlation occurs when two variables covary inversely; that is, when one decreases, the other increases. For example, as exercise increases body weight decreases.

Magnitude refers to the strength of the relationship found to exist between two variables. A correlation can range from a perfect positive correlation of 1.00 to a perfect negative correlation of 1.00. A correlation of zero means that there is no relationship between the two variables. It is generally accepted that correlations ranging between .10 and .30 are considered to be weak, .30 and .50, moderate, and greater than .50, strong; however, the final determination is based on the variables being examined. It is important to remember that magnitude is not dependent on or related to the direction of the correlation.

KEY TERMS

correlation coefficients: An estimate, ranging from 0.00 to +1.00, that indicates the reliability of an instrument; statistic used to describe the relationship among two variables

direction: The way two variables covary

magnitude: The strength of the relationship existing between two variables

FIGURE 13-11 Scatterplots of Correlational Relationships

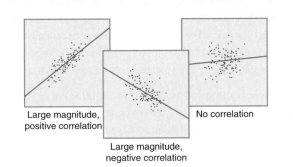

Large magnitude, positive correlation

Large magnitude, negative correlation

No correlation

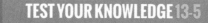

Match the following terms:

1. Range
2. Semiquartile range
3. Percentile
4. Standard deviation
5. *z* score
6. Coefficient of variation

a. Rank
b. Difference between maximum and minimum values
c. Measure of the average deviations of a value from the mean
d. Percentage comparing standard deviations when units of measure are different
e. Range of the middle 50% of data
f. Converted standard deviation to a standardized unit

How did you do? 1. b; 2. e; 3. a; 4. c; 5. f; 6. d

13.6 Inferential Statistics: Can the Findings Be Applied to the Population?

At the end of this section, you will be able to:

‹ Discuss the purpose of inferential statistical tests
‹ Explain how statistical testing is related to chance

When to Use Inferential Statistics

First, samples are analyzed using descriptive statistics. Then, if appropriate, inferential statistical tests can be conducted to: (1) make decisions about whether findings can be applied to the population, or in other words, to make inferences about the population based on the sample, and (2) test hypotheses. For some studies, the use of inferential statistics is not appropriate, and their use depends on the research questions being asked. Research questions that are descriptive would not require inferential statistics. For example, the research question "How often do nurses assess the use of herbal remedies by patients?" would best be answered by using descriptive statistics, such as frequencies, means, and standard deviations.

Using parameter estimation to determine inferences to the population is less common in nursing research; however, this approach is becoming more popular with the emphasis on evidence-based practice (EBP) in nursing and medicine (Borenstein, 1997; Straus, Richardson, Glasziou, & Haynes, 2010). Most frequently, these estimates are reported as *confidence intervals* (CIs). CIs are ranges established around means that estimate the probability of being

KEY TERM

confidence intervals: Ranges established around means that estimate the probability of being correct

correct (American College of Physicians—American Society of Internal Medicine, 2001; Hoekstra, Johnson, & Kiers, 2012). In other words, CIs estimate the degree of confidence one can have about the inferences. Researchers typically report confidence levels of 95% or 99%.

Use of inferential statistics to test hypotheses is best suited to research questions or hypotheses that ask one of two broad questions:

» Is there a difference between the groups?
» Is there a relationship among the variables?

Most experimental and quasi-experimental designs involve questions asking if there is a difference between the groups. For example, the use of inferential statistics to test the hypothesis "Patients who have uninterrupted sleep cycles have better wound healing than do patients who awaken throughout the night" would be appropriate. Research questions or hypotheses that ask about relationships among variables, such as "Is there a relationship between the number of hours of sleep and a score on a memory exam?" can also be tested using inferential statistics.

When deciding which statistical tests to use to analyze data, researchers must take into account many factors (Hayes, 1994). After considering whether the research questions or hypotheses involve groups or variables, the next most important factor researchers consider is the level of measurement. Whether variables are nominal, ordinal, interval, or ratio is important because some tests are appropriate for interval and ratio data but not for other levels of measurement. Other factors that can influence selection of inferential statistical tests include whether: (1) a probability sampling method was used, (2) the data are normally distributed, and (3) there is potential confounding of the variables. Nurses should keep in mind that the strongest inferences can be made when the level of measurement is interval or ratio, a probability sampling method was used, the sample size is adequate, and the data are normally distributed.

It's All About Chance

Regardless of the type of question being asked, the major unanswered question is: What is the likelihood that the findings could have occurred by chance alone? For example, suppose that you toss a coin 10 times, and each time it lands heads up. Could that happen by chance? Absolutely. Now suppose you flip it another 10 times and it lands with heads up every time. Although it is possible that a coin could land heads up 20 times in a row, this would be a rare occurrence. Would you begin to wonder if this were happening by chance or would you suspect that the coin is not fair? How many times would you want to toss the coin before you conclude that the coin is not fair?

FYI
Statistics enable nursing researchers to determine the probability that results are not a result of chance alone.

KEY TERMS

probability: Likelihood or chance that an event will occur in a situation

sampling error: Error resulting when elements in the sample do not adequately represent the population

Researchers ask the same types of questions when they analyze data using inferential statistics. They ask, "What is the probability that the findings were a result of chance?" *Probability* is the likelihood of the frequency of an event in repeated trials under similar conditions. Probability is the percentage of times that an event (e.g., "heads") is likely to occur by chance alone. Probability is affected by the concept of sampling error. *Sampling error* is the tendency for statistical results to fluctuate from one sample to another. There is always a possibility of errors in sampling, even when the samples are randomly selected. The characteristics of any given sample are usually different from those of the population. For example, suppose a fair coin was tossed 10 times for 10 different trials. A tally of the results in **Table 13-9** shows that the trials varied; but as expected, more of the trials were nearer 50% heads than 100% heads.

TABLE 13-9   Coin Toss Example

	Trial 1	Trial 2	Trial 3	Trial 4	Trial 5	Trial 6	Trial 7	Trial 8	Trial 9	Trial 10
0 Heads 10 Tails										
1 Head 9 Tails										
2 Heads 8 Tails						X				
3 Heads 7 Tails										
4 Heads 6 Tails		X					X			
5 Heads 5 Tails	X				X					X
6 Heads 4 Tails				X					X	
7 Heads 3 Tails								X		
8 Heads 2 Tails			X							
9 Heads 1 Tail										
10 Heads 0 Tails										

CRITICAL THINKING EXERCISE 13-3

When is there enough testing to make a decision?

TEST YOUR KNOWLEDGE 13-6

1. Inferential statistical tests are used to: (Select all that apply.)
    a. make assumptions about the population.
    b. describe the sample with means and standard deviations.
    c. test hypotheses by asking if there are differences between the groups.
    d. select a sample.
    e. determine whether results occurred by chance.

How did you do? 1. a, c, e

Researchers determine whether the results were obtained by chance using inferential statistical tests, sometimes known as tests of significance. Mathematical calculations are performed, usually by computers, to obtain critical values. These values are plotted on a normal distribution, and determinations of whether findings are *statistically significant* or *nonsignificant* are made. Statistically significant critical values fall in the tails of the normal distributions, usually three standard deviations from the mean or where about only 0.3% of the data occur. Thus, when critical values are in that area, researchers believe it is appropriate to claim that the findings did not happen by chance.

KEY TERMS

statistically significant: When critical values fall in the tails of normal distributions; when findings did not happen by chance alone

nonsignificant: When results of the study could have occurred by chance; findings that support the null hypothesis

13.7 Reducing Error When Deciding About Hypotheses

At the end of this section, you will be able to:

< Distinguish between type I and type II errors
< Describe alpha levels commonly used in nursing research

Researchers do many things to reduce error so that nurses can have confidence in findings. They reduce error by selecting designs that fit with research questions, controlling the independent variable, carefully measuring variables, and reducing threats to internal and external validity. They also take steps to reduce error when deciding whether a research hypothesis is supported or not supported.

When making decisions about hypotheses, researchers keep several principles in mind (Hayes, 1994). First, hypotheses are claims about the world. Second, decisions are made about null hypotheses, not research hypotheses. The purpose of inferential statistical tests is to determine whether the null hypothesis should be accepted or rejected. Third, it is important to remember that no matter how well errors are reduced or how powerful the findings are, nothing is ever proven. The most that can be claimed is that a research hypothesis is either supported or unsupported. Last, it is wise to understand that an empirical view is adopted and an assumption is made that there is a single reality in the physical world and that science can be used to discover the truth about reality.

For example, suppose a researcher is testing a new way to assess risk for skin breakdown over the sacrum. The researcher hypothesizes that prior to the presentation of redness, skin temperature will be increased. From an empirical viewpoint, it is assumed that skin temperature, redness, and sacrum are real entities and that in the real world one of four situations is true: prior to the appearance of redness over the sacrum, the skin temperature will be increased, unchanged, decreased, or varied. Now suppose that in the real world, the unknown truth is that skin temperature does increase before redness appears over the sacrum. After collecting and analyzing data, statistically significant results were obtained. The researcher decides to reject the null hypothesis, that there will be no difference in skin temperature before the appearance of redness, and the research hypothesis is supported. In this instance, unknown to the researcher, an error was not made. The claim of the original hypothesis, that skin temperature would be increased prior to the appearance of sacral redness, matches what actually happens in the world. The researcher rejected the null hypothesis, and it was indeed false. If nurses accumulated additional supporting evidence, findings would make their way into practice, and patients at risk for skin breakdown could be identified earlier.

Errors are avoided when researchers accept the null hypothesis when it is true. Consider this variation of the preceding example. The researcher hypothesizes that prior to the presentation of redness over the sacrum, skin temperature will be increased; however, in the real world there is no change in skin temperature over the sacrum prior to the appearance of redness. After collecting and analyzing data, the researcher finds that calculations from inferential statistical tests are nonsignificant and therefore the null hypothesis is supported. Although disappointed, the researcher accepts the null hypothesis and unwittingly avoids error because there is no temperature change in the real world. The goal of hypothesis testing is to accept true claims and reject false ones.

Type I and Type II Errors

The goal is to avoid the two kinds of errors that can be made when making decisions about null hypotheses. These errors are known as type I and type II errors. A *type I error* occurs when the researcher rejects the null hypothesis when it should have been accepted. In nursing, when the null hypothesis is wrongly rejected, the usual result is that the researcher makes false claims about the research hypothesis. Usually this means that the researcher claims that some treatment works or some relationship exists, when in actuality that is not the case. For example, in the previous examples, the researcher hypothesized that skin temperatures over the sacrum would be increased prior to the appearance of redness. Now suppose that in the real world, there is no change in the temperature; however, analysis of the data collected indicates that there is an increase of temperature. In other words, the researcher has obtained statistically significant results. This false finding could be the result of any number of errors, such as sampling bias and measurement error. The false finding could have happened by chance, just as it would be possible by chance to get 20 heads in a row when tossing a fair coin. The researcher, unaware about what is true in the world, rejects the null hypothesis based on the statistical analysis and claims that the research hypothesis is supported. This is a type I error. If nurses adopt this finding into practice, they will unnecessarily spend time measuring skin temperature because it would provide no indication of risk. If the practice of measuring skin temperature continued without evaluation of patient outcomes, it is possible that this type I error would never be discovered.

A *type II error* occurs when researchers accept the null hypothesis when it should have been rejected. In nursing, this type of error usually means that practice does not change when it should be changed. The opportunity to implement an effective treatment or claim the discovery of a relationship has been missed. Consider this variation of the previous example. The researcher still hypothesizes that sacral skin temperature is increased prior to the appearance of redness, and in the real world this is true. The researcher completes the analysis, which has statistically nonsignificant results. These nonsignificant results can be the result of error or chance. Based on the statistical analysis, the researcher is forced to accept the null hypothesis, unaware that the research hypothesis is true in the real world. A type II error has occurred, and nurses miss an opportunity to predict which patients are at risk for skin breakdown.

There are a few strategies for remembering type I and type II errors. One way is through the graphic representation in **Table 13-10**. One axis of the table

KEY TERMS

type I error: When the researcher rejects the null hypothesis when it should have been accepted

type II error: When the researcher inaccurately concludes that there is no relationship among the independent and dependent variables when an actual relationship does exist; when the researcher accepts the null hypothesis when it should have been rejected

CRITICAL THINKING EXERCISE 13-4

Individuals make decisions every day. They make decisions based on their assumptions about the world, only to find out later that the assumptions were incorrect. Can you think of times when you have made a type I error? What about a situation when a type II error was made?

TABLE 13-10	Type I and Type II Errors	
	The Null Hypothesis Is True in Real World	**The Null Hypothesis Is False in Real World**
Researcher Accepts the Null Hypothesis	No Error	Type II Error
Researcher Rejects the Null Hypothesis	Type I Error	No Error

represents whether the null hypothesis is true or false in the real world. The other axis represents the two decisions that can be made by researchers about the null hypothesis: to accept or to reject. The center boxes are then filled in as appropriate. No errors are made when a decision to accept a null hypothesis is made when it is true in the real world. Likewise, there is no error when a false null hypothesis is rejected. A type I error is made when researchers, obtaining statistically significant results, reject the null hypothesis when in fact it was true. A type II error occurs when researchers fail to obtain statistically significant results, and thus they accept the null hypothesis despite the fact that it is false. Another way to remember type I and type II errors is to think of the acronym RAAR (Gillis & Jackson, 2002). RAAR stands for the phrase: "Reject the null hypothesis when you should accept it, and accept the null hypothesis when you should reject it." The first two letters, RA, stand for type I error. The second two letters, AR, stand for type II error.

Level of Significance: Adjusting the Risk of Making Type I and Type II Errors

In health care, type I errors are considered to be more serious than type II errors are (Smith, 2012). It seems much more risky to claim that a treatment works when in reality it does not than to miss the opportunity to claim that a treatment works. For example, a researcher invents and tests a new device for measuring blood sugar. If a type I error is made, the researcher claims that the new device works when in reality it does not. Patients begin using the device, which inaccurately measures blood sugar. Because nurses evaluate the implementation of this new device, they eventually realize that the device is not effective as the researcher claimed. The type I error could result in accusations of harming diabetics with a fraudulent measuring device. Because patients who used the device might have been harmed, they might want to sue the researcher. However, if a type II error is made, the researcher throws away the device for measuring blood sugar even though in reality it is superior to other devices. In this situation, the researcher misses the opportunity to market the device and earn money, and diabetics miss the opportunity to benefit from the measuring device. Although neither scenario is desirable, most researchers would choose to miss the opportunity to make money rather than to harm patients and risk the legal implications.

Researchers must make decisions about how much risk they are willing to tolerate. When interventions are complex, expensive, invasive, or have many side effects, such as a new procedure for cardiac surgery, researchers are usually less willing to make type I errors. When interventions are simple, inexpensive, or noninvasive, such as a new teaching method, the tolerance for a type I error is increased.

Researchers use statistics to adjust the amount of risk involved in making type I and type II errors. It is helpful to remember that type I and type II errors have an inverse relationship. When type I error is increased, type II error is decreased. Risks for these errors are adjusted by selecting the *alpha level*, which is the probability of making a type I error. Alpha level is designated at the end of the tail in a distribution (see **Figure 13-12**). In nursing research, the alpha

> **KEY TERM**
>
> **alpha level:**
> Probability of making a type I error; typically designated as .05 or .01 at the end of the tail in a distribution

FIGURE 13-12   Placement of Alpha Level on Normal Distribution

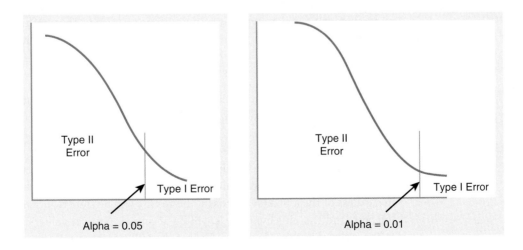

Alpha = 0.05

Alpha = 0.01

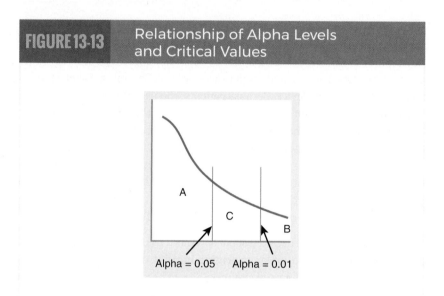

FIGURE 13-13 Relationship of Alpha Levels and Critical Values

levels are usually either .05 or .01. In the figure, the placement of the alpha level shows how type I and type II errors can be adjusted. In this example of a one-tailed test, the area under the curve to the left of the alpha level represents the amount of type II error. The area under the curve to the right of the line is the amount of type I error. Notice that when the alpha level is larger, there is more space to the right of the line than when the alpha level is smaller.

What are the implications of these alpha levels? When the alpha level is set at .05, it is likely that 5 times out of 100, the researcher would make a type I error by wrongly rejecting the null hypothesis. When .01 is used for the alpha level, a researcher would make a type I error only 1 time out of 100. Thus, alpha levels of .05 increase type I errors while reducing type II errors. In general, although alpha levels of .01 reduce type I errors, the likelihood of making a type II error increases. In nursing, .05 is used more commonly than .01 is.

Although the mathematical difference between these alphas is miniscule, the implications for decision making are great. **Figure 13-13** provides an illustration of how the acceptance or rejection of the null hypothesis is affected by the alpha level selected. When conducting statistical tests to test hypotheses, suppose there is a chance for three possible critical values. Note in Figure 13-13 that critical value "A" falls to the left of both alpha levels. Regardless of the alpha level chosen, the results will be statistically nonsignificant, and the null hypothesis will be accepted. Critical value "B" falls to the right of both alpha levels. The results will be statistically significant regardless of the alpha level selected. Now consider the position of critical

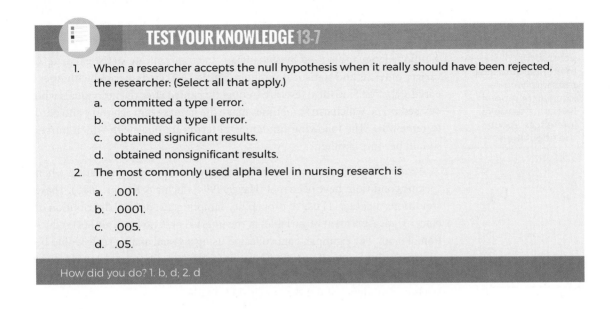

TEST YOUR KNOWLEDGE 13-7

1. When a researcher accepts the null hypothesis when it really should have been rejected, the researcher: (Select all that apply.)

    a. committed a type I error.
    b. committed a type II error.
    c. obtained significant results.
    d. obtained nonsignificant results.

2. The most commonly used alpha level in nursing research is

    a. .001.
    b. .0001.
    c. .005.
    d. .05.

How did you do? 1. b, d; 2. d

value "C." How would the decision about the null hypothesis be affected by either of these two alphas? If the alpha level is set at .05, the critical point would be significant and the null hypothesis would be rejected. However, if an alpha level of .01 is selected, the critical point would be nonsignificant, and the researcher would accept the null hypothesis. To avoid any temptation to select alpha levels that bias decision making, researchers must always state their selected alpha levels in the initial research proposal. Strong rationales for the one selected must also be provided.

13.8 Using Statistical Tests to Make Inferences About Populations

At the end of this section, you will be able to:

‹ Match common notations with associated statistical tests

‹ Identify common statistical tests as parametric or nonparametric

‹ Describe tests used to determine statistically significant differences between groups

‹ Discuss tests used to determine statistically significant differences among variables

‹ Assign commonly used statistical tests to examples based on type of research question and level of measurement

The Language of Inferential Statistics

A unique language is used by statisticians to communicate statistical data. A variety of terms and statistical symbols (**Table 13-11**) is associated with inferential statistics. Statistical tests are frequently named after the individuals who devised them, which can sometimes make the names seem arbitrary and hard to remember. The following fundamental terms are ones with which nurses should become familiar.

Parametric tests are used to make inferences about the population when specific conditions have been met (Hayes, 1994; Plichta & Kelvin, 2013). These conditions include: (1) use of probability sampling, (2) normal distribution of data, (3) measurement of variables at the interval or ratio level, and (4) reduction of error. For example, data collected using a visual analog scale would be analyzed using parametric tests. These important conditions make parametric tests especially powerful. When parametric tests are used, nurses can have high levels of confidence about the conclusions made.

TABLE 13-11	Statistical Symbols for Inferential Statistics

Symbol/Abbreviation	Definition
ANOVA	Analysis of variance
df	Degrees of freedom
F	Fisher's *F* ratio
ns	Nonsignificant
p	Probability
r	Pearson product–moment correlation
R	Multiple correlation
R^2	Multiple correlation squared
t	Computed value of *t* test
α	Alpha; probability of type I error
β	Beta; probability of type II error
Δ	Delta; amount of change
Σ	Sigma; sum or summation
X^2	Chi square

When all four conditions are not met, researchers must use less powerful tests known as *nonparametric* tests. Nonparametric statistics are used for interval data that do not have a normal distribution or for data that are nominal or ordinal in nature. Because these tests are considered to be less powerful, the level of confidence nurses have about making inferences about the population is not as strong as when parametric tests are used.

Another term used when talking about statistics is *degrees of freedom*. Degrees of freedom (*df*), based on the number of elements in a sample, are used to correct for possible underestimation of population parameters when performing mathematical equations. Specifically, *degrees of freedom* refers to the freedom of a variable's score to vary given the other existing variables' score values and the sum of these score values ($df = N - 1$) (Plichta & Kelvin, 2013). For example, suppose a data set consists of four scores: 1, 4, 4, and 7. Before any of these scores were collected, the researcher did not know what these scores would be. Each score was free to vary. This means that each score was independent from the other scores. Because there are four scores, there are four degrees of freedom. However, when the mean is calculated, one degree of freedom is lost. This is because after the mean is known, along with three of the scores, the fourth score is no longer free to vary. The fourth score can be calculated, and only one value will be correct. Therefore, the data set of four scores has three degrees of freedom, $n - 1$, because one degree of freedom is lost. Many inferential statistics include degrees of freedom in their calculations.

Another concept important in the language of inferential statistics is *sampling distribution* (Nieswiadomy, 2012; Plichta & Kelvin, 2013). In theory, an infinite number of samples can be drawn from a population. Some samples are more likely to be drawn than others are. For example, when sampling coin tosses, getting half heads and half tails when tossing a coin 20 times is far more likely than is tossing heads 20 times in a row. For many inferential tests, statisticians have calculated the likelihood of obtaining different samples and reported them in tables. When researchers perform certain inferential tests, they refer to these tables to find out whether their results are likely or unlikely. Results that are unlikely to occur as a result of chance are then considered to be statistically significant.

Nurses commonly see a number of inferential tests in the literature. Although the study of statistical tests can seem overwhelming to some individuals, to appraise evidence it might not be necessary to fully understand why each test is conducted and how the calculations are performed. Nurses should be able to discern that the correct tests were used to analyze data. This can be determined by focusing on two broad questions: (1) "What type of question is being asked by the researcher?" and (2) "What is the level of measurement being used to measure the variables?" Some inferential statistical tests commonly used in nursing research are listed in **Table 13-12**. Although it is beyond the scope of

KEY TERMS

nonparametric: Inferential statistics involving nominal- or ordinal-level data to make inferences about the population

degrees of freedom: A statistical concept used to refer to the number of sample values that are free to vary; *n* – 1

sampling distribution: A theoretical distribution representing an infinite number of samples that can be drawn from a population

TABLE 13-12   Inferential Tests Commonly Used in Nursing

| | What is the hypothesis asking? | | | | | |
| | Is there a difference between the groups? | | | | Is there a relationship among the variables? | |
What is the level of measurement?	1 Group	2 Groups — Related	2 Groups — Independent	> 2 Groups	2 Variables	> 2 Variables
Nonparametric — **Nominal**	✓ Chi square	✓ Chi square ✓ Fisher's exact probability test	✓ Chi square	✓ Chi square	✓ Phi coefficient ✓ Point biserial	✓ Contingency coefficient
Nonparametric — **Ordinal**	✓ Kolmogorov-Smirnov	✓ Sign test ✓ Wicoxin matched pairs ✓ Signed rank	✓ Chi square ✓ Median test ✓ Mann-Whitney U	✓ Chi square	✓ Kendall's Tau ✓ Spearman Rho	
Parametric — **Interval or Ratio**	✓ Correlated t (paired t)	✓ Correlated t (paired t)	✓ Independent t	✓ ANOVA ✓ ANCOVA ✓ MANOVA	✓ Pearson's r	✓ Multiple regression ✓ Path analysis ✓ Canonical correlation

Note: ANOVA = analysis of variance; ANCOVA = analysis of covariance; MANOVA = multivariate analysis of variance.

this text to elaborate on all the tests listed in the table, information about some of the most common tests is worth remembering. When answering questions about statistically significant differences between groups, nurses should be familiar with Chi square, *t* tests, and analysis of variance (ANOVA). They should also be familiar with Pearson's *r* and multiple regression, which are tests used to determine if there is a statistically significant correlation among the variables.

Testing for Differences Between Groups

As shown in Table 13-12, a variety of tests is used to analyze data for the purpose of determining if there is a statistically significant difference between the groups. When deciding which test to use, researchers must consider the number of groups to be included in the analysis and at what level variables were measured. Pilot studies frequently involve one group, whereas classic experiments and quasi-experiments can include two or more groups. Before analyzing data, researchers need to consider whether the groups are dependent or independent to select the correct tests to perform. For example, suppose a researcher is studying perceptions of health in married couples before and after a class about stress reduction. The researcher tests both men and women who are married to one another. Because individuals in a marriage have many characteristics in common, the data collected should be analyzed using inferential tests for dependent groups. Data from designs using subjects as their own controls, for example, measuring blood pressures before and after exercise, are also treated as data from dependent groups. More likely than not, researchers collect data from independent groups, for example, test scores from two groups of diabetic patients.

The Chi Square Statistic

Chi square is a very commonly used statistic (Hayes, 1994; Plichta & Kelvin, 2013). Calculated when analyzing nominal and ordinal data, it is a nonparametric test. One reason Chi square is used so often is because it is very useful for finding differences between the groups on demographic variables. For example, suppose that a researcher is studying the effect of aromatherapy on blood pressure and randomly assigns 200 individuals to one of two groups. The experimental group contains 54 women and 46 men, while the control group has 46 women and 54 men. By performing a Chi-square test, the researcher can determine whether the groups are alike on the extraneous variable of gender. If the groups are not significantly different on gender, it can be assumed that changes in blood pressure are more likely a result of the intervention than of gender.

When Chi-square statistics are used, the frequencies that are observed during the study are compared to the frequencies that would be expected to

KEY TERMS

t statistic:
Inferential
statistical test to
determine whether
a statistically
significant
difference between
groups exists

correlated t test:
A variation of the
t test used when
there is only one
group or when
groups are related;
paired t test

independent t test:
A variation of the
t test used when
data values vary
independently from
one another

**analysis of
variance:** Inferential
statistical test used
when the level of
measurement is
interval or ratio
and more than two
groups are being
compared

occur if the null hypothesis were true. Observed and expected frequencies are entered into contingency tables, and a Chi-square statistic is calculated. Using the calculated Chi-square statistic, the degrees of freedom, and the alpha level, researchers consult Chi-square tables to determine the critical value and judge whether the critical value is statistically significant. In the literature, notations for Chi square, such as $X^2 = 1.89$, $df = 1$, $p < .05$, appear reported with degrees of freedom and significance. Another reason Chi squares are frequently used is that they can be calculated without the use of computers. However, the sample size must be adequate because there must be at least five or more observed frequencies in each cell of the table. If this minimum is not met, then a variation of the Chi square, known as Fisher's exact probability test, is used.

The *t* Statistic

The *t statistic* is another inferential statistical test that is frequently reported in nursing research. Commonly known as the *t* test, or Student's *t* test, this parametric measure is used to determine whether there is a statistically significant difference between two groups (Hayes, 1994; Plichta & Kelvin, 2013).

There are two variations of the *t* test. One variation, known as the *correlated t test* or paired *t* test, is used when there are only two measurements taken on the same person (one group) or when the groups are related. For example, a paired *t* test would be used to assess for differences between subjects' morning and evening blood pressure readings. The other variation is known as an *independent t test* and is used when data values vary independently from one another.

In experimental and quasi-experimental designs, the *t* test is used to determine whether the means of two groups are statistically different. Suppose a researcher is measuring the effectiveness of applying ice for pain reduction in patients with a new cast applied for fracture of the tibia. The mean pain intensity rating for the experimental group, which received the ice application, is 5.6, whereas for the control group, which did not get the ice, it is 6.0. As with a Chi-square test, researchers calculate the *t* statistic and consult tables using the statistic, degrees of freedom, and alpha levels to find the critical value. The critical value is obtained and a decision about its statistical significance is made. In reports, the *t* test information provided includes *t*, indicating the statistical test done, number of degrees of freedom, actual *t* value obtained, and significance level, which is reported in the following manner: $t(2) = 2.54$, $p < .01$.

Analysis of Variance

Analysis of variance (ANOVA) is used when the level of measurement is interval or ratio and there are more than two groups or the variable of interest is measured more than two times (Hayes, 1994; Plichta & Kelvin, 2013). The broad question being answered is whether group means significantly differ from one another. Using ANOVA allows researchers to compare a combination of pairs of means while reducing the odds for a type I error. For example, suppose that a researcher is testing three different styles of education with adolescents who have asthma: peer, text messaging, and Web-based. There would be three different pairs of means to compare: peer to text messaging, peer to Web-based, and text messaging to Web-based. If *t* tests were conducted for each pair, the same null hypothesis would be tested three times, increasing the risk of a type I error. By using an ANOVA, researchers can compare the variations among the groups using one statistical test, thereby reducing the chances of making a type I error.

ANOVA and *t* tests are very closely related. When testing only two groups, the same mathematical answer would result whether an ANOVA or a *t* test were used. Using ANOVA, researchers calculate the *F* statistic, which is based on the *F* distribution using degrees of freedom. The greater the *F* statistic, the greater the variation between the means of the groups. Tables of the *F* distributions and degrees of freedom are also used. $F = 4.65$, $df = 2, 50$, $p < .05$ is an example of the notation that would be used to report an ANOVA. However, the *F* statistic indicates only that the null hypothesis can be rejected because there is a difference between the group means, but the *F* test alone does not tell which specific group differed. Instead, researchers have to conduct post hoc tests to determine where the significant difference occurred.

Two variations of ANOVA, analysis of covariance (ANCOVA) and multivariate analysis of variance (MANOVA), are also used in nursing research. ANCOVA is used to statistically control for known extraneous variables. For example, if a researcher believes that level of education affects the amount learned by the adolescents with asthma, the researcher may use ANCOVA to control for grade in school. When researchers have more than one dependent variable, they used MANOVA instead of ANOVA to analyze data.

Other Tests of Significance

Table 13-12 shows that a number of other inferential statistics can be used to determine whether there are statistically significant differences between groups. These include Kolmogorov-Smirnov test, sign test, Wilcoxin matched pairs test, signed rank test, median test, and Mann-Whitney U test (Hayes, 1994; Plichta & Kelvin, 2013). These tests are used when ordinal level data are involved; thus, they are categorized as nonparametric tests. Tests are selected based on considerations such as the number of groups being compared, the distribution pattern of the data (normal or skewed), and other nuances that can be found in the data.

Testing for Relationships Among Variables

To find whether there are relationships among variables, a variety of statistical tests is used to determine the significance of correlations (see Table 13-12). Decisions about which statistical tests to use are based on whether there are two variables or more than two variables. Consideration is also given to the level of measurement used. Understanding how decisions are made allows nurses to ascertain the quality of the findings.

Pearson's r

When researchers pose hypotheses about the relationships among variables, they are testing for the significance of the correlation coefficient. When two variables are measured at the interval or ratio level, they calculate the *Pearson's r* statistic, also known as the Pearson product–moment correlation (Hayes, 1994; Plichta & Kelvin, 2013). The degrees of freedom for this test are always $N - 2$, which means that the correlation coefficient can be affected by the sample size. It is possible for a small correlation coefficient to be statistically significant when there is a large sample. In the literature, the notation $r = .62, p < .01$ is used. This notation provides three important pieces of information about the two variables. First, the variables are related at a magnitude of .62, which is usually considered to be a moderate—or moderately strong—relationship. Second, the two variables have a positive relationship with each other because the value is positive. Third, the correlation is statistically significant. A statistically significant correlation is one that is significantly different from zero.

Small correlations can be statistically significant because it does not take much variation to be significantly different from a correlation of zero (Nieswiadomy, 2012). Therefore, researchers can use a variation of Pearson's r that determines the percentage of variance shared by two variables, which provides more meaningful information. By squaring the coefficient (r^2), the overlap, or shared variance, is computed. A helpful way to think about variance is to think of a pie chart. The entire pie chart represents all the variables that can contribute to changes in the dependent variable. Each r^2 indicates how large a section of the pie chart that variable earns. With this information, knowledge of one variable can be used to predict the value of the other variable. For example, suppose that a correlation coefficient of .23 was obtained for the variables self-esteem and weight gain. Squaring .23 equals .0529. This is interpreted to mean that self-esteem accounts for about 5% of weight gain. Thus, the researcher would know that other variables must also contribute to weight gain.

Multiple Regression

A change in one variable is usually the result of many factors. Thus, when researchers want to study the relationship of many independent variables on one dependent variable, they use *multiple regression* analysis (Hayes, 1994; Plichta & Kelvin, 2013). Calculations such as these have become much more sophisticated with the use of computers because computers can perform simultaneous calculations. Like Pearson's *r*, multiple regression is used when variables are measured at the interval or ratio level. For example, suppose a researcher wants to determine which factors best predict an anorexic adolescent's success at maintaining a weight in the normal range. Independent variables might include self-esteem, social support, anxiety, and locus of control. In this situation, a multiple regression will be performed.

There are different approaches to performing multiple regression based on the way in which the predictor variables are entered into the analysis. One common approach to multiple regression is known as step-wise. This approach is used to find the smallest number of independent variables that account for the greatest proportion of variance in the outcome variable (Pedhazur, 1982). For example, in a study of adolescents with anorexia, a researcher might find that self-esteem, anxiety, and locus of control account for 24% of the variance in weight gain and that social support does not make any significant difference in weight gain. Researchers can use another approach to multiple regression know as hierarchical regression. This approach is typically used when the importance of variables has been specified in theories. For example, suppose it is proposed in a theory about anorexia in adolescents that locus of control is the most important factor, followed by self-esteem and then anxiety. Based on this theory, the researcher would be able to specify the order the independent variables are to be entered into the equations. As in step-wise multiple regression, the amount of variance that is significant is reported.

Other Tests of Significance

Because all variables are not measured at interval and ratio levels, there are other tests of significance that can determine whether changes in variables are significant (Hayes, 1994; Plichta & Kelvin, 2013). When nominal data are involved, statistics such as phi coefficients, point biserials, and contingency coefficients are reported. Researchers use Kendall's Tau, Spearman Rho, and discriminate function analysis to analyze ordinal-level data. There are also very sophisticated methods for testing and predicting the strength and direction of relationships among multiple variables. These analytic methods, such as linear structural relationships or structural equation modeling, are useful ways to use data to test theories.

KEY TERM

multiple regression: Inferential statistical test that describes the relationship of three or more variables

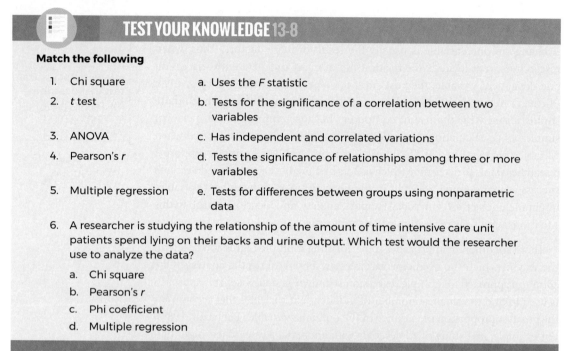

TEST YOUR KNOWLEDGE 13-8

Match the following

1. Chi square
2. *t* test
3. ANOVA
4. Pearson's *r*
5. Multiple regression

a. Uses the *F* statistic
b. Tests for the significance of a correlation between two variables
c. Has independent and correlated variations
d. Tests the significance of relationships among three or more variables
e. Tests for differences between groups using nonparametric data

6. A researcher is studying the relationship of the amount of time intensive care unit patients spend lying on their backs and urine output. Which test would the researcher use to analyze the data?

   a. Chi square
   b. Pearson's *r*
   c. Phi coefficient
   d. Multiple regression

How did you do? 1. e; 2. c; 3. a; 4. b; 5. d; 6. b

13.9 What Does All This Mean for EBP?

At the end of this section, you will be able to:

< Interpret data reported in statistical tables
< Differentiate between statistical significance and clinical significance
< Appraise data analysis sections of an article

When reading research articles, nurses must assume that mathematical calculations were done accurately because raw data are not included. What nurses should appraise is that the correct tests were performed. Table 13-12 is a helpful tool for appraising the analysis sections of articles.

Nurses should also appraise data presented in tables to determine whether conclusions drawn by researchers are supported by the findings. Although many readers frequently skip over the tables when reading research articles, this is not a good practice. The tables contain evidence on which practice changes can be made, and for this reason they may be one of the most important components of the report. Nurses need to acquire skill at reading and interpreting tables. Some hints for doing so are presented in **Box 13-1**.

BOX 13-1	Tips for Reading Statistical Tables

Be familiar with symbols used.

Read the title of the table first.

Pay attention to the labels of columns and rows.

Observe when headings for subsamples and subscales are indented.

Follow columns carefully both horizontally and vertically.

Attend to significant findings.

Alpha levels are either reported with a notation or under the table with an asterisk (*).

Pay attention to superscript or footnote markings.

Do not skip tables, because information can be clearer after studying a table.

Recognize that there can be typos and math errors.

Remember that subsamples may be omitted from the table (i.e., sample indicates total subjects and number of women, leaving reader to calculate number of men).

It is also important to differentiate between statistical significance and clinical significance. For example, suppose a drug lowered cholesterol levels on average from 195 to 178. Analysis indicated that this decrease was statistically significant; however, because any cholesterol value below 200 is considered to be within normal range, there is no clinical significance to this finding. In another example, consider an experimental study involving guided imagery. Children in the guided imagery group had average pain ratings of 4.2, while children in the control group had average pain ratings of 5.2. Although the difference between these means is not statistically significant, it may be clinically significant to have pain ratings a whole point lower. Furthermore, because guided imagery was noninvasive and inexpensive and children reportedly enjoyed it, it might be worth incorporating as a practice intervention. When appraising evidence, it is wise for nurses to keep in mind that statistical significance and clinical significance are different.

Appraising the results section of research reports can be challenging. An understanding of the material presented in this chapter can assist you in meeting this challenge. Information in **Box 13-2** and **Figure 13-14** should be considered when evaluating data analysis.

FYI

Although many readers frequently skip over the tables when reading research articles, this is not a good practice. Data presented in tables may contain evidence on which practice changes can be made, and thus may be one of the most important components of a report.

BOX 13-2 Questions for Appraising Analysis of Data

1. What statistics were used to describe the characteristics of the sample? What statistics were used to analyze the data that were collected? Were the statistics appropriate for the level of measurement?
2. Were measures of central tendency provided? If so, which ones were used? Are they the most appropriate? How sensitive to outliers is the measure reported?
3. Were measures of variation/dispersion provided? Were standard deviations reported for each mean that was reported?
4. What was the distribution of the data? Were data normally distributed? Was skewness or kurtosis discussed?
5. What statistics were used to determine differences between the groups? Were the results significant?
6. What statistics were used to express relationships among variables of interest? What was the magnitude and direction of the relationship? Was it significant?
7. Are all the hypotheses addressed in the analysis section of the report?
8. Is the selected level of significance appropriate for the purpose of the study and the types of analyses being conducted?
9. Do the tables and graphs agree with the text? Are they precise and do they offer economy of information?
10. Are the results understandable and presented objectively?

FIGURE 13-14

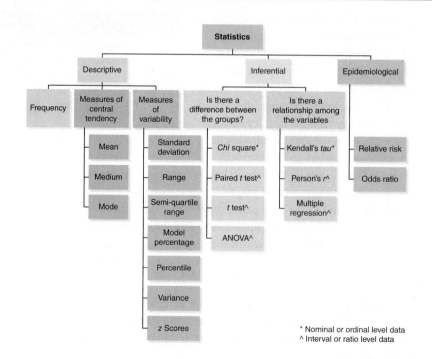

* Nominal or ordinal level data
^ Interval or ratio level data

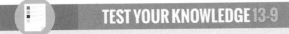

True/False

1. Nurses should determine that researchers are using the correct statistical tests to analyze data.
2. Data contained in tables are an important source of evidence for practice.
3. All statistically significant findings have clinical significance.
4. Reading the table after the text is a helpful strategy that can improve comprehension of ideas.

How did you do? 1. T; 2. T; 3. F; 4. T

13.10 Keeping It Ethical

At the end of this section, you will be able to:

‹ Discuss ethical considerations when conducting statistical analyses

All researchers hope that their hypotheses will be supported. Researchers develop a passion for their topics that keeps them invested in their research. However, researchers must use care when analyzing data and selecting alpha levels. It is best if decisions about which statistical tests to conduct and which alpha levels to use are made prior to implementing the study. These decisions are usually presented, with strong rationales for the decisions, in the proposal for the study. Although there are situations when it is appropriate to conduct additional statistical tests, it is unethical for researchers to "go fishing" for evidence to support their hypotheses.

Editors and research conference planners who review studies are faced with making decisions about which studies warrant dissemination. Studies with significant findings are much more likely to be accepted for presentation or publication. Because nonsignificant findings have an important role in making decisions about practice, decision makers, such as conference planners and journal publishers, need to give more consideration to studies with nonsignificant findings.

Ignoring incidental findings that are pertinent to decision making is also unethical. Incidental findings are findings that were not purposefully sought. A dilemma can occur when an intervention is found to be effective, but incidental findings, such as side effects or risks, are found to be associated with the intervention. It is possible for researchers to report additional analyses comparing risks and benefits. Reporting adverse effects is necessary so that professionals and patients can make informed choices. Researchers should also report incidental findings when findings have clinical significance or are interesting and indicate a need for further research.

CRITICAL THINKING EXERCISE 13-5

Imagine that manuscripts for 10 different studies conducted about the effect of massage on the oxygen saturation of infants in the neonatal intensive care unit are sent to a variety of journals. Only one study had significant findings, and it was accepted for publication. If none of the other nine studies were accepted for publication, what evidence would be available to nurses for EBP? How might practice be affected if all 10 studies were published?

TEST YOUR KNOWLEDGE 13-10

Which of the following are unethical?

1. Selecting an alpha of .05 so that the research hypothesis is supported when it would not be if the alpha were set at .01.

2. Publishing articles about studies with nonsignificant findings.

3. Including information about incidental findings, especially when they involve side effects or risks.

How did you do? 1. Unethical; 2. Ethical; 3. Ethical

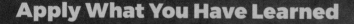

Apply What You Have Learned

The EBP committee is nearly done analyzing the evidence. Complete the outcomes column in the grid by adding information about the quantitative designs. When available, report the pre- and post-hand hygiene compliance rates so that you can determine which interventions were most effective.

RAPID REVIEW

» Statistics are used to describe numerical outcomes and the probabilities derived from calculations on raw data.

» There are two types of statistics: descriptive and inferential. Descriptive statistics explain characteristics of variables found in a sample. Inferential statistics are the basis for predictions about the phenomenon.

» Univariate analysis involves only one variable at a time and includes frequency distributions, measures of central tendency, shape of the distribution, and measures of variability.

» Bivariate analysis is conducted to describe relationships between two variables.

» Frequencies may be grouped or ungrouped data describing how often a variable is found to occur. Line charts, bar graphs, pie charts, histograms, and scattergrams are ways frequencies can be depicted.

» The mode, median, and mean are measures of central tendency. In a normal distribution, they are all the same value.

» A normal distribution is a bell-shaped curve that is symmetric around the mean. Asymmetric distributions are known as skewed and have either positive or negative directions.

» Data with little variability are considered to be homogenous, whereas data with wide variations are considered to be heterogeneous.

» Measures of variability include the range, semiquartile range, percentile, standard deviation, z scores, and coefficient of variation.

» The Rule of 68–95–99.7 is a way of describing the percentage of scores falling within specific standard deviations of the mean.

» Correlation coefficients are used to describe the relationship between two variables.

» Inferential statistics are used to estimate population parameters and test hypotheses.

» CIs describe the probability of being correct.

» When selecting which statistical tests to use, researchers must consider the type of question being asked and the level of measurement. The null hypothesis is statistically tested and is rejected when significant findings occur. Research hypotheses are supported but never proven.

» Probability is the likelihood of a frequency of an event in similar trials under similar conditions and indicates how probable it is that the results were obtained by chance. Sampling error is the tendency for statistics to fluctuate from one sample to another and forms the basis of probability.

» Type I errors occur when researchers reject the null hypothesis when it should have been accepted. Type II errors occur when researchers accept the null hypothesis when it should have been rejected.

» Alpha levels of either .05 or .01 are typically used in nursing research. Alpha levels affect the amount of risk involved for making type I and type II errors.

» Parametric tests are more powerful than nonparametric tests are because they are used with interval or ratio level data.

» To test for differences between groups, researchers can use Chi square, *t* test, and ANOVA.

» To test for relationships among variables, Pearson's *r* and multiple regression can be used.

» To apply findings to EBP, nurses must be able to interpret statistical tables, differentiate between clinical and statistical significance, and appraise data analysis.

» To maintain ethical integrity, researchers should select statistical tests and alpha levels in advance and report incidental findings. It is as important to disseminate nonsignificant findings as it is to disseminate significant findings.

REFERENCES

American College of Physicians—American Society of Internal Medicine. (2001). Primer on 95% confidence intervals. *Effective Clinical Practice, 4*, 229–231. Retrieved from http://ecp.acponline.org/sepoct01/primerci.pdf

Borenstein, M. (1997). Hypothesis testing and effect size estimation in clinical trials. *Annals of Allergy, Asthma, and Immunology, 78*, 5–11.

Gillis, A., & Jackson, W. (2002). *Research for nurses: Methods and interpretation.* Philadelphia, PA: F. A. Davis.

Harper, D. (2013). Statistics. *Online Etymology Dictionary.* Retrieved from http://www.etymonline.com/index.php?term=statistics

Hayes, W. L. (1994). *Statistics.* Boston, MA: Wadsworth.

Hoekstra, R., Johnson, A., & Kiers, H. A. L. (2012). Confidence intervals make a difference: Effects of showing confidence intervals on inferential reasoning. *Educational and Psychological Measurement, 72*(6), 1039–1052.

Nieswiadomy, R. M. (2012). *Foundations of nursing research* (6th ed.). Upper Saddle River, NJ: Pearson Education.

Pedhazur, E. J. (1982). *Multiple regression in behavioral research: Explanation and prediction* (2nd ed.). Philadelphia, PA: Harcourt Brace.

Plichta, S. B., & Kelvin, E. (2013). *Munro's statistical methods for health care research* (6th ed.). Philadelphia, PA: Wolters Kluwer/Lippincott Williams & Wilkins.

Smith, C. J. (2012). Type I and type II errors: What are they and why do they matter? *Phlebology, 27*(4), 199–200.

Straus, S. E., Richardson, W. S., Glasziou, P., & Haynes, R. B. (2010). *Evidence-based medicine: How to practice and teach EBM* (4th ed.). Edinburgh, Scotland: Churchill Livingstone.

CHAPTER OBJECTIVES

At the end of this chapter, you will be able to:

- Compare and contrast ways that qualitative data are analyzed
- Discuss the benefits of Computer Assisted Qualitative Data Analysis Software to assist with managing qualitative data
- Describe how researchers draw conclusions from the data and verify them
- Recognize the common ways data are presented in reports
- State why qualitative research is evaluated differently from how quantitative research is evaluated
- Define trustworthiness in terms of credibility, transferability, dependability, and confirmability
- Describe strategies for evaluating qualitative research
- Describe key ethical issues in qualitative research

KEY TERMS

auditability
axial coding
coding
Computer Assisted
   Qualitative Data
   Analysis Software
   (CAQDAS)
confessionist tales
confirmability

credibility
data reduction
data saturation
dependability
impressionist tales
member checks
negative case analysis
open coding
peer debriefing

personal narrative
qualitative data analysis
realist tales
reflexivity
replicated
representativeness
transferability
triangulation
trustworthiness

CHAPTER 14

What Do the Qualitative Data Mean?

Kristen L. Mauk

14.1 Qualitative Data Analysis

At the end of this section, you will be able to:

‹ Compare and contrast ways that qualitative data are analyzed
‹ Discuss the benefits of Computer Assisted Qualitative Data Analysis Software to assist with managing qualitative data

What Is Qualitative Data Analysis?

Qualitative data analysis is a much less straightforward process than quantitative data analysis is. Using words versus numbers to explain phenomena is both more subjective and more labor intensive. Qualitative data analysis has been described as being "directed by few standardized guidelines" (Polit & Beck, 2012), and there are many acceptable methods to analyze the data. Sandelowski (1995) pointed out that although data analysis and interpretation often occur simultaneously in qualitative research, they should be considered distinct processes. "Qualitative analysis is a means to knowledge production" (Sandelowski, 1995, p. 373) that involves the breakdown, categorization, and prioritization of data into a useful system. She described data analysis as having two major parts: getting a sense of the whole and developing a system. According to Strauss and Corbin (1998), data analysis is "the process of breaking down, examining, comparing, conceptualizing, and categorizing data" (p. 57). Bogdan and Biklen (2006) described data analysis in two stages: analysis (systematically arranging the data) and interpretation.

Miles and Huberman (1994) defined qualitative analysis as having three "concurrent flows of activity: data reduction, data display, and conclusion drawing/verification" (p. 10). Although each of these definitions differs somewhat, there is agreement that data analysis involves some type of process in which data are managed, organized, arranged, or prioritized.

Unfortunately, qualitative research is still often viewed as less essential or of less significance than quantitative research is. Certainly, it is usually ranked lower on most hierarchies of evidence. Recent evidence suggests that despite the progress in qualitative methods, published qualitative studies use methods inconsistently, terminology is not uniform across studies, and rigor may still be lacking in some studies (Ball, McLoughlin, & Darvill, 2011). Researchers can demonstrate rigor in this type of research by addressing the evaluation strategies that will be discussed in this chapter.

Managing the Data

Researchers begin analysis by examining data. Remember that qualitative researchers may have mounds of data from numerous pages of transcribed interviews and field notes. This large amount of data must be reduced or broken into manageable units (Houghton, Murphy, Shaw, and Casey, 2015; Ganapathy, 2016). Because the nature of qualitative research is thick description, "the purpose of analysis is to organize the description so that it is manageable" (Patton, 1990, p. 430). Remember that data gathering and analysis may be occurring simultaneously, with ideas and results enlightening subsequent data collection and interaction with participants (Clissett, 2008).

Coding and Data Reduction

Line-by-line *coding* was historically a common way to begin data analysis and one by which many new researchers learned about this process. It involves reading transcripts line by line and attaching labels to each line. Coding is done to categorize the data into groups. Line-by-line coding done by hand, as many novice researchers do to gain practice, is tedious and frustrating work and not always as fruitful as one would like. Stepping back and taking in the whole data set by thorough reading and rereading prior to considering the grouping of data into meaningful and manageable units should precede any type of systematic coding.

There are many ways to approach coding, or labeling. Some researchers use a note card system with labels, filing key quotes under the basic codes, while others handwrite codes into the margins in a complicated hierarchy according to a codebook they have developed. Color coding is another option, as is the use of computer software, but ultimately researchers come up with their own systems by which to organize the data into manageable units.

Tesch (1990) believed that traditional hand coding resulted in more data instead of less, and that *data reduction* is a better alternative. Miles and Huberman (1994) stated that "data reduction refers to the process of selecting, focusing, simplifying, abstracting, and transforming the data that appear in written-up field notes or transcriptions" (p. 10). Data reduction is part of analysis, and the researcher must make decisions about which data are most representative of the entire story being told. As researchers choose which patterns or categories best present the most essential chunks of the data, they become the tool for data analysis and interpretation.

There is no perfect process for coding data, and there is no wrong process either. Ganapathy (2016) suggested that coding is essentially a personal filing system, and this is why there is no exact way to code data. As a result, the knowledge and skill of the qualitative researcher take on such great significance and importance in qualitative research.

Traditional *open coding* (Corbin & Strauss, 1990, 2008) is one way to describe the first step in grouping the data into categories that seem logical. Researchers should always leave an audit trail by keeping a log of their ongoing thoughts and ideas about the naming and assigning of categories to the data so that they can later examine why certain labels were chosen and others discarded. *Axial coding* (Corbin & Strauss, 1990, 2008) takes the analysis process further and requires researchers to compare the categories and labels, defining and exploring relationships among them.

After the data have been organized by basic coding, Marshall and Rossman (2011) suggest that the next step is to generate categories, themes, and patterns. Researchers must search for categories of meaning that best express "relevant themes, repeating ideas or language, and patterns of belief linking people and settings." Codes might be connected through a common theme. There might be patterns across and within the themes. Researchers look at how codes overlap and how themes and patterns emerge in relationship to each other. The analysis process is done with the end result in mind: to stay true to the data and best represent the story or phenomenon being studied.

After the data are categorized and themes emerge, researchers need to pull everything together to paint a picture of the underlying truths revealed by the data. This pulling together of the evidence into a meaningful report that can be communicated to others is another challenge. As Sandelowski (1995) stated, "Qualitative analysis also has artistic dimensions that are often inchoate and incommunicable, involving playfulness, imaginativeness, and creativity" (p. 375).

KEY TERMS

data reduction:
The simplification of large amounts of data obtained from qualitative interviews or other sources

open coding:
The grouping of qualitative data into categories that seem logical

axial coding:
The analysis of categories and labels after completion of open coding

The following examples were taken from interviews with stroke survivors (Easton, 2001). The examples provide some raw data from which you can derive some ideas or common threads. In the first example, what do you perceive? Are any important concepts, ideas, or themes expressed? What was the participant trying to convey?

> Well I know one of the therapists, physical therapists here at the campus, uh, I talked to her about it and then she says, oh, she says, it may never get all right. It was sorta a jolt for me. (p. 148)

Compare the next example with the previous and see whether you notice any similarities or differences. If so, what are they? Are the different participants in these interviews saying anything that might lead you to believe they had similar experiences?

> That, uh, you know, just get up and go do what you were gonna do. But that was just a flashing—and then we realized that, uh, we can't do that no more. (p. 148)

Look at one more quote from yet another stroke survivor. Are there any similarities between this participant's ideas and those of the other two cited previously? If so, what are they?

> I was home probably, oh, I had been to the SOS meeting, and after listening and watching some of the people there, I realized I may never get back everything. (p. 148)

In the previous examples, one might observe some common threads such as *a sense of loss* or *realizing that things may not be the same as before the stroke*. These snippets of data are examples of those that researchers might identify as containing codes or ideas. Using the ideas found within the data as codes, researchers compile lists of codes and then return to the data again and again to categorize data into organized units. Remember that analysis occurs while data collection is still in progress. When common ideas begin to emerge, the analysis should be used to adapt future interviews and direct and focus the data collection process. This entire process of data analysis and interpretation can be compared to discovering and putting together the pieces of a puzzle to form a meaningful picture that best represents the essence of the story told by the participants.

Sandelowski (1995) recommended some alternative strategies to traditional coding for developing a system to manage the data. She suggested extracting the facts and looking for story lines, topics, and content in addition to reduction of the data. Facts are those items of data that are not subject to debate, that are "givens," and later may be important for establishing the context of the research. While capturing the data in a systematic way, Sandelowski's approach avoids line-by-line coding. The aim is to think of the data as telling a story. Researchers approach the data by trying to identify the main points of the story or the major idea. Sandelowski suggested making a list that captures all the topics present in the data, much like the major plot points in each scene of a play.

In a more recent work, Sandelowski, Leeman, Knafl, and Crandell (2013) proposed a new method of data analysis and interpretation called data extraction. Sandelowski and colleagues summarized this method by stating that "findings are transformed into portable statements that anchor results to relevant information about sample, source of information, time, comparative reference point, magnitude and significance and study-specific conceptions of phenomena" (p. 1428). This method allows for a more accurate contextual view of the data.

It is always best to try to use the language of the participants for formulating labels for codes, themes, or patterns. Qualitative researchers, in efforts to remain true to the data, select words that reflect the participants' language and ideas, even often using those native terms as key labels for the data. For example, in Easton's (2001) stroke survivor study, a major subconcept early in the stroke recovery process was labeled the *mirage of recovery*, using a term coined by Veith (1988), an author of one of the books used in the theoretical development for the framework of the study. Veith used this term in reference to the optimistic and unrealistic assurances given to her by physicians that she would recover from her stroke with no residual effects. The quotations in **Box 14-1** are direct quotes from face-to-face interviews with stroke survivors whose average time at the interview since their stroke was 5 years. Do these quotes illustrate any similar ideas that may have supported Easton's label of the mirage of recovery?

Computer Software

Software can assist researchers in managing qualitative data. Just as statistical software helps to manage and manipulate numbers, software for qualitative data

---

BOX 14-1   Quotes from Stroke Survivors

"I always expected it to go away."

"I didn't think it was going to be very bad. I thought it was just going to be a mild stroke. . . . I thought I'd be recovered before I went home."

"Even after 3 years, I can't help but believe that, eh, your, that's always a little progress . . . and I can't help but believe that it's all gonna go away."

"I always thought I would [recover]. I had a feeling that if I tried hard enough, I could beat it."

"I had a neurologist tell me, he said 6 weeks . . . but then . . . he [another doctor] said 9 months."

"He [the doctor] said that this was all on the left side, and I should have complete recovery, that's what he said."

Reproduced from Easton, K.L. (1999). The Post-stroke journey: From agonizing to owning. *Geriatric Nursing, 20*(2), 70–76. Copyright 1999, with permission from Elsevier. http://www.elsevier.com

KEY TERM

Computer Assisted Qualitative Data Analysis Software (CAQDAS):
Computer software that assists in the management, coding, grouping, and analysis of qualitative data

helps to manage multitudes of words. The software available today falls into several categories that include word processing, text, analysis, grouping and linking, and displaying relationships. The type of software researchers choose is determined by what they intend to do with the data and how the data will be displayed or managed.

Although software can be extremely helpful in managing large amounts of data, it does not do the work of coding for the researcher. Qualitative researchers are still responsible for analyzing and labeling the data. Software programs can help with the sorting and grouping of data so that researchers can view similar statements or categories in a systematic way. This is often referred to as computer-assisted qualitative data or qualitative data analysis software (Cope, 2014; Houghton et al., 2015), or more currently it is known as Computer Assisted Qualitative Data Analysis Software (CAQDAS) (University of Surrey, 2017a). A basic word processor, such as Microsoft Word, generally serves as the initial data entry software. That is, the interviews or field notes are transcribed from audiotapes into a word processing document. Such software itself is a useful tool and works well for simple data analysis. However, if the study is large and will result in copious amounts of data, it is wise to investigate the benefits of *Computer Assisted Qualitative Data Analysis Software (CAQDAS).*

There are so many analysis programs on the market today that the University of Surrey (2017a) developed the CAQDAS project aimed to provide "practical support, training and information in the use of a range of software programs designed to assist qualitative data analysis" (para. 1). The CAQDAS networking project also provides a forum for researchers to discuss qualitative issues with the use of software and promotes discussion among researchers using qualitative methods.

Software assists researchers to label statements within the transcriptions, group them into categories, and then make interpretations or inferences. Some of the more popular software packages include Roter Interaction Analysis System (RIAS) (Cope, 2014), ATLAS.ti V5, HyperRESEARCH, NVivo, Dedoose, and C.A.T. (Boston University Information Services and Technology, 2017). These programs have enormous searching capabilities to help researchers look through hundreds of pages of text to find items of specific data, group data, and make charts and graphs, as well as many other features (University of Surrey, 2017b). Researchers must compare the features of each program and decide which to use depending on the type of qualitative methods employed. Qualitative researchers may also use a variety of tools or apps to manage data.

Likewise, Ethnograph (Qualis Research, 2008) is a software program for the analysis of text-based data that is highly regarded by qualitative researchers, particularly those doing ethnography. Ethnograph was first introduced in 1985 and has continued to be developed in various forms. The major categories in Ethnograph 6.0 include creating and managing data files, coding data files, the codebook, master list, family tree, and analytic writing. Ethnograph allows text-based data to be imported directly and was one of the pioneer programs for management and analysis of qualitative data.

Although software can be helpful, qualitative packages are generally cumbersome to learn and require a commitment on the part of researchers to master the software to maximize its usefulness. Data entry and coding are still time consuming and tedious. The greatest benefit to such software is the ability to group, compare, and contrast data more efficiently because of easier accessibility after all data are entered. Software is also helpful when preparing written reports of the data and selecting quotations or collapsing data for presentations, although some researchers find that basic word processing software is sufficient for these purposes.

TEST YOUR KNOWLEDGE 14-1

1. Put the following in the correct order:
   a. Pull together evidence into a meaningful report
   b. Code line by line
   c. Transcribe interviews
   d. Group coded data to generate categories, themes, and patterns

True/False

2. Computer software programs used to analyze qualitative data automatically generate themes based on participants' words.
3. There are many different strategies for coding data.
4. Analysis of data in qualitative research is done simultaneously with data collection.

How did you do? 1. c, b, d, a; 2. F; 3. T; 4. T

14.2 Qualitative Data Interpretation

At the end of this section, you will be able to:

< Describe how researchers draw conclusions from the data and verify them
< Recognize the common ways data are presented in reports

FYI

The interpretation of qualitative data should provide evidence for practice; the results of the study must be reported with sufficient rigor and details about the methods used to establish trustworthiness of the findings so that readers can have confidence that the results represent suggestions for best practice. There are three common approaches to reporting qualitative data: realist tales, confessionist tales, and impressionist tales.

Sandelowski (1995) distinguished between analysis and interpretation of data by stating:

> In contrast, qualitative interpretation is the knowledge produced: the end-product of analysis where the researcher construes or renders the analyzed data in such a way that something new is created that is different from, yet faithful to, that data in its original form. (p. 372)

In other words, data analysis is the means to an end, with the final outcome being a useful piece of research that can be applied in practice. It is important for researchers to be mindful of the language used to ensure that the message is accessible and usable to a broad range of readers and so that strategies for the point of care can be implemented (Sandelowski & Leeman, 2012). Thus, one could say that the interpretation of qualitative data provides evidence for practice. This is the evidence of words.

Drawing and Verifying Conclusions

As the data are being analyzed, researchers are also drawing some conclusions that are continually tested and modified, discarded, or verified. So, how does one figure out what all the data and codes mean? How do researchers know that codes they have chosen to use are correct? **Table 14-1** lists five levels of qualitative

TABLE 14-1   Five Levels of Qualitative Data

Level of Data	Summary
A priori framework	Data analyzed according to a preexisting framework; lowest level of data; provides no new knowledge
Descriptive	Researcher develops labels for data categories but does not explicate relationships among the categories; useful for devising lists of descriptors on a topic
Developing a synthesis	Researcher explains and explores relationships among themes with logical integration
Increased complexity and case variance	Researcher explains variations and negative case examples of the research; a step beyond developing a synthesis
A product that comprehensively explains a complex human phenomenon	The level of research that is considered to be the gold standard; provides an explanation of a phenomenon with depth and breadth as to increase others' understanding and advance the science

Data from Jacelon, C. S., & O'Dell, K. K. (2005). Analyzing qualitative data. *Urologic Nursing, 25,* 217–220; Kearney, M. (2001). Focus on research methods: Levels and applications of qualitative research evidence. *Research in Nursing and Health, 24,* 145–153.

data (Jacelon & O'Dell, 2005; Kearney, 2001) that range from simple to most complex. To address this question of what the data mean, one could start with the simplest level of research analysis and merely describe the phenomenon. As the levels progress to more complex, researchers become increasingly engaged in exploration, explanation, and synthesis. Qualitative researchers should strive for a product that meets level 5 in Table 14-1 and provides the most useful level of information aimed at positively influencing nursing practice.

For practical purposes, Miles and Huberman (1994) suggested 13 tactics for generating meaning from data. These are summarized in **Table 14-2**. Using strategies such as these, qualitative researchers extract the most important points from large amounts of data to form a logical conclusion.

To verify the conclusions drawn, Miles and Huberman (1994) suggested several other strategies. These include checking for researcher effects or bias

TABLE 14-2   Strategies for Generating Meaning

Strategy	Summary
Noting patterns, themes	Items that "jump out" at you; commonalities
Seeing plausibility	When categories make sense, feel right, fit
Clustering	Clumping or grouping data into categories
Making metaphors	Making comparisons with things that people identify with
Counting	Looking at number of times, recurrence
Making contrasts/comparisons	Comparing cases with practical significance
Partitioning variables	Unbundling variables as needed; separating variables that should not be clumped together
Subsuming particulars into the general	Asking whether a specific thing really stands alone, or does it belong in a more general category
Factoring	Identifying general themes to see which go together
Noting relations among variables	Describing the effects of one variable on another and any relationships among concepts
Finding intervening variables	Identifying the variables that go together only with the help of an additional variable to facilitate
Building a logical chain of evidence	Defining causal links that make logical sense when viewed as a whole
Making conceptual/theoretical coherence	Moving from constructs and interrelationships to theories that can be predictive

Modified from Miles, M. B., & Huberman, A. M. (1994). *Qualitative data analysis*. Thousand Oaks, CA: Sage.

KEY TERMS

representativeness:
The degree to
which elements of
the sample are like
elements in the
population

replicated: When
another researcher
has findings similar
to a previous study

realist tales: A
real-life account of
the culture being
studied presented
in a third-person
voice that
clearly separates
researchers from
participants

**confessionist
tales:** Qualitative
researchers'
personal accounts
that provide
insight about data
collection and
scientific rigor

**impressionist
tales:** Qualitative
researchers'
storytelling
and personal
descriptions about
the experiences of
conducting studies

that might have been introduced by the researcher's presence among the participants. Researchers must ask themselves if their presence may have influenced the participants to act any differently, and if so, how? Researchers should also check for *representativeness*. This means that researchers should challenge their assumption that the participants included in a study indeed represent the group. In addition, all cases that do not fit the typical profile that emerged from the data should be examined. These extreme or negative cases should be analyzed to see why they are not represented by the researchers' findings. Such exceptional cases should be few and able to be logically explained.

Confirmation of a study's findings is enhanced if the findings can be *replicated*. This means that if another researcher can essentially do the same study with similar results, this helps to validate the original researcher's findings. Another strategy is to get feedback from the study participants about how well the results represent what they actually experienced. Having the participants themselves confirm the findings of the study lends credibility to the results.

Writing Reports

Another challenge of qualitative research is reporting the results. Traditional formats for reporting quantitative research do not fit well with most qualitative studies, and many authorities have suggested that qualitative reports focus much more on detailed description and integration of the discussion of methods (Houghton et al., 2015). A typical report of qualitative research would follow a format similar to that presented in **Box 14-2**. Traditional reports contain an introduction, explanation of the significance of the project, a review of the relevant literature, description of methods, findings, discussion, and conclusions. However, there are several ways in which qualitative research may be presented, and researchers should carefully choose the strategy for presentation that best represents what they are trying to convey. Thought should be given to creatively reporting findings if it would enhance the ability of nurses to better apply the research in practice. That said, the results of the study must be reported with sufficient rigor and details about the methods used to establish trustworthiness of the findings so that readers can have confidence that the results represent suggestions for best practice.

Although there are several ways to approach the reporting of qualitative data, Van Manen (1988) identified three that are often referred to when considering how to write the report: *realist tales, confessionist tales*, and *impressionist tales*. Realist tales are the most common and were used by ethnographers such as Margaret Mead (Marshall & Rossman, 2011). When using this approach, researchers write a real-life account of the culture being studied and present it by using a third-person voice, clearly separating researchers from the participants

BOX 14-2	Example of Standard Components of a Qualitative Research Report

Title page

Abstract

Introduction

Aim or purpose of the study

Review of literature

Methods
    Sample
    Setting
    Data collection methods
    Data analysis methods

Findings or results

Discussion
    Nursing implications
    Limitations of study

Conclusions
    Questions that arose
    Recommendations for future research

in the study. The focus is on the many details about the group, and there is very little description of methods. The researcher is almost invisible (Miles & Huberman, 1994). Scholarly journals or monographs are common places to publish this type of writing. Peer-reviewed articles are standard and respected types of articles, but they have been criticized for being dull and boring. Whatever strategy for reporting the data is used, the discussion should always reflect the data and be true to the data (Houghton et al., 2015).

Confessionist tales are more personalized accounts in which the writer gives insight into the process of data collection and shows the scientific rigor of the field methods. The confessionist tale is written from the researcher's viewpoint with personal authority and thick description (Van Manen, 1988).

Impressionist tales allow researchers to chronicle their experiences "in a type of auto-ethnography" (Marshall & Rossman, 2011). Researchers speak more personally about the experiences of conducting the study, and they are participant observers versus disconnected realists. These reports are often more like storytelling and help the reader relive the experience.

Whichever voice researchers choose to use when reporting the results of the study, the decision should be made with the goal of communicating results in the most useful manner. Reports should be written with the audience in mind.

If the audience is nursing students, the focus will be different from a focus for registered nurses who are working on their master's degrees and different still if the readers are interdisciplinary team members outside of nursing.

Patton (1990) stated that the most important aspect of reporting is focus. When writing qualitative research reports, researchers must take care to include enough detail but not too much so as to preclude the major purpose of communicating useful, evidence-based information that influences practice. "Sufficient description and direct quotations should be included to allow the reader to enter into the situation and thoughts of the people represented in the report. Description should stop short, however, of becoming trivial and mundane" (Patton, 1990, p. 430). Sandelowski summarized her view by saying, "I think one of the hallmarks of a good qualitative researcher is someone who writes in a very accessible way for particular audiences" (Morse, 1994, p. 280).

Some differences in reporting formats among the four major types of qualitative research should also be noted. In phenomenological research, researchers can use realist tales, confessionist tales, or impressionist tales when writing. The choice depends on the audience and certainly on the sample size. If the sample is small, perhaps a storytelling approach would best convey the participants' experiences. The *personal narrative*, as a way of conveying the meaning of experiences, has recently received increased attention. Gaydos (2005) suggested that nurses can use their intuition to assist key informants who are ready to tell their stories in a type of cocreation of a personal narrative by using memories and metaphors. "The experience of creating a self story with a nurse can be healing, as the self story is heard by a caring person, memories are understood in new ways, and the self story is both confirmed and recreated" (Gaydos, 2005, p. 254). This may represent yet another way to report information about lived experience.

Grounded theory, conversely, is often presented more traditionally because it seeks to communicate a process that the researcher has discovered, lending itself to a more detached, analytic mode of reporting. So, although one could use a variety of voices in reporting qualitative data, it is key to focus the report to the audiences and choose the best approach to communicate with that audience.

With ethnography, researchers often choose the realist voice, but perhaps the impressionist tale would be better to describe information about a certain concept with a different culture. For example, if a researcher was studying death and burial practices of an unknown tribe in the jungle, perhaps a storytelling approach would be the most effective way to communicate the message learned from the research. Henderson (2005) suggested that dramaturgy (a description of the scene or social situation that is similar to a play) be included in field notes and reported in conjunction with ethnography to better explain the societal context of social activity.

KEY TERM

personal narrative: A way of conveying the meaning of experiences through storytelling

CRITICAL THINKING EXERCISE 14-1

You have just finished helping with a qualitative research study on homeless people in the rural Midwest, in which you assisted with data collection. The research team has discovered some essential health-related information about the homeless people living in the vicinity of your university. The lead researcher asks your opinion about how the research should be presented for publication. She wants the information to be targeted to nurses and nursing students. How should the article be written for the target audience? What suggestions would you make about the best way to present this information to students? How could information be disseminated to promote evidence-based practice (EBP) or to improve the community outreach efforts of your university?

In historical research, the typical voice is the realist because the data are usually obtained from documents. Miller and Alvarado (2005) suggested that documents could be used as commentary and as actors in qualitative research. Reports using documents would include more talk and observation. Certainly, with this approach, one might choose a different voice to present the results or at least take a more creative approach to reporting.

TEST YOUR KNOWLEDGE 14-2

1. Which of the following are strategies for drawing and verifying conclusions? (Select all that apply.)
   a. Checking for representativeness
   b. Ignoring negative cases
   c. Being sensitive to bias
   d. Confirming findings through replication

2. Match the following:
   a. Real-life account using third-person voice   1. Realist tales
   b. Speaking as a participant observer about the experience 2. Confessionist tales
   c. Emphasizing scientific rigor in the method   3. Impressionist tales

How did you do? 1. a, c, d; 2. a. 1, b. 3, c. 2

14.3 Qualitative Data Evaluation

At the end of this section, you will be able to:

< State why qualitative research is evaluated differently from how quantitative research is evaluated
< Define trustworthiness in terms of credibility, transferability, dependability, and confirmability
< Describe strategies for evaluating qualitative research

Standards for Evaluating Qualitative Data

As with quantitative research, certain standard criteria are accepted for evaluating qualitative studies. These were developed because quantitative criteria such as internal validity, external validity, generalizability, reliability, and objectivity were for evaluating numbers and did not fit well when evaluating words. It is expected that qualitative studies be conducted with extreme rigor because of the potential for subjectivity that is inherent in this type of research. In addition to addressing ethical issues, such as informed consent and use of data, qualitative researchers are guided by the requirements for establishing *trustworthiness* of the study. This is a more difficult task when dealing with words and people than numbers and statistics. Lincoln and Guba (1985) proposed a different set of criteria with unique terminology that is appropriate for evaluation of qualitative research. These criteria are still considered to be a gold standard to establish trustworthiness or rigor of a study (Houghton, Casey, Shaw, & Murphy, 2013).

Establishing Trustworthiness

Trustworthiness refers to the quality, the authenticity, and the truthfulness of findings in qualitative research. It relates to the degree of trust, or confidence, readers have in the results. Trustworthiness can be established by meeting four criteria (Lincoln & Guba, 1985): *credibility, transferability, dependability,* and *confirmability*. **Box 14-3** provides a summary of strategies for meeting these criteria. By maintaining an audit trail, researchers can demonstrate whether these criteria are met. *Auditability* means that records maintained by the researcher can be examined by others. For example, just like an auditor reviews financial records to ensure ethical business practices are used, peer reviewers can evaluate documents from qualitative studies to judge the trustworthiness of findings. When another researcher can follow the audit trail, that researcher should arrive at the same or similar conclusions. If contradictions about the conclusions exist, then the trustworthiness of the study could be called into question.

Credibility

Credibility in qualitative research is akin to internal validity in quantitative research. To meet the criterion of credibility, the research must be shown to be authentic and truthful. The results should make sense and be believable. There are many strategies to help establish and evaluate credibility. Researchers should use well-established research methods and describe them with sufficient detail so the study can be replicated. If a similar study can show similar results using another method, credibility is supported.

Good interviewing skills help to establish credibility of the data. Shenton (2004) suggested that specific questions be asked of participants to ensure that

BOX 14-3	Strategies to Establish Trustworthiness of a Study

Credibility
Use of well-established research methods
Prolonged engagement
Triangulation
Thick description
Detailed interviews
Data saturation
Peer debriefing
Member checks
Constant comparison
Negative case analysis
Reflexivity (reflective journaling)

Confirmability
Audit trail
Peer debriefing
Member checks
Self-reflection of the researcher evidenced by journals

Dependability
Audit trail
Peer debriefing
Coding checks that show agreement
Uniformity of responses across subjects
Ability to relate previous research findings to the current study

Transferability
Clear explanation of the boundaries/limitations of the study
Thick description
Checking for representativeness of the data
Audit trail

Data from Houghton, C., Casey, D., Shaw, D., & Murphy, K. (2013). Rigour in qualitative case-study research. *Nurse Researcher, 20*(4), 12–17.

KEY TERMS

auditability: When another researcher can clearly follow decisions made by the investigator, arriving at the same or comparable conclusions

data saturation: In qualitative research, the time when no new information is being obtained and repetition of information is consistently heard

peer debriefing: A technique used in qualitative research in which the researcher enlists the help of another person, who is a peer, to discuss the data and findings

they are giving the truth and not misleading researchers during interviews. Likewise, Kuper, Lingard, and Levinson (2008) recommended asking several key questions when evaluating a qualitative research report. These included, "Was the sample appropriate for the research question?" "Were data collected and analyzed appropriately?" "Are the methods clear?" "Can the results be transferred to the reader's own setting?" and "Do the researchers address ethical considerations?"

Data saturation, when no new information is being provided by participants, should be achieved. When evaluating qualitative research for credibility, readers should be able to see that researchers used *peer debriefing* to ensure that

KEY TERMS

member checks: A strategy used in qualitative studies when the researcher goes back to participants and shares the results with them to ensure the findings reflect what participants said

negative case analysis: A qualitative strategy involving the analysis of cases that do not fit patterns or categories

triangulation: Use of different research methods in qualitative research to gather and compare data

reflexivity: Using a journal to record thoughts, ideas, and decisions during qualitative data gathering

truth emerged from the data. Peer debriefing provides researchers with another professional's opinion and views of the data. A peer who does the debriefing should be at the same educational and positional levels as the researcher and should be considered a colleague but not a supervisor or boss.

Using the constant comparison method, researchers may choose to do *member checks* in which participants are asked to confirm the results as data collection progresses. Another strategy, *negative case analysis*, includes analyzing cases that do not seem to fit the patterns or categories that emerge and exploring the reasons for this. Other strategies involve keeping a reflective journal that details thoughts and ideas as they emerge and relating the research findings of others' studies to one's own. In addition, researchers should have appropriate expertise, skills, and established credentials to carry out the study. "The presence of the researcher is integral and should be acknowledged" (Barham, 2013, para. 5). All of these strategies are used to both establish and evaluate credibility.

Triangulation is another way to promote credibility of qualitative research. This strategy uses different research methods to gather and compare data. Two ways that triangulation helps to establish credibility include confirming the data and ensuring completeness of the data. So, if data gathered through various methods or sources are found to be consistent, the credibility of the research is promoted (Houghton et al., 2013). Additionally, *reflexivity*, or reflective journaling, also promotes credibility of findings by demonstrating the researcher's thoughts during the entire process. The researcher records thoughts, ideas, and decisions during data gathering and refers to them throughout the analysis and when developing themes and deriving patterns from the data.

Transferability

Transferability relates to external validity, generalizability, or fittingness of the data (Miles & Huberman, 1994). Although the purpose of qualitative research is not specifically to generalize, it is necessary to note the significance of the study with relation to its importance in helping understand a phenomenon in different contexts or situations. For example, a qualitative study uncovers themes about the lived experience of waiting for a heart transplant. Nurses working with transplant patients would need to consider whether these findings are transferable to individuals waiting for another type of organ transplant. Certainly, if the findings of a study are congruent with existing research or theoretical frameworks, this supports transferability. Other strategies used to meet this criterion include providing a clear explanation of the limitations of the study, giving thick descriptions of the study context and setting, leaving a paper trail that can be followed, checking that the data are representative in most cases, and making suggestions for other settings to test the findings. In addition, if the study is sufficiently described so that it can be replicated, transferability is supported.

Dependability

Dependability in qualitative research is similar to reliability in quantitative research. This means that the study should be consistent over time and that enough observations were made to show this consistency. Dependability is supported when coding checks show that there is agreement within and among the concepts and themes. When existing theories can be tied to new findings, dependability is enhanced. Review by peers or colleagues, as with peer debriefing, also supports dependability. There should be a logical consistency between responses of participants that carries over into the coding and analysis procedures. The audit trail should show rigor of research method with multiple journals being used to record thoughts, decisions, and reflections about the data and coding procedures.

> **FYI**
>
> The standard criteria accepted for evaluating quantitative data (internal validity, external validity, generalizability, reliability, and objectivity) fit well for evaluating numbers, but not words, the basic unit of qualitative data. Establishing the trustworthiness of qualitative data is particularly challenging because of the potential for subjectivity that is inherent in this type of research; however, it can be achieved by meeting four criteria: credibility, transferability, dependability, and confirmability.

Confirmability

Confirmability in qualitative research is most like objectivity in quantitative research. *Neutrality* refers to the findings of the research versus the researcher (Sandelowski, 1986). Some subjectivity is inherent in qualitative methods because the researcher is the instrument for data gathering as well as analysis and interpretation. It is when any potential biases are not recognized or accounted for that confirmability may be in question. Member checks and peer debriefing may help researchers remain true to the data. Methods of the study should be described completely with an audit trail clearly detailing all aspects of the study. The self-reflections of researchers should be recorded in journals. Record keeping must be accurate. Data should make sense and appear to be real and authentic.

In summary, qualitative researchers should consciously address the four criteria that are the standard for establishing trustworthiness. Nurse researchers should review the strategies for meeting these criteria and build them into the research plan. Journaling, good record keeping, recording detailed field notes with thick descriptions, and recognizing sources of bias are essential to meet these criteria. In addition, scientific and ethical standards for rigor in qualitative research must be maintained to provide the best possible believability and trustworthiness for the study.

CRITICAL THINKING EXERCISE 14-2

Compare and contrast each of the four criteria of trustworthiness of a qualitative study with what you have learned about the criteria for evaluating quantitative studies. How are they alike? How are they different? What is your understanding of the reasons behind using different measures to evaluate qualitative versus quantitative research?

TEST YOUR KNOWLEDGE 14-3

1. Which of the following are criteria for establishing trustworthiness? (Select all that apply.)
   a. Credibility
   b. Reliability
   c. Confirmability
   d. Inferability
2. Which of the following are techniques used by qualitative researchers? (Select all that apply.)
   a. Peer review
   b. Member checks
   c. Data saturation
   d. Audit trails

How did you do? 1. a, c; 2. b, c, d

14.4 Keeping It Ethical

At the end of this section, you will be able to:

< Describe key ethical issues in qualitative research

Numerous ethical issues are inherent in qualitative research. Some issues arise during the initial phases of planning a research study, and others arise during implementation. Certain ethical issues are of note during data analysis, interpretation, and evaluation. Miles and Huberman (1994), still considered a standard resource for qualitative data analysis, recommended that specific ethical issues be given particular attention. These are summarized in **Table 14-3**.

Many of the ethical issues posed in Table 14-3 can be addressed by establishing trustworthiness of the research project. Researchers should be able to defend and explain why a study is significant and describe what it adds to EBP.

Potential risks to participants should be carefully weighed against benefits, and justifications for decisions should be made. Researchers should be competent to carry out proposed studies and have the necessary skills and expertise to interpret findings and convey them for use in practice.

Because qualitative research deals with unique human situations that are largely interpreted by researchers, issues related to scientific rigor seem to be always present. It is essential, then, that qualitative researchers take every care to ensure anonymity and confidentiality of study participants. In sharing

TABLE 14-3	Ethical Issues to Consider in Qualitative Research

Issue	Ask Yourself (Implications for Nursing)
Worthiness of the project	Is this a worthwhile project to pursue? Does it have value? What will it add to nursing knowledge?
Competence boundaries	Am I adequately prepared to conduct this study? If not, what would I need to become so, or whom can I get to assist me?
Informed consent	Have I obtained informed consent from participants? Did I explain the purpose, risks, and benefits of the study and allow time for questions?
Benefits, costs, and reciprocity	Does the cost/benefit ratio make sense? Is it fiscally responsible?
Harm and risk	Is there minimal harm or risk to participants? Have any potential effects been explained to participants?
Honesty and trust	Have I established trust and been honest with participants?
Privacy, confidentiality, and anonymity	Have I received institutional review board approval? How have I ensured privacy, confidentiality of responses, and anonymity of participants will be maintained? Have I met criteria for training in protection of human subjects?
Intervention and advocacy	Do I advocate for the right when I observe wrong behavior of other researchers? Can my subjects count on me to put their interests above my own? Do I avoid any real or perceived conflict of interest?
Research integrity and quality	Do I adhere to accepted standards of practice and embrace scientific integrity? Am I absolutely true to the data to avoid fraud and deception in analysis? Have I considered every aspect of evaluating trustworthiness of the data?
Ownership of data and conclusions	Have I clarified who owns my work and the results of it? Who has access to the data, and have I protected the data, and thus my subjects, sufficiently?
Use and misuse of results	Have I taken adequate care to avoid interventions and persuasion instead of remaining in the role of the researcher? Have my findings been sufficiently described so as not to be misinterpreted or misused by others for their own purposes?
Conflicts, dilemmas, and trade-offs	Have I examined all of the possible ethical dilemmas that could arise, or have arisen, from my data collection and analysis? Have I thought of my position related to these possible dilemmas and how I would handle them? Have I taken steps to avoid any possible conflict of interest related to the study?

Modified from Miles, M. B., & Huberman, A. M. (1994). *Qualitative data analysis*. Thousand Oaks, CA: Sage.

FYI

Certain ethical issues are of note during data analysis, interpretation, and evaluation; they can be addressed by establishing trustworthiness of the research project. Researchers should be able to defend and explain why a study is significant, describe what it adds to EBP, and carefully weigh potential risks to participants against benefits.

people's words and thoughts, the potential for inappropriate disclosure of personal information is greater than in studies where numbers and statistics form the descriptions. Careful explanations of how data will be used and how participants' identities will be protected must be given to participants. Researchers must make certain to honor these obligations. Participants must be able to trust that if they share their innermost thoughts with researchers, researchers will do what has been promised with regard to protecting privacy and safeguarding personal data. Details of the study must be carefully planned in advance so that even the smallest matter is not left to chance.

Qualitative researchers have an inherent obligation and contract with participants to use data in the way that has been specified, to analyze data with an open mind, and to be true to the data when reporting findings. For example, when using ethnography as a method, researchers must address challenges such as avoiding bias when studying cultural groups different from their own and finding how best to obtain informed consent among these groups (Lipson, 1994). The American Anthropological Association (2016), in its statement on Ethnography and Institutional Review Boards, stated that "the ethnographer bears the responsibility of ensuring that the participants are fully informed of the intent of the ethnographic research, how the participants' information contributes to the research, and the anticipated risks and benefits the participants may expect to occur as a result of their agreement to participate in the research" (p. 3).

When the research findings further nursing science and translate into better care and outcomes for study participants, or those like them, then researchers can be assured that an important task has been accomplished. If this goal is kept in mind while maintaining the expected rigor of this type of research, researchers are much less likely to violate ethical standards.

TEST YOUR KNOWLEDGE 14-4

True/False

1. Qualitative researchers do not need to obtain informed consent because they participate in the process.

2. Qualitative researchers often assign code names to participants to protect participants' privacy.

3. There is no harm or risk associated with participation in qualitative research because data are typically collected through interviews.

How did you do? 1. F; 2. T; 3. F

Apply What You Have Learned

The EBP committee has almost completed entering information into the grid. To conclude the analysis, report the findings from Jackson et al. (2014). Because this is a qualitative study, it is appropriate to indicate the themes in the column for outcomes.

RAPID REVIEW

» In qualitative research, data collection, data analysis, and data interpretation often occur simultaneously.

» Data analysis involves coding data into manageable units. This can involve data reduction, open coding, or axial coding.

» Coded data are used to generate categories, themes, and patterns.

» Themes, using the language of the participants, paint a meaningful picture of the phenomenon.

» Computer software programs, such as CAQDAS, can assist researchers in organizing and managing data.

» Interpretations of qualitative data strive to produce a description of complex phenomena.

» Qualitative research reports have a format different from quantitative reports. Authors use one of three approaches: realist tales, confessionist tales, or impressionist tales.

» Criteria used to evaluate quantitative studies cannot be applied when evaluating qualitative studies. Qualitative studies are trustworthy when strategies have been used to meet the criteria of credibility, transferability, dependability, and confirmability.

» Maintaining confidentiality and protecting anonymity are especially important when conducting qualitative studies. Researchers have an obligation to remain true to the data during analysis and interpretation.

REFERENCES

American Anthropological Association. (2016). Statement on ethnography and institutional review boards. Retrieved from http://www.americananthro.org/Participate AndAdvocate/Content.aspx?ItemNumber=1652

Ball, E., McLoughlin, M., & Darvill, A. (2011). Plethora or paucity: A systematic search and bibliometric study of the application and design of qualitative methods in nursing research 2008–2010. *Nurse Education Today, 31*(3), 299–303.

Barham, L. (2013). Hearing voices: Engaging with personal narratives obtained in interviews in qualitative research: Methodological considerations. Retrieved from http://www.eera-ecer.de/ecer-programmes/conference/8/contribution/21950/

Bogdan, R. C., & Biklen, S. K. (2006). *Qualitative research for education: An introduction to theory and methods* (5th ed.). New York, NY: Pearson.

Boston University Information Services and Technology. (2017). Qualitative data analysis software comparison. Retrieved from http://www.bu.edu/tech/services/cccs/desktop/distribution/nvivo/comparison/

Clissett, P. (2008). Evaluating qualitative research. *Journal of Orthopaedic Nursing, 12*(3), 99–105.

Cope, D. G. (2014). Computer-assisted qualitative data analysis software. *Oncology Nursing Forum, 41*(3), 322–323.

Corbin, J., & Strauss, A. L. (1990). Grounded theory research: Procedures, canons, and evaluative criteria. *Qualitative Sociology, 13*(1), 3–21.

Corbin, J., & Strauss, A. L. (2008). *Basics of qualitative research* (3rd ed.). Los Angeles, CA: Sage.

Easton, K. L. (2001). *The post-stroke journey: From agonizing to owning.* Unpublished doctoral dissertation, Wayne State University, Detroit, MI.

Ganapathy, M. (2016). Qualitative data analysis: Making it easy for nurse researchers. *International Journal of Nursing Education, 8*(2), 106–110.

Gaydos, H. L. (2005). Understanding personal narratives: An approach to practice. *Journal of Advanced Nursing, 49*(3), 254–259.

Henderson, A. (2005). The value of integrating interpretive research approaches in the exposition of healthcare context. *Journal of Advanced Nursing, 52*, 554–560.

Houghton, C., Casey, D., Shaw, D., & Murphy, K. (2013). Rigour in qualitative case-study research. *Nurse Researcher, 20*(4), 12–17.

Houghton, C., Murphy, K., Shaw, D., & Casey, D. (2015). Qualitative case study data analysis: An example from practice. *Nurse Researcher, 22*(5), 8–12.

Jacelon, C. S., & O'Dell, K. K. (2005). Analyzing qualitative data. *Urologic Nursing, 25*, 217–220.

Jackson, C., Lowton, K., & Griffiths, P. (2014). Infection prevention as "a show": A qualitative study of nurses' infection prevention behaviours. *International Journal of Nursing Studies, 51,* 400–408.

Kearney, M. (2001). Focus on research methods: Levels and applications of qualitative research evidence. *Research in Nursing and Health, 24*, 145–153.

Kuper, A., Lingard, L., & Levinson, W. (2008). Critically appraising qualitative research. *British Medical Journal, 337*, a1035.

Lincoln, Y. S., & Guba, E. G. (1985). *Naturalistic inquiry.* Newbury Park, CA: Sage.

Lipson, J. G. (1994). Ethical issues in ethnography. In J. M. Morse (Ed.), *Critical issues in qualitative research methods* (pp. 333–356). Newbury Park, CA: Sage.

Marshall, C., & Rossman, G. B. (2011). *Designing qualitative research.* Thousand Oaks, CA: Sage.

Miles, M. B., & Huberman, A. M. (1994). *Qualitative data analysis.* Thousand Oaks, CA: Sage.

Miller, F. A., & Alvarado, K. (2005). Incorporating documents into qualitative nursing research. *Journal of Nursing Scholarship, 37*, 348–353.

Morse, J. M. (1994). *Critical issues in qualitative research methods.* Newbury Park, CA: Sage.

Patton, M. Q. (1990). *Qualitative evaluations and research methods.* Newbury Park, CA: Sage.

Polit, D., & Beck, C. T. (2012). *Essentials of nursing research: Methods, appraisal, and utilization* (9th ed.). Philadelphia, PA: Lippincott Williams & Wilkins.

Qualis Research. (2008). The Ethnograph 6.0 Quick Tour Guide. Retrieved from http://www.qualisresearch.com/DownLoads/E6QuickTour.pdf

Sandelowski, M. (1986). The problem of rigor in qualitative research. *Advances in Nursing Science, 8*(3), 27–37.

Sandelowski, M. (1995). Qualitative analysis: What it is and how to begin. *Research in Nursing and Health, 18,* 371–375.

Sandelowski, M., & Leeman, J. (2012). Writing usable qualitative health research findings. *Qualitative Health Research, 22,* 1404–1413.

Sandelowski, M., Leeman, J., Knafl, K., & Crandell, J. L. (2013). Text-in-context: A method for extracting findings in mixed-methods mixed research synthesis studies. *Journal of Advanced Nursing, 69*(6), 1428–1437.

Shenton, A. K. (2004). Strategies for ensuring trustworthiness in qualitative research projects. *Education for Information, 22,* 63–75.

Strauss, A., & Corbin, J. (1998). *Basics of qualitative research: Techniques and procedures for developing grounded theory.* Thousand Oaks, CA: Sage.

Tesch, R. (1990). *Qualitative research: Analysis types and software tools.* New York, NY: Falmer Press.

University of Surrey. (2017a). Choosing an appropriate CAQDAS package. Retrieved from https://www.surrey.ac.uk/sociology/research/researchcentres/caqdas/support/choosing/

University of Surrey. (2017b). What is the CAQDAS networking project? Retrieved from http://www.surrey.ac.uk/sociology/research/researchcentres/caqdas/

Van Manen, M. (1988). *Tales of the field: On writing ethnography.* Chicago, IL: University of Chicago Press.

Veith, I. (1988). *Can you hear the clapping of one hand?: Learning to live with a stroke.* Berkeley, CA: University of California Press.

At the end of this chapter, you will be able to:

- < Describe strategies that individuals use to reduce uncertainty when making decisions
- < Explain how findings from quantitative designs contribute to evidence
- < Discuss characteristics that should be appraised when evaluating qualitative and quantitative designs
- < Rank pieces of evidence using a rating system
- < Explain the development and use of clinical practice guidelines
- < Discuss reasons why nurses should follow agency policies even when they conflict with evidence

active rejection
adoption
AGREE II
case control studies
clinical practice guidelines
cohort studies

descriptive studies
evidence hierarchies
GRADE
levels of evidence
meta-analyses
passive rejection

pilot
randomized controlled trials
rejection
systematic review
uncertainty

CHAPTER 15

Weighing In on the Evidence

Carol O. Long

15.1 Deciding What to Do

At the end of this section, you will be able to:

‹ Describe strategies that individuals use to reduce uncertainty when making decisions

Evidence-based nursing is the process whereby nurses make clinical decisions that integrate the best available research with clinical relevance and incorporate the patient's preferences, values, and circumstances (Melnyk & Fineout-Overholt, 2015). This assumes that sufficient evidence or research is clinically relevant, methodologically sound, and of scientific merit (Straus, Glasziou, Richardson, & Haynes, 2011). Some practice decisions are made by a committee responsible for overseeing policies and procedures in the clinical setting. Other decisions can be made when circumstances warrant a timely decision. For example, a patient may have an unusual complication that is not addressed by the current protocol. Healthcare providers may collaborate after securing evidence about an innovative treatment, and, after consulting with the patient, they may decide to implement it.

How do clinicians make decisions? There are really only two options: *adoption* or *rejection* of the innovation. Individuals aim to select the option about which they are the least uncertain. "Uncertainty is the degree to which a number of alternatives are perceived with respect to the occurrence of an event and the relative probability of these alternatives" (Rogers, 2003, p. 6). Individuals typically adopt an innovation when *uncertainty* is reduced. When there is a significant amount of uncertainty about a new innovation, individuals generally reject adopting the innovation.

FYI

Clinicians must decide to adopt or reject innovations through reducing the uncertainty of an innovation. One strategy that individuals use to reduce uncertainty during the decision-making process is to try a portion of the innovation or adopt the innovation on a trial basis, which is called a pilot.

KEY TERMS

adoption: Applying an innovation to practice

rejection: Decision not to adopt an innovation

uncertainty: Degree to which alternatives are perceived relative to the occurrence of an event and the probability of these alternatives

pilot: A small study to test a new intervention with a small number of subjects before testing with larger samples; adopting an innovation on a trial basis

Individuals use different strategies to reduce uncertainty during the decision-making process (Rogers, 2003). Sometimes individuals may decide to try a portion of the innovation or adopt the innovation on a trial basis, which is called a *pilot*. For example, a new infusion pump may be piloted on one unit to determine its efficiency before implementing the new model throughout the facility. In some cases, a trial of a new idea by peers and their recommendations are sufficient to affect a decision about adoption. Respected individuals are often asked to endorse innovations as a marketing strategy. Offering free samples, a frequent practice among pharmaceutical companies, is another strategy that can facilitate the adoption of an innovation. Demonstrations can also be effective in furthering the adoption of innovations.

There are two kinds of rejection: active and passive (Rogers, 2003). Just because an innovation is adopted for a period of time, there are no guarantees that rejection will not occur. *Active rejection* involves active decision making after a pilot and purposefully deciding not to adopt the innovation. For example, in the pilot testing of the new infusion pump, nurses reported that alarms sounded for no reason, requiring more time to monitor infusions. Therefore, it was decided not to adopt the new infusion pumps in the facility. *Passive rejection* is when there is no consideration given to adopting the innovation. In essence, no decision is ever made and old practices are continued.

Culture plays an important role in the decision-making process. In some cultures, it is common for decisions to be made collectively. For example, married women in an Asian village attended a presentation by a government change agent about intrauterine devices (IUDs). At the conclusion of the presentation, 18 women voted to adopt this method of birth control. They immediately went to a nearby clinic to have an IUD inserted (Rogers, 2003). In some cultures, such as mainstream America, individual goals supersede the goals of the group and a vote described above would be rare.

TEST YOUR KNOWLEDGE 15-1

1. Which of the following strategies reduce uncertainty during decision making? (Select all that apply.)
   a. Pilot testing
   b. Reviewing samples
   c. Listening to the opinions of peers
   d. Relying on intuition

How did you do? 1. a, b, c

15.2 Appraising the Evidence

At the end of this section, you will be able to:

< Explain how findings from quantitative designs contribute to evidence
< Discuss characteristics that should be appraised when evaluating qualitative and quantitative designs
< Rank pieces of evidence using a rating system

Does the Study Provide Good Evidence?

Determining the relevance of the evidence requires skill in analyzing research studies. These skills include techniques used for determining the strength, significance, and relevance of the evidence. There are five steps for evaluating and implementing evidence-based practice (EBP), which are listed and briefly described in **Table 15-1** (deGroot, van der Wouden, van Hell, & Nieweg, 2013). Although each step requires solid analytical skills and application of good research methods, the steps are especially important for weighing the evidence. When appraising, nurses need to ensure that the first two steps, ask and acquire, were thoroughly executed.

After specific literature about the research question has been collected, a rigorous evaluation is conducted. The mere fact that an individual study has been published in a peer-reviewed journal does not ensure that the findings are sound (Watson, 2012). During appraisal, the study design, how the research was conducted, and the data analysis are all scrutinized to ensure that the study was sound. **Box 15-1** presents questions that should be considered when examining individual studies.

KEY TERMS

active rejection: Purposefully deciding not to adopt an innovation

passive rejection: Lack of consideration given to adopting an innovation; hence, old practices are continued

TABLE 15-1	Five-Step Approach for Evidence-Based Nursing Practice
Ask	Identify the research question. Determine whether the question is well constructed to elicit a response or solution.
Acquire	Search the literature for preappraised evidence or research. Secure the best evidence that is available.
Appraise	Conduct a critical appraisal of the literature and studies. Evaluate for validity and determine the applicability in practice.
Apply	Institute recommendations and findings and apply them to nursing practice.
Assess	Evaluate the application of the findings, outcomes, and relevance to nursing practice.

Modified from de Groot, M., van der Wouden, J. M., van Hell, E. A., & Nieweg, M. B. (2013). Evidence based practice for individuals for groups: Let's make a difference. *Perspectives on Medical Education, 2,* 216–221.

| **BOX 15-1** | Questions to Consider When Appraising Nursing Studies |

Introduction

1. Does the introduction demonstrate the need for the study?
2. Is the problem clearly and concisely identified?
3. Is the problem presented with enough background material to acquaint the reader with the importance of the problem?
4. Is the purpose of the study clearly stated?
5. Are the terms and variables relevant to the study clearly defined?
6. Are the assumptions clearly and simply stated?
7. If appropriate to the design, are hypotheses stated?
8. Does the study use a theoretical framework to guide its design?

Review of the Literature

1. Is the review of the literature (ROL) relevant to the problem?
2. Is the ROL adequate in terms of the range and scope of ideas, opinions, and points of view relevant to the problem?
3. Is the ROL well organized and synthesized?
4. Does the ROL provide for critical appraisal of the contribution of each of the major references?
5. Does the ROL conclude with a summary of the literature with implications for the study?
6. Is the ROL adequately and correctly documented?

Methods

1. Is the research approach appropriate?
2. Was the protection of human subjects considered?
3. Are the details of data collection clearly and logically presented?
4. Are the instrument(s) appropriate for the study both in terms of the problem and the approach?
5. Are the instrument(s) described sufficiently in terms of content, structure, validity, and reliability?
6. Is the population and the method for selecting the sample adequately described?
7. Is the method for selection of the sample appropriate?
8. Is the sample size sufficient?
9. Is attrition of sample reported and explained?
10. Does the design have controls at an acceptable level for the threats to internal validity?
11. What are the limits to generalizability in terms of external validity?

Results

1. Is the presentation of data clear?
2. Are the characteristics of the sample described?
3. Was the best method(s) of analysis selected?
4. Are the tables, charts, and graphs pertinent?

Discussion

1. Are the results based on the data presented?
2. Is the evidence sufficient to draw conclusions?
3. Are the results interpreted in the context of the problem/purpose, hypothesis, and theoretical framework/literature reviewed?
4. Are the conclusions and generalizations clearly stated?
5. Are the limitations of the findings clearly delineated?
6. Are the generalizations within the scope of the findings or beyond the findings?
7. Does the study contribute to nursing knowledge?

Quantitative Designs

By this point, you are familiar with quantitative methods and are ready to learn to apply your knowledge about research principles to make decisions about the evidence. A critical appraisal of quantitative studies is necessary for nurses to determine the validity, reliability, statistical significance, clinical importance, and applicability of the findings (University of Alberta, 2008a).

When appraising *meta-analyses*, nurses should establish whether well-designed studies that fit with the research question are included. Both published and unpublished studies should be included. One must be confident that the literature was systematically searched to obtain an adequate sample size. There should be evidence that statistical findings from the studies were merged to identify incongruencies and similarities of findings among the studies.

Other kinds of studies that nurses are likely to appraise are *randomized controlled trials* (RCT). *RCT* sometimes also stands for randomized clinical trials. Studies of this type can be found in the nursing literature and are especially important to the advancement of EBP. Studies showing that a treatment has a greater effect, rather than studies showing a small effect, weigh more heavily in the appraisal. Sample sizes are typically large, and often patients are recruited from multiple sites. Studies are strengthened by using strategies such as blinded designs, ensuring that interventions are controlled, and showing that patient groups were similar at the beginning of the trial (University of Alberta, 2008b). Reviewers should determine whether there is bias by using the five Cs approach for evaluation: contamination, crossover, compliance, cointervention, and count, that is, attrition (Attia & Page, 2001). Results should be readily applicable to patients with similar clinical and demographic backgrounds.

Cohort studies, sometimes known as quasi-experimental studies, examine a large sample of the population and observe changes in characteristics over time. Like RCTs, there are two groups: one that receives the treatment and one that does not. Then both groups are followed for a period of time related to the outcome of interest. Cohort studies are considered to be less rigorous than RCTs are because subjects are not randomly assigned to groups; therefore, the two groups may vary on other characteristics, and the controls may be difficult to identify. Cohort studies may be retrospective or prospective.

Case control studies compare two groups: those who have a specific condition and those who do not have the condition. This type of research usually focuses on rare disorders or disorders where there is considerable time between exposure or treatment and the onset or change in outcome. In case control studies, fewer subjects are needed than in cross-sectional studies. The disadvantages of

KEY TERMS

meta-analyses: Scholarly papers that combine results of studies, both published and unpublished, into a measurable format and statistically estimate effects of proposed interventions

randomized controlled trials: Experimental studies that typically involve large samples and are conducted in multiple sites

cohort studies: Quasi-experimental studies using two or more groups; epidemiological designs in which subjects are selected based on their exposure to a determinant

case control studies: A type of retrospective study in which researchers begin with a group of people who already had the disease; studies that compare two groups: those who have a specific condition and those who do not have the condition

case control studies include the potential for confounding variables, bias (recall and selection), and difficulty in selecting the control group.

Descriptive studies aim to provide information about a phenomenon. They are nonexperimental in design and most often lack an independent variable. They are often used when little is known about the phenomenon. Correlational and survey designs fall into this category of research. These types of studies may have large or small samples, be cross-sectional or longitudinal, and typically report means, standard deviations, and frequencies. Correlations are reported if the purpose of the study is to determine relationships.

Qualitative Designs

Qualitative nursing research provides a valuable contribution to building nursing theory and understanding the practice of nursing. Qualitative studies have not been highly regarded in the growing field of EBP. Traditionally, it has been difficult for many individuals to accept qualitative findings because the criteria to determine scientific rigor are so different from the criteria for quantitative methods. However, the contributions of qualitative research should not be underestimated because findings provide the patient perspective, which is an important component of EBP.

When nurses appraise qualitative studies, they should evaluate several characteristics. The qualitative method selected should be appropriate for the research question. Unlike quantitative research, samples tend to be small, and nurses should determine that researchers report reaching saturation. Scientific rigor should be maintained through orderly and detailed data collection. Strong evidence is generated when analyses are systematic, rigorous, and auditable (Thorne, 2000). Conclusions should be grounded in the data.

Ranking the Evidence

Decisions should not be based on one piece of evidence. Nurses need to examine all the evidence to make recommendations about practice changes. You may think that this will be difficult to do; however, it is usually easier than appraising an individual study. There are predetermined scales, known as *evidence hierarchies*, that guide decisions for ranking studies. Because authors are typically very clear in their descriptions of their studies, it is usually easy to rank the evidence correctly. In EBP, there are a variety of ways to rate evidence. These rating systems have been designed by professional organizations or expert panels. **Figure 15-1** provides a rating system that is commonly used in nursing to make decisions about evidence.

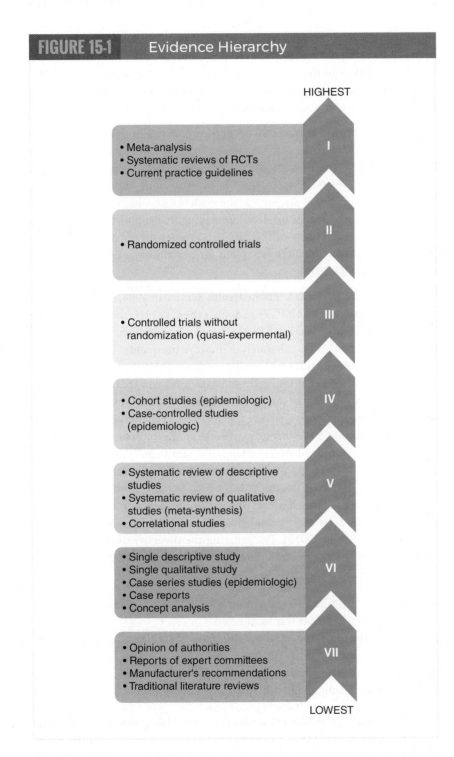

FIGURE 15-1   Evidence Hierarchy

HIGHEST

I
- Meta-analysis
- Systematic reviews of RCTs
- Current practice guidelines

II
- Randomized controlled trials

III
- Controlled trials without randomization (quasi-expermental)

IV
- Cohort studies (epidemiologic)
- Case-controlled studies (epidemiologic)

V
- Systematic review of descriptive studies
- Systematic review of qualitative studies (meta-synthesis)
- Correlational studies

VI
- Single descriptive study
- Single qualitative study
- Case series studies (epidemiologic)
- Case reports
- Concept analysis

VII
- Opinion of authorities
- Reports of expert committees
- Manufacturer's recommendations
- Traditional literature reviews

LOWEST

Although the rating system in Figure 15-1 provides a commonly encountered method for rating evidence, you will likely come across other useful rating scales. Regardless of the scale selected, they all have in common ranking/rating systems to stratify the evidence by quality. Several notable rating scales are presented so that you can become familiar with alternative approaches.

Members of the Canadian Task Force on Preventive Health Care (CTFPHC) were some of the first to generate *levels of evidence* (Centre for Evidence-Based Medicine, 2013). The recommendations that typically accompany clinical practice guidelines (CPGs) are graded by examining the risk versus the benefit and the quality or strength of the evidence on which the information is derived. Reviewers focus on decision making that supports evidence over consensus. Current efforts of the CTFPHC center on preventive care and health policy with guidelines generated for practitioners to use in clinical practice (CTFPHC, 2016).

First convened by the U.S. Public Health Service in 1984, the U.S. Preventive Services Task Force (USPSTF) adopted the CTFPHC methodology. The USPSTF is currently sponsored by the Agency for Healthcare Research and Quality (AHRQ). AHRQ's mission is to improve the quality, safety, efficiency, and effectiveness of health care for all Americans. AHRQ provides administrative, research, technical, and communication support for the USPSTF. The USPSTF evaluates scientific studies related to clinical preventive services and makes recommendations based on explicit criteria, generally intended for use in preventive care and the primary care setting. Recommendations provide information about the evidence, allowing clinicians to make informed practice decisions. The USPSTF grades the strength of the evidence as "A" (strongly recommends), "B" (recommends), "C" (no recommendation for or against), "D" (recommends against), or "I" (insufficient evidence to recommend for or against) while considering a balance of benefit and harm for the preventive service (USPSTF, 2013). Recognizing the diversity of rating systems, AHRQ identified three relevant domains and elements for systems to grade the strength of the evidence (USPSTF, 2008).

1. *Quality:* The aggregate of quality rating for individual studies, predicted on the extent to which bias was minimized
2. *Quantity:* The magnitude of effect, numbers of studies, and sample size or power
3. *Consistency:* For any given topic, the extent to which similar findings are reported using similar and different study designs

AHRQ's mission is to support quality of care and EBP, most notably through its 11 Evidence-based Practice Centers (EPCs) throughout the United States. The EPCs are awarded 5-year contracts to review relevant scientific materials

CRITICAL THINKING EXERCISE 15-1

Read the following description and determine how you would rank this study using the rating system in Figure 15-1.

The purpose of this experimental study was to test the efficacy of two interventions for mothers and their adolescents in delaying initiation of sexual intercourse for youth who are not sexually active and encouraging the use of condoms among sexually active youth. Adolescents (*N* = 582) and their mothers were randomly assigned to one of two groups (Dilorio et al., 2006).

on clinical, behavioral, organizational, and financial topics to produce evidence reports and technology assessments (AHRQ, 2002, 2016). EPCs also conduct research on methodology and *systematic reviews*, and evidence-based reports are added to the AHRQ website on a regular basis (AHRQ, n.d.).

The Cochrane Collaboration, founded in 1993, is an international not-for-profit organization that is dedicated to disseminating information about the effects of health care worldwide. The Cochrane Collaboration has several resources at the disposal of evidence-based practitioners, one of them being the Cochrane Database of Systematic Reviews, published on a continuous basis from the Cochrane Library (http://www.cochranelibrary.com/). The Cochrane Collaboration is best known for its comprehensive evidence-based summaries written in an easy-to-read style. Existing Cochrane Reviews are updated regularly, keeping pace with the fast-paced healthcare environment.

The Joanna Briggs Institute (2014) is an international not-for-profit research organization that is part of the School of Translational Science at the University of Adelaide, South Australia. Its central mission is to evaluate health outcomes for the client and community from an economic and clinical perspective. The institute also focuses on the evaluation of research. It identifies topics for systematic review, plans the review, and uses expert panels and reviewers to publish systematic reviews. With more than 70 collaborating entities, the Joanna Briggs Institute has an international presence, providing the best clinical evidence at the point of care. Factors such as feasibility, meaningfulness, effectiveness, and appropriateness are some of the aspects that are critiqued. The Joanna Briggs Institute (2011) uses these factors to grade recommendations used in CPGs and gives them numbered levels. The institute has an array of resources to appraise the research evidence, assist in the process of conducting a systematic review, and facilitate thematic analysis of primary data.

Clearly, there are many evidence rating and grading schemes. There is controversy about which scheme provides the best evaluation. Yet deciding on one universal rating scheme may not be feasible. Grades of Recommendations,

KEY TERM

systematic reviews: Rigorous and systematic syntheses of research findings about clinical problems

Assessment, Development, and Evaluation, known as *GRADE*, has been an international effort to develop a universal system of evaluation (The GRADE Working Group, 2017). The mission has been to consolidate the forces of many reputable organizations and agencies, such as AHRQ, the Centers for Disease Control and Prevention, the World Health Organization, and many other professional societies within the United States and abroad (http://www .gradeworkinggroup.org). GRADE is closely aligned with the Cochrane Collaboration. The GRADE system ranks the strength and quality of evidence into four levels: (1) high, (2) moderate, (3) low, and (4) very low. The recommendation is either (1) strong or (2) weak. Criteria of the GRADE system can be accessed at http://www.gradeworkinggroup.org. The GRADE Working Group has developed a free software application that uses a systematic approach to grade the evidence and create a summary table with the findings.

When weighing evidence, nurses may be involved in discussions that involve determining the clinical significance of the findings (Straus et al., 2011). Questions about diagnosis, therapy, prognosis, causation, harm, and etiology can be discussed. Examples are provided in **Table 15-2**. It would not be unusual for the discussion to include concepts such as relative risk, relative risk reduction, absolute risk reduction, numbers needed to treat, and odds ratio. Definitions of these terms are provided in **Box 15-2**. This content is included so that you can become familiar with the terminology, not so that you become adept at performing calculations.

It should be noted that not all the rating systems discussed include a way to rank qualitative studies. Melnyk (2004) noted that EBP must consider the inclusion of qualitative studies when reviewing studies of merit, and those qualitative studies should assume a step on the hierarchy ladder. The research findings

TABLE 15-2	Common Clinical Questions
Diagnosis	Queries the selection and interpretation of diagnostic tests
Therapy	Examines therapeutic treatment(s) for healthcare problems and their efficacy, cost, and potential harm
Prognosis	Evaluates the course of treatment over time, any complications, and overall prognosis
Causation/harm/etiology	Looks at the causes of disease, including iatrogenic causes, potential harm, and benefits
Other	Questions may be written related to prevention, clinical examinations, cost, point of contact, or patient/client data

Modified from Straus, S. E., Glasziou, P., Richardson, W. S., & Haynes, R. B. (2011). *Evidence based medicine: How to practice and teach it* (4th ed.). Edinburgh, Scotland: Elsevier.

BOX 15-2   Definitions of Clinically Significant Statistics

Relative risk *(RR)* is the risk of the outcome in the treated group (Y) compared to the risk in the control group *(X)*. $RR = Y / X$

Relative risk reduction *(RRR)* is the percentage reduction in risk in the treated group (Y) compared to the control group *(X)*. $RRR = 1 - Y / X \times 100\%$

Absolute risk reduction (ARR) is the difference in risk between the control group (X) and the treatment group (Y). $ARR = X - Y$

Numbers needed to treat *(NNT)* is the number of patients that must be treated over a given period of time to prevent one adverse outcome. $NNT = 1 / (X - Y)$

Odds ratio *(OR)* is the odds of an experimental patient suffering an event compared to a patient in the control group or the odds of risk.

Modified from Straus, S. E., Glasziou, P., Richardson, W. S., & Haynes, R. B. (2011). *Evidence based medicine: How to practice and teach it* (4th ed.). Edinburgh, Scotland: Elsevier.

---

that emerge from qualitative research are valued because they incorporate the "patients' voice into evidence based process" (p. 142). As such, qualitative research deserves a place in the hierarchy of evidence although it may not be considered equivalent to quantitative research findings.

TEST YOUR KNOWLEDGE 15-2

1. Which of the following would be considered when appraising quantitative studies? (Select all that apply.)

    a. Representativeness of the sample

    b. Trustworthiness

    c. Sample size

    d. Control over extraneous variables

2. Which of the following would be considered when appraising qualitative studies? (Select all that apply.)

    a. Validity and reliability

    b. Audit trail

    c. Thick description

    d. Participants are experienced in the phenomenon

3. Place the following kinds of evidence in order from highest to lowest.

    a. Meta-analyses

    b. Case studies

    c. RCTs

    d. Cohort studies

    e. Expert opinions

How did you do? 1. a, c, d; 2. b, c, d; 3. a, c, d, b, e

15.3 Clinical Practice Guidelines: Moving Ratings and Recommendations into Practice

At the end of this section, you will be able to:

‹ Explain the development and use of clinical practice guidelines

Various professional associations and other clinical entities have developed *clinical practice guidelines* to be used in practice settings. The National Guideline Clearinghouse (NGC), under the auspices of the AHRQ and the U.S. Department of Health and Human Services (http://www.guidelines.gov), hosts a myriad of these documents. Nurses can purchase other guidelines through professional associations. The NGC is a public resource for evidence-based practice guideline summaries that provide inclusion criteria, attributes of the guideline, a glossary, the classification scheme, and summary of the content development.

Most guidelines have a standard format and therefore provide similar information. Most often they identify the names of the reviewers or development team or a listing of the background of experts who served on the panel plus any disclosures. The method of review is generally presented, such as the number of citations, databases searched, and other means to capture relevant research and secondary sources of interest. Panel members typically review findings and reach consensus about best practice. Usually limitations of the review are listed, which may include exclusions of certain topics tangential to the guidelines or issues that were beyond the scope of the review, such as issues related to legal matters, economics, or healthcare system issues. Recommendations by the panel members form the basis of CPGs. Appendixes often contain the rating scales used to evaluate the evidence, tables, and figures. Often a disclaimer is included that notes that recommendations serve as guides and are not to be used in lieu of "critical thinking, sound judgment, and clinical experience" (American Geriatrics Society, 2009, p. 1333).

Clinical practice guidelines are just that: guidelines. CPGs offer an evaluation of the quality of the relevant scientific literature and an assessment of the likely benefits and harms of a particular treatment (Institute of Medicine [IOM], 2011, p. 1). As such, they serve as useful tools to direct clinical practice. They typically include all relevant process and outcome measures that would be indicated for the average patient with a specific diagnosis or treatment problem. Guidelines provide an easy-to-read consolidation of research findings.

Algorithms or decision trees are used in some guidelines to demonstrate a stepwise process for resolving a specific clinical problem. Although evidence-based CPGs specify good clinical practice, healthcare providers may not be using them to their maximum potential. Clinicians, patients, and healthcare systems stand to benefit when guidelines are easy to follow and widely used.

Although guidelines may appear to be comprehensive, they do not include all of the variables that clinicians encounter when managing patient conditions or treatments. Guidelines are unable to address unique patient characteristics. Social, psychological, emotional, spiritual, environmental, and biomedical factors are not considered in the guidelines. Using guidelines can result in making generalizations that can be problematic. Guidelines provide a general approach to clinical management based on scientific evidence, but caution must be exercised when applying them to individual patients.

Heath (2005) warned about the use of CPGs as an "instrument of surveillance" (p. 269), whether it is for financial reward, measures of quality, punitive action, or ethical or legal considerations. Manipulation of guidelines for such purposes should be considered carefully because their primary intent is to describe best practice for the typical patient. Nurses must be aware that guidelines may also contain bias and therefore must critically evaluate them. The IOM (2011) recommended that CPGs need to be trustworthy or of high quality for healthcare practitioners to improve decision making and effect quality outcomes. CPGs need to show transparency in how recommendations are derived and rated, allowing for external review and timely updating.

To remedy some of the concerns about bias, the Appraisal of Guidelines Research and Evaluation (*AGREE II*) instrument was developed as part of an international collaborative of researchers and policymakers. The instrument provides a standard framework for the development and implementation of CPGs. A checklist of 23 items across six different quality domains provides a useful tool for the generation and evaluation of guidelines (AGREE Collaboration, 2009; **Table 15-3**). The AGREE II instrument is generic and can be applied to all types of CPGs. It is based on evidence-based geriatric nursing protocols (Levin & Jacobs, 2012). A tutorial is available to learn how to use the tool and is useful for teaching EBP nursing in the classroom or clinical setting (Levin, Ferrara, & Vetter, 2012). The instrument and tutorials can be accessed at http://www.agreetrust.org/resource-centre/agree-ii-training-tools/.

CPGs will continue evolving because of the momentum generated by EBP. Evidence is more available because of the increased capacity to search

TABLE 15-3	Domains of Quality in the AGREE II Instrument
Domain 1	Scope and purpose of the guidelines
Domain 2	Stakeholder involvement
Domain 3	Rigor of development
Domain 4	Clarity and presentation
Domain 5	Applicability
Domain 6	Editorial independence

Data from AGREE Collaboration. (2013). *Appraisal of guidelines for research and evaluation II (AGREE II) instrument.* Retrieved from http://www.agreetrust.org/wpcontent/uploads/2013/06/AGREE_II_Users_Manual_and_23-item_Instrument_ENGLISH.pdf

the literature. Computerization capabilities are allowing information from guidelines, such as algorithms or decision tools, to be loaded into the personal digital assistants of practicing nurses. Others, such as insurers, attorneys, and ethicists, will be interested in guideline development.

CRITICAL THINKING EXERCISE 15-2

Think about your last clinical experience. What practice guidelines would have been helpful? Where might you find these guidelines? Do you think the staff would be receptive to your using clinical guidelines on the unit?

TEST YOUR KNOWLEDGE 15-3

True/False

1. Patient care must follow clinical guidelines exactly.
2. A panel of experts synthesizes evidence to make recommendations for clinical guidelines.
3. Nurses should evaluate clinical guidelines because they may be biased.

How did you do? 1. F; 2. T; 3. T

15.4 Keeping It Ethical

At the end of this section, you will be able to:

‹ Discuss reasons why nurses should follow agency policies even when they conflict with evidence

When weighing evidence, nurses need to remember that there are no perfect studies; therefore, there are always limitations of the evidence. Even though systematic reviews are highly regarded, they may not provide all the answers a researcher would like to have or that the clinician might want to know. Evidence might support a certain treatment or intervention, but one must remember that the literature might not report all aspects that were tested. For example, the use of case reports might reveal harm from a pharmaceutical agent, such as an adverse drug reaction. A systematic review might ensue to appraise harmful consequences of the pharmaceutical agent. However, because negative trials typically never make it to publication, the information would not be uncovered during a systematic review. Similarly, the evidence derived from research might be perceived to be ironclad, without exception or deviation. This cannot be further from the truth. Clinicians must examine the evidence within the context of the question, and consequently, the answer that is revealed. Nurses must incorporate several sources of evidence at the bedside: the individual patient experience, the clinical experience, and policy or cost considerations (Rycroft-Malone, 2003). Questions that nurses can ask are (Straus et al., 2011):

» Are our patients enough like those in the study so that results can apply?
» Is the treatment feasible in our setting?
» What are the potential benefits and harms from the treatment for our patients?
» What are our patients' values and expectations about the treatment and the outcomes?

Generalizability is always a concern when deciding how to apply evidence to practice. Application of evidence to practice relies on findings and recommendations generated from samples. Individual patients may not have the same characteristics as study subjects, and this raises concern for nurses when considering the adoption and application of the evidence to the point of care.

Gray (2005) suggested that the path from the evidence to utilization in practice can be value laden and raise ethical concerns. For example, recommendations for specific diagnostic screenings, such as routine cancer testing for specific age groups or genders, may be scientifically justified based on incidence and

FYI

Nurses who engage in activities that promote EBP, such as journal clubs and policy committees, may find that even after diligently reviewing the evidence, practice changes are not implemented. Nurses need to follow agency policy and act as change agents to effectively bring the evidence to the point of care.

prevalence rates and other population characteristics. In a perfect world of unlimited resources, a full battery of cancer screening tests could begin at age 21 and be done annually thereafter. However, in the real world with limited resources and potential harm from repeated screening, it would be difficult to justify this standard of screening. Using resources for routine, comprehensive cancer screening at age 21 would be considered foolish and wasteful. Clinical decisions are ultimately derived from choices that are influenced by the needs and values of the population. Even when practice is based on evidence, other factors might affect clinical decision making.

An ethical dilemma may arise if agency policy conflicts with evidence. Nurses who engage in activities that promote EBP, such as journal clubs and policy committees, may find that even after diligently reviewing the evidence, practice changes are not implemented. But for legal reasons, nurses need to follow agency policy and act as change agents to effectively bring the evidence to the point of care.

TEST YOUR KNOWLEDGE 15-4

True/False

1. Decisions about clinical practice are based solely on evidence.
2. If a conflict exists between evidence and facility policy, the nurse should implement procedures based on the evidence.

How did you do? 1. F; 2. F

RAPID REVIEW

» When weighing the evidence, clinicians can either adopt or reject an innovation. Innovations are adopted when uncertainty is reduced.

» There are two kinds of rejection: active and passive.

» Appraisal involves reviewing the design, sampling methods, and data analysis.

» Quantitative designs must be appraised to ensure that appropriate conclusions are drawn.

» Qualitative research is appraised for scientific rigor, systematic analysis, and conclusions that are grounded in data.

» Evidence hierarchies provide a meaningful way to rank research studies based on scientific rigor and the levels of evidence: CPGs, meta-analyses, systematic reviews, RCTs, cohort studies, case control studies, descriptive studies, qualitative studies, expert opinions, and case studies.

» A variety of professional organizations and clinical entities have developed rating systems that provide a systematic way to rate risks, benefits, quality, and strengths of the evidence. An international collaboration proposes to use the GRADE system as a single standard.

» CPGs provide recommendations for practice based on a thorough review of evidence conducted by expert panel members. Because CPGs might have bias, the AGREE II instrument assists nurses in evaluating guidelines.

» Nurses must consider other factors aside from evidence that influence clinical decision making.

Apply What You Have Learned

The EBP committee has been meeting regularly to analyze evidence and is now able to make recommendations for best practice. Of course, if you were on an actual EBP committee, there would be much more evidence about hand hygiene that you would need to consider. We have provided only a sample of evidence for you throughout this exercise. When making a policy decision in clinical practice, you would need to consider all of the evidence. In this exercise, first examine each study to determine whether the study is valid by considering the questions presented in Box 15-1. Then, use the rating system described in Figure 15-1 to assign each piece of evidence a ranking. Make a decision about the evidence, and write a nursing policy that you think will increase compliance with hand hygiene. Be sure to consider the feasibility (organizational and individual barriers) of your policy. A template is included within this text's digital resources that serves as an example of a format that can be used to standardize the way policies are written in a healthcare facility. Use this template to record your policy.

REFERENCES

Agency for Healthcare Research and Quality. (n.d.). EPC evidence-based reports. Retrieved from http://www.ahrq.gov/research/findings/evidence-based-reports/index.html

Agency for Healthcare Research and Quality. (2002). *Systems to rate the strength of scientific evidence* (Evidence Report/Technology Assessment No 47. AHRQ Pub. No. 02-E016). Retrieved from http://archive.ahrq.gov/clinic/epcsums/strengthsum.pdf

Agency for Healthcare Research and Quality. (2016). Evidence-based practice centers (EPCs). Retrieved from http://www.ahrq.gov/research/findings/evidence-based -reports/centers/index.html

AGREE Collaboration. (2013). *Appraisal of guidelines for research and evaluation II (AGREE II) instrument.* Retrieved from http://www.agreetrust.org/wp-content /uploads/2013/10/AGREE-II-Users-Manual-and-23-item-Instrument_2009 _UPDATE_2013.pdf

American Geriatrics Society. (2009). The pharmaceutical management of persistent pain in older persons. AGS Panel on Persistent Pain in Older Persons. *Journal of the American Geriatrics Society, 57,* 1331–1346.

Attia, J., & Page, J. (2001). A graphic framework for teaching critical appraisal of randomized controlled trials. *Evidence Based Medicine, 6,* 68–69.

Canadian Task Force on Preventive Health Care. (2016). History. Retrieved from http://canadiantaskforce.ca/about-us/history/

Centre for Evidence-based Medicine. (2013). Oxford Centre for Evidence-based Medicine: Levels of evidence. Retrieved from http://www.cebm.net/index.aspx ?o=1025

de Groot, M., van der Wouden, J. M., van Hell, E. A., & Nieweg, M. B. (2013). Evidence-based practice for individuals for groups: Let's make a difference. *Perspectives on Medical Education, 2,* 216–221.

Dilorio, C., Resnicow, K., McCarty, F., De, A. K., Dudley, W. N., Wang, D. T., & Denzmore, P. (2006). Keepin' it R. E. A. L.! Results of a mother–adolescent HIV prevention program. *Nursing Research, 55*(1), 43–51.

The GRADE Working Group. (2017). GRADE. Retrieved from http://www.grade workinggroup.org/

Gray, J. A. (2005). Evidence-based and value-based healthcare. *Evidence-based Healthcare and Public Health, 9,* 317–318.

Heath, I. (2005). The use and abuse of guidelines. *Evidence-based Healthcare and Public Health, 9,* 268–269.

Institute of Medicine. (2011). *Clinical practice guidelines we can trust.* Washington, DC: Author.

Joanna Briggs Institute. (2014). *Reviewers' manual 2014 edition.* Retrieved from http://joannabriggs.org/assets/docs/sumari/ReviewersManual-2014.pdf

Levin, R. F., Ferrara, L., & Vetter, M. J. (2012). Evaluating clinical practice guidelines. In R. F. Levin & H. R. Feldman (Eds.), *Teaching evidence-based practice in nursing* (2nd ed., pp. 133–137). New York, NY: Springer.

Levin, R. F., & Jacobs, S. K. (2012). Developing and evaluating clinical practice guidelines: A systematic approach. In M. Boltz, E. Capezute, T. Fulmer, & D. Zwicker (Eds.), *Evidence-based geriatric nursing protocols for best practice* (4th ed., pp. 1–10). New York, NY: Springer.

Melnyk, B. M. (2004, Second Quarter). Evidence digest. *Worldviews on Evidence-based Nursing,* 142–145.

Melnyk, B. M., & Fineout-Overholt, E. (2015). *Evidence-based practice in nursing and healthcare: A guide to best practice* (3rd ed.). Philadelphia, PA: Lippincott Williams & Wilkins.

Rogers, E. M. (2003). *Diffusion of innovations* (5th ed.). New York, NY: Free Press.

Rycroft-Malone, J. (2003). Consider the evidence. *Nursing Standard, 17*(45), 21.

Straus, S. E., Glasziou, P., Richardson, W. S., & Haynes, R. B. (2011). *Evidence based medicine: How to practice and teach it* (4th ed.). Edinburgh, Scotland: Elsevier.

Thorne, S. (2000). Data analysis in qualitative research. *Evidence Based Nursing, 3*, 68–70.

University of Alberta. (2008a). Introduction to evidence based medicine. Retrieved from http://www.ebm.med.ualberta.ca/EbmIntro.html

University of Alberta. (2008b). Therapy/prevention article appraisal guide. Retrieved from http://www.ebm.med.ualberta.ca/Therapy.html

Watson, R. (2012). Peer review under the spotlight in the UK. *Journal of Advanced Nursing, 68*(4), 718–720.

Implementation

Innovations are not helpful if they are not adopted.

At the end of this chapter, you will be able to:

- Identify evidence-based practice (EBP) models
- Discuss barriers to application of evidence to practice
- Discuss strategies for creating change to support EBP
- Describe strategies for engaging others in change
- List Kotter's eight phases of change
- Discuss dilemmas that can be encountered during change

barriers
change
change phases model

conduct and utilization of research in nursing (CURN)
cost-benefit ratio

Iowa model for EBP to promote quality care
journal club
Nursing Quality Indicators
Stetler model

CHAPTER 16

Transitioning Evidence to Practice

Maria Young

16.1 Evidence-Based Practice Models to Overcome Barriers

At the end of this section, you will be able to:

‹ Identify evidence-based practice (EBP) models
‹ Discuss barriers to application of evidence to practice

By now you should have an understanding of EBP. As you recall, trial and error, educated guesses, and intuition are all useful in contributing to a nurse's experience that guides practice, but these processes or behaviors do little to provide the stronger evidence needed to achieve positive patient outcomes. In today's rapidly changing, highly complex healthcare environment, patient outcomes based on evidence provide the foundation for safe, quality patient care. So, how do we take the evidence and apply it to the point of care? What EBP models have the potential to increase our use of research to guide care? What are the barriers to applying evidence to practice? What elements are necessary if nurses are to create a practice culture that is committed to and supports evidence-based processes, policies, and actions? Answers to these questions are examined in this chapter as well as strategies to create an EBP setting.

Evidence-Based Practice Models

EBP is nothing new to nurses. Florence Nightingale, through her use of meticulous record keeping and data analysis, was able to demonstrate that mortality rates decreased when sanitary methods were improved (Riddle, 2006). By using the data she had gathered, Nightingale developed interventions that, when applied to medical and surgical patients, reduced mortality rates caused by unsanitary conditions. In general, the term *EBP* describes a model of care whereby nurses, using current evidence or research knowledge, make decisions using clinical expertise and patient preferences to guide patient care (Melnyk & Fineout-Overholt, 2015). The University of Minnesota (n.d.) has on its website the following definition of evidence-based care: "Evidence-Based Practice is the thoughtful integration of the best available evidence coupled with clinical expertise."

Clinical practice based on evidence would seem to be an important goal for nurses, yet many nurses acknowledge that they do not incorporate research findings into their practices (Malik, McKenna, & Plummer, 2016; Warren et al., 2016). Why this is so has been explored by many researchers (Hommelstad & Ruland, 2004; Pettengill, Gillies, & Clark, 1994; Retsas, 2000; Rutledge, Greene, Mooney, Nail, & Ropka, 1998; Sitzia, 2001) and is a topic that remains under continued examination (French, 2002).

Several models have emerged and serve as the foundation for evidence-based nursing practice. Some models are the *conduct and utilization of research in nursing (CURN)* project, the *Stetler model*, and the *Iowa model for EBP to promote quality care*.

CURN

The CURN project was one of the earliest attempts to increase the use of research in practice by registered nurses (RNs). It was a 5-year project awarded to the Michigan Nurses' Association by the Division of Nursing in the 1970s and focused on helping nurses transition research findings into their practice settings (Polit & Beck, 2016). An outcome of the CURN project was a realization that practicing nurses would use research only if it had been widely disseminated and was relevant to their practice (Horsely, Crane, & Bingle, 1978). The CURN project moved nursing practice from customs, opinions, and authority to searching for the best research available and integrating the evidence with a nurse's clinical expertise, patient preferences, and existing resources (Polit & Beck, 2016).

To appreciate the importance of the CURN project, consider that in the 1970s nurses engaged in practice behaviors solely because "we've always done it this way." For example, consider the practice of restraining patients by tying them to their beds or chairs to prevent falls. It has only been through research studies examining this practice that nurses now know that although tying patients to beds or chairs may have prevented falls, it also predisposed patients to other injuries, such as strangling, as they tried to get out of the restraints. Because 30–50% of patient falls result in injury, the need to conduct research and disseminate the findings about the prevention of patient falls remains a priority (the Joint Commission, 2015). Without the work of the CURN project, an understanding of how nurses embrace and use research in their clinical practice might not have occurred.

The Stetler Model

Whereas the CURN project has given nurses insight into how and why nurses embrace research in clinical practice, the Stetler model (Stetler, 2001) focuses on how individual practitioners adopt research findings at the bedside. Originally developed in 1976 as the Stetler/Merram model for research utilization, this model can be used to systematically integrate research into practice. The model was updated to facilitate examination of both the product and process of research. Products of research are things such as research findings. An example is that 9 out of 10 dentists recommend a certain chewing gum for their patients who chew gum. The process of research tells how to go about solving a problem. For example, nurses on a busy medical-surgical unit want to explore why they have noticed an increase in patient falls. They begin to examine the problem by conducting a chart audit of all the patients who have fallen in the past year. Next they determine whether there are any common factors. When the common factors are identified, a list of risk factors is developed that can guide interventions to reduce the number of falls. These nurses are engaging in a process of research. As evidenced in these examples, both product and process are important to facilitate EBP.

Because Stetler's model (2001) is prescriptively designed, it provides practitioners with step-by-step instructions for integrating research into practice and is useful to help nurses deliver safe patient care. In the updated version of the model (see **Figure 16-1**), Stetler provides a traditional graphic accompanied by a narrative of the five phases of the model.

In the first phase of the model, known as the preparation phase, Stetler (2001) encourages nurses to be very clear about the purpose, the context, and the sources of any research evidence. Questions to be answered include what are the issues, who are the stakeholders, and how will we define our outcomes? Questions such as these assist nurses to be very purposeful in their thinking when making decisions about EBP.

The second phase of the model is the validation phase. In this phase, nurses analyze the evidence to determine whether it is sufficient and credible to use in the practice setting. You should be familiar with techniques, such as creating a grid to summarize and weigh research articles, that are important for successfully progressing through this phase.

The third phase, also called the comparative evaluation/ decision making phase, is when nurses engage in labeling, condensing, organizing, and attributing meaning to all the assembled evidence. Questions that could be considered during this phase are: Do you have all the data needed to make a good decision? Is the evidence that you have uncovered reliable? How strong is the evidence for any recommendations being made? For example, you may not want to make a practice change if the only evidence came from a nonpeer-reviewed journal and was based

FIGURE 16-1 Stetler Model of Research Utilization to Facilitate EBP

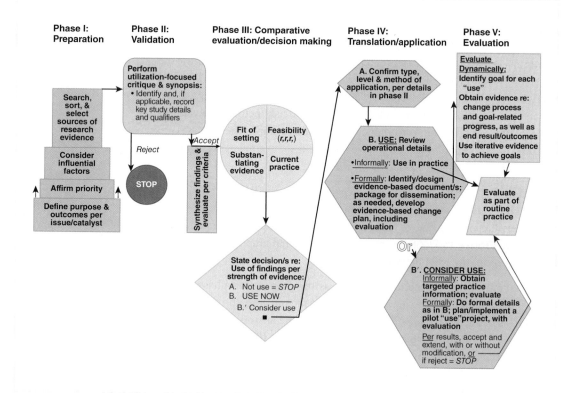

FIGURE 16-1   *Continued*

Phase I: Preparation	Phase II: Validation	Phase III: Comparative evaluation/decision making	Phase IV: Translation/application	Phase V: Evaluation
Purpose, context, & sources of research evidence:	Credibility of findings & potential for/ detailed qualifiers of application:	Synthesis & decisions/ recommendations per criteria of applicability:	Operational definition of use/actions for change:	Alternative types of evaluation:
• Potential Issues/ Catalysts = a problem, including unexplained variations or less-than-best practice; or routine update of knowledge; or validation/ routine revision of procedure, policy, etc; or innovative program goal	• Critique & synopsize essential components, operational details, and other qualifying factors, per source	• Synthesize the cumulative findings:	• Types = cognitive, symbolic &/or instrumental	• Evaluation can be formal or informal, individual or institutional
		• *Logically organize & display the similarities and differences across multiple findings, per common aspects or sub-elements of the topic under review*	• Methods = informal or formal; direct or indirect	• Consider cost-benefit of various evaluation efforts
	• *See instructions for use of utilization-focused review tables to facilitate this task; fill in the tables for group decision making or potential future synthesis*	• *Evaluate degree of substantiation of each aspect/sub-element; reference any qualifying conditions*	• Levels = individual, group, or department/ organization	• Use RU as a process to enhance credibility of evaluation data
• Affirm perceived problems with internal evidence		• Evaluate degree & nature of other criteria: feasibility (r,r,r = risk, resources, readiness); pragmatic fit; & current practice	• Direct instrumental use: change individual behavior (vis-à-vis assessment; plan/ intervention options; implementation details; &/or evaluation); or change policy, procedure, protocol, algorithm, program components, etc.	• For both dynamic & pilot evaluations, include two types of evaluative information:
• Focus on high priority Issues	• Critique systematic reviews			
• Decide if need to form a team or involve formal "structures"/key stake-holders	• Reassess fit of individual sources	• Make a decision whether/what to use:	• Cognitive use: validate current practice; change personal way of thinking; increase awareness; better understand or appreciate condition/s or experience/s	• *formative, regarding actual implementation & goal progress*
	• Rate the level & quality of each evidence source per a "table of evidence"	• *Can be a personal practitioner-level decision or a recommendation to others*	• Symbolic use: develop position paper or proposal for change; persuade others regarding a way of thinking	• *summative, regarding Phase I outcomes and goal results*
• Consider other influential internal and external factors, such as beliefs, resources, or timelines		• *Judge the strength of this decision; indicate if primarily "research-based" or, per use of supplemental information, "evidence-based"; qualify the related level of strength of decision/ recommendations per related table*	CAUTION: Assess whether translation/ product or use goes beyond actual findings/evidence:	
	• Differentiate statistical and clinical significance		• *Research evidence may or may not provide various details for a complete policy, procedure, etc.; indicate this fact to users, and note differential levels of evidence therein*	
• Define desired, measurable outcome/s Seek out systematic reviews	• Eliminate noncredible sources			
	• End the process if there is no evidence or if there is clearly insufficient credible research evidence that meets your need	• *For formal recommendations, determine degree of stakeholder consensus*	• Formal dissemination & change strategies should be planned per relevant research (Include Dx analysis):	
		• If decision = "Not use" research findings:	• *Simple, passive education is rarely effective as an isolated strategy. Consider multiple strategies, e.g., interactive education, opinion leaders, educational outreach, audit, etc.*	
• Determine need for an explicit type of research evidence, if relevant		• *May conduct own research or delay use until additional research is done by others*	• *Consider implementation models (e.g., Kitson or PRECEDE)*	
• Select research sources with conceptual fit		• *If still decide to act now, e.g., on evidence of consensus or another basis for practice, STOP use of model but consider need for planned change and evaluation*	• Consider need for appropriate, reasoned variation	
			• <u>WITH B,</u> where made a decision to use in the setting:	
		• If decision = "Use/Consider Use," can mean a recommendation for or against a specific practice	• *With formal use, may need a dynamic evaluation to effectively implement & continuously improve/refine use of best available evidence*	
			• <u>WITH B',</u> where made a decision to consider use & thus obtain additional, pragmatic information before a final decision	
	See Stetler et al. (1998) for noted tables, reviews, & synthesis process.		• *With formal consideration, need a pilot project*	NOTE: Model applies to all forms of practice, i.e., educational, clinical, managerial, or other
			• *With a pilot project, must assess if need IRB review, per relevant institutional criteria*	

on the manufacturer's recommendations because this may not be very strong evidence. Many associations define beforehand what level of evidence to require when identifying evidence-based standards, guidelines, or recommendations. For instance, the American Association of Critical-Care Nurses defines levels of evidence as follows:

» *Level A:* Evidence includes meta-analysis of multiple controlled studies or systematic review of RCTs with results that consistently support a specific action, intervention, or treatment.
» *Level B:* Evidence includes well-designed controlled studies, both randomized and nonrandomized, with results that consistently support a specific action, intervention, or treatment.
» *Level C:* Recommendations are based on qualitative studies; systematic reviews of qualitative, descriptive, or correlational studies; integrative reviews; or randomized controlled trials with inconsistent results.
» *Level D:* Recommendations are based on peer-reviewed professional organizational standards, with clinical studies to support recommendations.
» *Level E:* Recommendations are based on theory-based evidence from expert opinion or multiple case reports, and level M are manufacturer's recommendations only.
» *Level M:* Manufacturer's recommendations only (Peterson et al., 2014).

By the end of this third phase in the Stetler model, a decision is made about whether to use the evidence to guide practice.

In the fourth phase, the challenge is to translate or apply the research in the practice setting (Stetler, 2001). For many organizations this may be easier said than done. For example, consider the difficulties encountered when integrating into practice knowledge about discharge planning for patients with heart failure (HF). While many nurses understand the concept of discharge planning and the practice of beginning discharge planning upon admission, the ability to develop processes that support discharge are lacking as demonstrated by all-cause readmissions of 10–50% for this patient population (Joynt & Jha, 2011). This illustrates how difficult it can be to adopt innovations in a social system. When applying research to practice, it is important for nurses to think carefully about how the evidence will be communicated, disseminated, and applied. In this example, relevant questions to consider include who will be responsible for implementing HF guidelines into practice, what resources (time, money, personnel) are available to operate the program, and how will the success of the program be measured? Change is at the heart of this phase.

In the fifth and final phase of the Stetler model (2001), nurses evaluate the outcomes of the change in practice. Continuing with the example of HF discharge planning, questions from the fourth phase provide a means for evaluating how well research is applied to practice. In the fourth phase it was decided that practice should be based on the knowledge that patients respond best to HF discharge advice when they are hospitalized because of symptoms related to HF and when they indicate they are ready to make changes. Practice was altered to have nurses assess patient readiness to make changes and immediately provide written and verbal HF management information. The success of this practice change can be evaluated by comparing how often patients are given HF management information with how many of them are being readmitted for symptoms of HF.

> **FYI**
>
> By understanding barriers to creating EBP, nurses are better able to anticipate potential problems when initiating research activities in clinical practice. Barriers to applying research to practice include organizational culture, nurses' belief systems related to practice, and research-related barriers.

The Iowa Model

The Iowa model for EBP to promote quality care is a systematic method that explains how organizations change practice (see **Figure 16-2**). Originally a research utilization model, it has been updated recently to include more emphasis on EBP and renamed the Iowa model of evidence-based practice to promote quality care (Titler et al., 2001). In this model nurses consider the following questions: Is the topic a priority for the organization? Is there a sufficient research base? Is change appropriate for adoption for practice? By considering these questions, nurses address many of the same issues as in the Stetler model (2001), such as the need to gather relevant research, identify outcomes to be achieved, apply the research to practice, and evaluate the application of the research to practice.

Barriers to Connecting Research and Practice

By understanding *barriers* to creating EBP, nurses are better able to anticipate potential problems when initiating research activities in clinical practice. Several studies have examined barriers to applying research to practice and have found organizational culture, nurses' belief systems related to practice, and research-related barriers as some of the reasons why integration of research findings is difficult for practicing nurses at the point of care (Malik, McKenna, & Plummer, 2016; Warren et al., 2016).

Organizational Culture

That health care is practiced in a rapidly changing, highly complex environment is no surprise to nurses. Nurses are constantly challenged to provide patients with high-quality, safe care with limited resources. How successful nurses are at delivering high-quality patient care can depend on how

> **KEY TERM**
>
> **barriers:** Factors that limit or prevent change

FIGURE 16-2 The Iowa Model of Evidence-Based Practice to Promote Quality Care

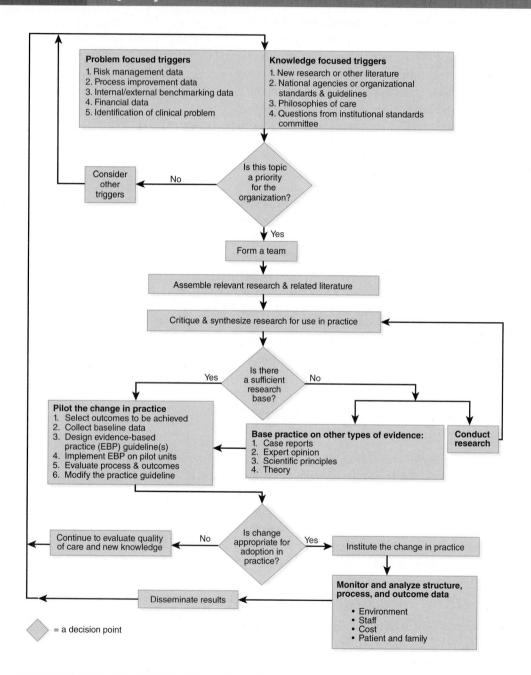

effective professional organizations are in fostering nurses' abilities to develop and initiate interventions aimed at safe patient care. Funk, Tornquist, and Champagne (1995) identified several organizational characteristics necessary to create and sustain an evidence-based culture: (1) adequate resources for research activities, (2) support and encouragement for inquiry, and (3) an expectation for staff to engage in research activities. The Institute of Medicine (2004) report called for organizational leaders to "incorporate multiple academic and other research-based organizations to support HCOs [healthcare organizations] in the identification and adoption of evidence-based management systems" (p. 155). This is good news to nurses who have often practiced in environments that seldom recognized the need for, nor appreciated, the evidence needed for best practice.

Within the nursing profession there is evidence of changing expectations, as noted by the development of *Nursing Quality Indicators* (Press Ganey National Database of Nursing Quality Indicators® (NDNQI®), 2016). These indicators show the outcomes of nursing care and are meant to address patient safety and quality of care. Organizations committed to quality assurance collect data on the following clinical indicators:

Staffing and workforce indicators
Pressure injury prevalence
Patient falls
Resistant prevalence
Catheter-associated urinary tract infection
Central line catheter-associated bloodstream infections
Pediatric peripheral intravenous infiltration rate
Pediatric pain assessment, intervention, reassessment cycle
Patient volume and flow
Nurse turnover
Ventilator-associated pneumonia
Ventilator-associated events
Psychiatric physical/sexual assault rate
RN education/specialty certification
Discharge care coordination
Hospital readmission rates
Care coordination

> **KEY TERM**
>
> **Nursing Quality Indicators:** Outcomes of nursing care, identified by the American Nurses Association, that address patient safety and quality of care

CRITICAL THINKING EXERCISE 16-1

Why do nurses seem reluctant to incorporate research findings into their practice? The next time you are on a clinical unit, ask the staff how they apply research findings in their practice.

Nurses are expected to use the best evidence available to achieve the best patient outcomes possible (Krugman, 2003). Many organizations have come to appreciate the link between EBP and positive patient outcomes as a result of changing reimbursement policies. Third-party payers are demanding the implementation of policies, processes, and practices that have the greatest potential to contribute to the best outcomes. When organizations support EBP, the potential exists to balance costs as well as benefits to patients (Wurmser, 2009). The reason this balance is important has to do with the limited resources being experienced in health care today. Payers, in an effort to conserve their expenditures, are interested in knowing where their dollars are being spent. They want to know what patients are getting for their money (Wurmser, 2009). This does not mean payers are interested only in the dollar value; they are also interested in the quality of the care. In other words, a balance needs to be achieved between quality and cost of care. If the cost is low but patients are continually being readmitted because they did not receive appropriate care in the beginning, nothing would be gained. Conversely, high cost does not necessarily translate into quality care.

Nurses' Belief Systems Related to Practice

Nurses are no different from most humans when asked to make changes. For many people, change is difficult. Some might react by outright refusal to change. Others pretend to go along with the change but in reality are not in favor of it. Some totally embrace the change. Studies indicate that nurses from around the world generally have a positive attitude toward research (Akerjordet, Lode, & Severinsson, 2012; Moreno-Casbas, Fuentelsaz-Gallego, Miguel, Gonzalez-Maria, & Clarke, 2011), but they often feel that there are significant barriers. Some nurses, while having been exposed to research in their basic programs, have in the ensuing years done little with the knowledge they gained in school. For others, no formal instruction related to research was required, making the ability to read, understand, and analyze research a skill that was never developed (Polit & Beck, 2016). Creating educational opportunities for nurses to learn about EBP will help to overcome this barrier.

Research-Related Barriers

Research-related barriers make it difficult for the nurse at the point of care to understand, interpret, and/or use the research. Because the ability to replicate a study and achieve the same results means a nurse can have greater confidence in applying the evidence to practice, it would seem there is a need to conduct and disseminate research findings in a way that bedside nurses can understand. Unfortunately, this is not the case because, for most practicing nurses, the complex statistics and research jargon act as barriers to understanding research articles (Moreno-Casbas, 2011; Polit & Beck, 2016). The authors suggest that there are no perfect studies, and nurses would be wise to consider research findings as they engage in EBP.

TEST YOUR KNOWLEDGE 16-1

1. Which of the following described the use of research by RNs?
   a. Stetler model
   b. Iowa model
   c. CURN
   d. Institute of Medicine Report
2. Which of the following are ANA Nursing Quality Indicators? (Select all that apply.)
   a. Pressure injury prevalence
   b. Patient satisfaction with pain management
   c. Staffing and workforce indicators
   d. Ventilator-associated pneumonia

How did you do? 1. c; 2. a, c, d

16.2 Creating Change

At the end of this section, you will be able to:

‹ Discuss strategies for creating change to support EBP
‹ Describe strategies for engaging others in change
‹ List Kotter's eight phases of change

The key to transitioning evidence to practice is to reframe thinking about organizational culture, knowledge about research, attitudes about research, and skills in using research. Change is at the heart of reframing our thinking to make decisions about EBP.

What Is Change?

Change is a process that creates an alteration in a person or the environment. Fullan (2001) defined change as a "double-edged" sword (p. 1). For many people change represents excitement and challenge, while for others change is feared and avoided. Just as we needed to understand the barriers to research utilization, we now need to understand how change can affect EBP. On one

KEY TERM

change: A process that creates an alteration in a person or environment

hand, if nurses are in organizations that operate from a philosophy of "we have done it this way for years," one can expect change to be painful. On the other hand, it can be equally disturbing if one is in an organization that seems to change with the seasons. So, what is the solution? Prepare, prepare, prepare, or as Fullan noted, it is about strategizing. Think of EBP as a process. By using some of the models described in this chapter, nurses can strategize about how to embed evidence into practices, processes, and policies. You can learn more about the change process by reading the works of Beer, Eisenstat, and Spector (1990), Hammel (2002), and Kotter (1996).

Engaging Others in Change

One place to start engaging others in transitioning to EBP is to conduct an assessment of the practice environment. In conducting the assessment, nurses may find it helpful to include as many of their colleagues as possible.

Box 16-1 provides an example of a tool for assessing the practice environment. Although this tool is by no means an exhaustive list of questions, it provides the reader with an understanding of the types of questions to be

---

BOX 16-1 Assessment of Practice Environment

Date of Assessment:_____

Practice Environment Being Assessed:_____

Answer as many of the following questions as possible. The more complete the answers, the better the quality of the assessment.

1. What types of patients do you take care of on your unit?
2. What is the average daily census on the unit?
3. What care delivery model do the nurses on the unit use to care for patients?
4. What is the staffing mix on the unit? How many RNs, LPNs, aides?
5. How are practice errors reported?
6. Who is responsible for reporting practice errors?
7. What are the top three practice errors reported on your unit?
8. When errors are identified, what is done to correct the error?
9. Where is the policy and procedure manual on your unit?
10. How easy is it for you to access the policy and procedure manual?
11. How often are policies and procedures updated in your organization?
12. Who is responsible for updating policies and procedures?
13. How much input do staff nurses have related to creating or revising policy and procedure?
14. What are the quality initiatives in place on the unit at present?
15. How well is the unit doing related to the quality initiatives?
16. How are the results of quality initiatives communicated to staff?

CRITICAL THINKING EXERCISE 16-2

Identify a nurse on your clinical unit who has a skill for creating tables in a computer program. Who would be good at collecting and organizing data? Find another nurse who has a talent for public speaking. Try to include as many colleagues as possible.

asked to gain a complete picture of a practice environment. After the data are collected, decide whether a problem exists. To illustrate this concept, recall the medical-surgical unit where the nurses perceived an increase in patient falls. Suppose when the data were examined, patient falls appeared actually to have decreased. One would have a difficult time convincing colleagues on the unit, much less nursing administrators, that there was a need to change practice, process, or policy. From this scenario it would seem that another important activity to engage others in transitioning evidence to practice is the need to be able to demonstrate that a problem exists.

What if you did not have this skill related to creating and communicating a problem statement? What could you do next? One approach that might be considered is to develop competencies related to data collection and problem identification. Identify someone on the unit or within the organization who collects, organizes, and presents the data and problem well. You can recognize these colleagues by their job title or because you understand the issues and data when listening to their presentations. Some job titles are clinical nurse specialist, process improvement specialist, or data abstractor specialist. Another way to develop abilities to gather, organize, and present data is to volunteer to help a more experienced nurse or volunteer to participate on an organization's process improvement committee. Through such collaboration, two things are accomplished. First, a better understanding of the process can be gained. Second, you develop a collegial relationship with someone who can assist you in the future.

A *journal club* is another technique to engage others in transitioning evidence to practice (Gardner et al., 2016). Traditionally, one or two articles about a topic are provided to nurses in the club. Nurses gather to discuss the content in the articles. In many organizations, journal clubs take the form of brown bag lunches, nursing grand rounds, or unit-based potlucks. These gatherings provide a relaxed atmosphere where nurses can be exposed to practice issues and current evidence and ask questions. For some individuals, it is easier to ask questions and challenge assumptions with those they interact with on a daily basis. For others, a more formal structure to the inquiry and learning process may be necessary. With the advances in technology, journal clubs are developing online (Chan et al., 2016) or you can take a hybrid approach by

KEY TERM

journal club:
A strategy for disseminating research among nurses by discussing articles in a small group

having some structured discussions online, coupled with face-to-face meetings (Wilson et al., 2015). If you do not feel comfortable taking the lead on this, ask a nurse manager, nurse educator, advanced practice nurse (APN), or nursing administrator in your organization for help.

Many of the preceding examples for engaging others in the change process were at one time voluntary. However, in today's current healthcare environment, meeting established outcomes is mandatory and influences an organization's financial bottom line where payers reimburse based on those outcomes. For example, the American College of Cardiology (ACC) and the American Heart Association have strong evidence for how to treat patients with HF and myocardial infarcts. The ACC has developed guidelines that have demonstrated improved patient outcomes when the guidelines are followed. Payers are evaluating the effect of these guidelines on patient outcomes. Organizations that have initiated practice, process, and policy changes are recognizing that high-quality, low-cost care that patients receive means better patient outcomes with increased reimbursements. Organizations are changing by using standardized order sets where practice guidelines are embedded into physician orders or nursing care plans, care maps, clinical pathways, or electronic documentation systems. Care maps and clinical pathways tend to be multidisciplinary in nature and outline for practitioners how a patient's hospital stay will proceed within a particular diagnosis. With the advent of the electronic documentation system, best practice interventions are identified as pop-up screens or highlighted electronic reminders. Healthcare providers are expected to follow the guidelines. Care maps or clinical pathways, although not mandatory, are effective means to incorporate EBP.

Making Change Happen

What can we say about change? Because individuals do not view the concept of change in the same manner, identifying strategies to make change less frequent or less frightening for others is desirable. Constant organizational change can be stressful. Think how you would feel if every 6 months the policies related to charting changed. It would be frustrating to learn a new way of charting so frequently. Conversely, never making any changes or making changes very slowly can also be frustrating. Much has been written about the change process. John Kotter (1996) is known for his work on change. He proposed an eight-step process that has been described as a top-down transformation process (Fullan, 2001). Although not widely noted in the nursing literature, Kotter's eight *change phases model* is useful here because of its simplicity. The phases of the model are as follows: establish urgency, create a coalition, develop a vision and strategy, communicate the vision, empower broad-based action, generate short-term wins, consolidate improvements and produce more change, and anchor new approaches (**Figure 16-3**).

KEY TERM

change phases model: An eight-phase process to describe organizational change

FIGURE 16-3   Phases of Change Model

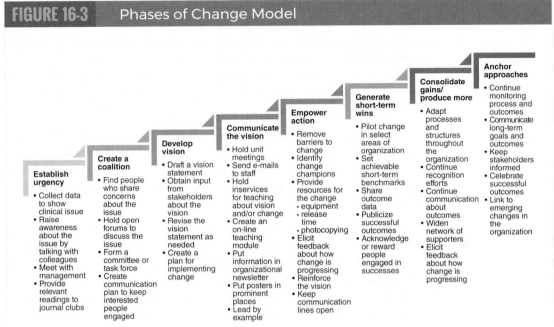

Kotter's model (1996) can be applied to clinical situations. For example, suppose there is a desire to develop a policy about patients leaving the unit to smoke, but a consensus cannot be reached about what the policy should be. Because there is no policy, nurses do not feel that they have the authority to stop patients from leaving the unit. Frustration builds after repeated attempts to create a policy are unsuccessful.

How could this situation be changed? Using Kotter's model of change (Kotter, 1996), the first phase is to create a sense of urgency. One strategy to accomplish this is to collect data about the problem. Data can be a powerful tool for creating a sense of urgency by communicating the scope of an issue. For example, suppose you learn that an organization's all-cause read-mission rate for HF patients is 25%. This high rate is problematic because patient satisfaction decreases for patients who experience frequent readmissions and organizations are not reimbursed for readmissions. It is important for an organization to understand why this is occurring and to reduce the rate of readmission. In your work to understand why HF patients are being readmitted, you realize the discharge process may not be as complete as it needs to be. Now consider how much strength could be added to the description of the problem if colleagues from other units were engaged in collecting data. By taking the time to collect data about an issue and present it to others, a sense of urgency is created.

Communicating the sense of urgency often results in the development of a coalition, the second phase of Kotter's model (1996). A coalition is a group of colleagues who share similar thoughts and a vision for change. In the example about the HF discharge process for patients, a coalition is created when colleagues recognize the potential impact on patient readmission rates in the creation of a discharge process. A benefit of creating a coalition is the collaboration and cooperation that arise.

A cohesive group sharing similar thoughts and ideas can work toward developing a vision and strategy for change, the third phase of Kotter's model (1996). Through the process of collaboration and cooperation of the coalition members, a clear vision and strategy have the greatest potential of being developed.

After the vision and strategy for change have been developed, the group must communicate the vision to others. Communicating the vision is the fourth phase of the model (Kotter, 1996). Often, it seems that change is not possible because communication has not been clear. Unclear communication can lead to misunderstandings and misconceptions about the change that is being suggested, resulting in unnecessary resistance. Communication then becomes an important phase of the change process. Good communication contributes to the potential to gain increased support to change the policy.

Creating a sense of urgency, building a coalition, developing a vision and strategy, and communicating a vision do not cause a policy, process, or practice to change. Kotter (1996) described this fifth phase as empowering broad-based action. The diversity of the coalition should be considered. A diverse group of members from the nursing unit can help develop, communicate, and sustain the vision for a policy, process, or practice change. The sustained support of the group is needed to ensure that the new policy is understood and followed. Empowering broad-based action means that members from all departments have a responsibility and accountability for the success or failure of any policy, practice, or process. To understand this idea further, suppose the proposed HF discharge process has been approved. The process requires that physicians write recommendations for their patients to monitor their weight, make a follow-up appointment with the physician, follow a low-sodium diet, take medications as prescribed, know what to do if symptoms get worse, and know what type of activity is allowed. The process requires that nurses and other ancillary staff members, from the perspective of their disciplines, teach patients about HF. Other healthcare providers also have a responsibility to notify nurses if they become aware of a patient's intent or inability to embrace the recommended plan of care for the management of HF upon discharge. If the HF discharge process was considered only a nursing process, then the needed change would be less likely to occur.

When a variety of healthcare providers is empowered, there is a greater chance for success. Succeeding in some aspect of any proposed change becomes the focus for Kotter's (1996) sixth phase of the change process, which is to generate short-term wins. This could mean recognizing individuals on the unit who embrace the new process. Tell them how much you appreciate their support of the new process, policy, or practice. For example, a dietician begins to routinely visit HF patients in order to assess their knowledge of low-sodium diets. This action represents a short-term win. By acknowledging the dietician's effort, the opportunity exists to reinforce the change. Each time someone on the healthcare team role models the desired practice change, a short-term win is created.

> **FYI**
>
> Constant organizational change can be stressful, and never making any changes or making changes very slowly can also be frustrating. It is essential to identify strategies that make change desirable to others. An effective strategy is to implement change in phases: establish urgency, create a coalition, develop a vision and strategy, communicate the vision, empower broad-based action, generate short-term wins, consolidate improvements and produce more change, and anchor new approaches.

Kotter's (1996) seventh phase involves consolidating the improvements. Each time changes can be articulated, there is a greater chance of producing more change. In the HF discharge process, for example, each time all members of the healthcare team are united in their efforts to enforce the new process, success has been achieved. Each success builds on previous successes, perpetuating adherence to the process. Consolidating improvements that produce more change also creates a sense of teamwork.

The more successes the healthcare team can recognize, the stronger the practice becomes, essentially anchoring the change in practice. The process of anchoring the change is the last, or eighth, phase of the process (Kotter, 1996). Although identified as the last phase, it should not be considered unimportant. If change does not become anchored, thus transforming practice behaviors, then all of our energies have been wasted. The need to consider how change will be anchored is an aspect that must be considered and identified early in the change process. You may want to remember this and make sure you think about how you will anchor a practice behavior change.

From this discussion it should be apparent to you how the concepts of engaging others in the change process and Kotter's (1996) strategies for change are intertwined. Depending on the type of evidence we wish to transition to the bedside, it is important for you to identify and know the stakeholders in the change process.

Stakeholder Involvement

Whenever you consider a practice change, it is important to consider the stakeholders. Identification of stakeholders is important because it allows for clarification of the purpose of the proposed change, decreases

BOX 16-2   Stakeholder Identification Tool

The following list of questions, when answered, may help to identify many of the stakeholders to any proposed change of practice, process, or policy.

1. What is the proposed change?
2. Does it affect practice, process, or policy?
3. What are the components of the practice, process, or policy?
4. What is the setting and context for the practice, process, or policy?
5. What is the history behind the practice, process, or policy?
6. What is the structure and administrative design of the practice, process, or policy?
7. Who participates in the practice, process, or policy?
8. Who sponsors the practice, process, or policy?
9. Are there any groups that will be excluded by the practice, process, or policy?
10. Who are the direct beneficiaries of the practice, process, or policy?
11. Are there any indirect beneficiaries of the practice, process, or policy?
12. Does the proposed change to practice, process, or policy create opportunities for any particular group(s)?
13. Do any particular groups stand to lose power as a result of the proposed change to practice, process, or policy?
14. Is there a funding group for the proposed change to practice, process, or policy?

misunderstandings related to the change, and facilitates implementation of the change. **Box 16-2** presents an example of a questionnaire that can be used to identify stakeholders. The following illustrates how implementing a change without collaborating with stakeholders can have negative results. Nurses on a busy medical-surgical unit have discovered that many patients are not being assessed in the morning. This is causing some difficulty for patients because physicians need morning assessments completed so they can make treatment changes. Upon further examination it is discovered that the physical therapy department, in an effort to balance their staffing and workload, has changed its routine and staff are now coming to the unit first thing in the morning before the nurses have had a chance to assess the patients. Nurses on the unit voice their concerns, but change does not occur, and the physical therapy staff continues with the new schedule.

What factors contribute to some of the negative outcomes associated with the physical therapy scheduling change? Had the physical therapy staff identified all the stakeholders, they might have discovered that their proposed practice change would affect patient care negatively. Because patients were being taken out of their rooms before breakfast, nurses were unable to complete morning assessments; thus, physicians did not have the information to make decisions about treatment options. The only group that benefited from the change was the physical therapy department, which was able to balance its staffing and workload. When input from stakeholders is not solicited, mistrust can develop among healthcare providers, often putting patients in the middle of the feuding disciplines.

TEST YOUR KNOWLEDGE 16-2

1. Which of the following are ways to engage others in transitioning evidence to practice? (Select all that apply.)
    a. Journal club
    b. Collaborating with an APN
    c. Developing care maps
    d. Maintaining status quo
2. Put Kotter's eight phases of change in order.
    a. Develop a clear vision
    b. Anchor the change
    c. Create a coalition
    d. Empower people to clear obstacles
    e. Establish a sense of urgency
    f. Consolidate and keep moving
    g. Secure short-term wins
    h. Share the vision

How did you do? 1. a, b, c; 2. e, c, a, h, d, g, f, b

16.3 Keeping It Ethical

At the end of this section, you will be able to:

‹ Discuss dilemmas that can be encountered during change

One must compare the benefits of any proposed change to the potential cost that might be incurred as a result of that change (resulting in a *cost-benefit ratio*). Sadly, many individuals in health care think about cost only in terms of dollars and cents. Although the financial bottom line cannot be ignored, other kinds of cost must be considered such as time, personnel, patient preferences, and relationships. If changes are made to practice, process, and policy without considering other aspects of cost, change may be inadvertently sabotaged.

To illustrate this point, consider how health care has changed to a system of reimbursement based on a patient's length of stay (LOS). Suppose a patient

KEY TERM

cost-benefit ratio: Comparison of benefits to potential costs that might result from change

is admitted to the hospital with HF, and the insurance will pay $10,000 for his care. It costs the hospital $10,000 to provide 6 days of care for this type of patient. If the patient stays for 6 days, the hospital breaks even. If the patient goes home in fewer than 6 days, the hospital profits because it still receives $10,000. If the patient stays longer than 6 days, the extra costs of providing care such as salaries, food, and supplies are assumed by the hospital.

Some nurses decide to approach administration and change the care process whereby HF patients are discharged in 4 days. Is this a good idea? Will patients be ready to go home in 4 days? HF patients often need several days for medications to work. They also need education related to diet and activity. Some patients are so weak that they need the services of physical therapy. The proposed decrease in LOS for HF patients means that the physical therapist would need to see patients within 24 hours of admission. Will HF patients be too sick during that time to benefit from a physical therapy evaluation? Patients who are discharged before they are ready are at risk for being readmitted just days after discharge, potentially adding cost and compromising quality of care. Readmissions can result in patient and family dissatisfaction and mistrust of healthcare providers and the healthcare system. This example illustrates how one simple change, discharging HF patients 2 days early, has the potential to increase cost while expected benefits are not realized. To achieve the most positive benefits, it is important to examine all aspects of any proposed change.

Apply What You Have Learned

Now that the policy has been written and has received the necessary administrative approvals, the EBP committee must devise an implementation plan. Use strategies identified in this chapter to create your plan, being sure to consider communication channels, equipment needs, and any education that the staff might need. Include what outcomes you measure to know if the intervention increases hand hygiene compliance.

RAPID REVIEW

» Three models serve as a foundation for EBP: CURN, Stetler model, and Iowa model.

» Barriers to EBP include organizational culture, nurses' belief systems, and research-related barriers.

» The National Database of Nursing Quality Indicators® addresses patient safety and quality of nursing care.

» Change is a process that results in an alteration. Some individuals adapt well to change, whereas others resist it.

» Strategies for transitioning evidence to practice include forming a journal club, creating a care map, and collaborating with an APN.

» Kotter's model outlines eight phases of change that can be used to guide the process.

» Journal clubs can be face-to-face, online, or hybrid.

» The cost-benefit ratio must be examined when planning for change because dilemmas can arise when changing practices, processes, and policies.

REFERENCES

Akerjordet, K., Lode, K., & Severinsson, E. (2012). Clinical nurses' attitudes towards research, management, and organizational resources in a university hospital: Part 1. *Journal of Nursing Management, 20,* 814–823.

Beer, M., Eisenstat, R. A., & Spector, B. (1990). Why change programs don't produce change. *Harvard Business Review, 68,* 158–166.

Chan, T. M., Thoma, B., Radecki, R., Topf, J., Woo, H. H., Kao, L. S., . . . Lyn, M. (2015). Ten steps for setting up an online journal club. *Journal of Continuing Education in the Health Professions, 35*(3), 148–154.

French, P. (2002). What is the evidence on evidence-based nursing? An epistemological concern. *Journal of Advanced Nursing, 37*(3), 250–257.

Fullan, M. (2001). *Leading in a culture of change.* San Francisco, CA: Jossey-Bass.

Funk, S. G., Tornquist, E. M., & Champagne, M. T. (1995). Barriers and facilitators of research utilization: An integrative review. *Nursing Clinics of North America, 30*(3), 395–407.

Gardner, K., Kanaski, M. L., Knehans, A. C., Salisbury, S., Doheny, K. K., & Schirm, V. (2016). Implementing and sustaining evidence based practice through a nursing journal club. *Applied Nursing Research, 31,* 139–145.

Hammel, G. (2002). *Leading the revolution? How to thrive in turbulent times by making innovation a way of life.* New York, NY: Plume.

Hommelstad, J., & Ruland, C. (2004). Norwegian nurses' perceived barriers and facilitators to research use. *AORN Journal, 79*(3), 621–634.

Horsely, J. A., Crane, J., & Bingle, J. D. (1978). Research utilization as an organizational process. *Journal of Nursing Administration, 8*, 4–6.

Institute of Medicine. (2004). *Keeping patients safe: Transforming the work environment of nurses.* Washington, DC: National Academies Press.

The Joint Commission. (2015). Preventing falls and fall related injuries in health care facilities. *Sentinel Event Alert, 55.* Retrieved from http://www.jointcommission.org /assets/1/18/SEA_55.pdf

Joynt, K. E., & Jha, A. K. (2011). Who has higher readmission rates for heart failure, and why? Implications for efforts to improve care using financial incentives. *Circulation: Cardiovascular Quality and Outcomes, 4*(1), 53–59.

Kotter, J. (1996). *Leading change.* Boston, MA: Harvard Business School Press.

Krugman, M. (2003). Evidence-based practice: The role of staff development. *Journal for Nurses in Staff Development, 19*, 279–285.

Malik, G., McKenna, L., & Plummer, V. (2016). Facilitators and barriers to evidence-based practice: Perceptions of nurse educators, clinical coaches and nurse specialists from a descriptive study. *Contemporary Nurse, 52,* 544–554.

Melnyk, B., & Fineout-Overholt, E. (2015). *Evidence-based practice in nursing and health care: A guide to best practice* (3rd ed.). Philadelphia, PA: Lippincott Williams & Wilkins.

Moreno-Casbas, T., Fuentilsaz-Gallego, C., Gil deMiguel, A., Gonzáles-Mariá, E., & Clarke, S. P. (2011). Spanish nurses' attitudes towards research and perceived barriers and facilitators of research utilisation: A comparative survey of nurses with and without experience as principle investigators. *Journal of Clinical Nursing, 20,* 1936–1947.

Peterson, M. H., Barnason, S., Donnelly, B., Hill, K., Miley, H., Riggs, L., & Whiteman, K. (2014). Choosing the best evidence to guide clinical practice: Application of AACN levels of evidence. *Critical Care Nurse, 34*(2), 58–68.

Pettengill, M. M., Gillies, D. A., & Clark, C. C. (1994). Factors encouraging the use of nursing research findings. *Image: Journal of Nursing Scholarship, 26*, 143–147.

Polit, D. F., & Beck, C. T. (2016). *Nursing research principles and methods: Generating and assessing evidence for nursing practice* (10th ed.). Philadelphia, PA: Lippincott Williams & Wilkins.

Press Ganey National Database of Nursing Quality Indicators® (NDNQI®). (2016). *Nursing-sensitive quality indicators.* Chicago, IL: Press Ganey Associates, Inc.

Retsas, A. (2000). Barriers to using research evidence in nursing practice. *Journal of Advanced Nursing, 31*, 599–606.

Riddle, L. (2006). *Biographies of women mathematicians: Florence Nightingale.* Retrieved from http://www.agnesscott.edu/Lriddle/WOMEN/nitegale.htm

Rutledge, D. N., Greene, P., Mooney, K., Nail, L., & Ropka, M. (1998). Barriers to research utilization for oncology staff nurses and nurse managers/clinical nurse specialists. *Oncology Nursing Forum, 25*, 497–506.

Stetler, C. B. (2001). Updating the Stetler model of research utilization to facilitate evidence-based practice. *Nursing Outlook, 49*, 272–279.

Titler, M. G., Kleiber, C., Steelman, V., Rakel, B., Budreau, G., Everett, L. Q., . . . Goode, T. (2001). The Iowa model of evidence-based practice to promote quality care. *Critical Care Nursing Clinics of North America, 13*(4), 497–509.

University of Minnesota. (n.d.). Evidence-based practice: An interprofessional tutorial. Retrieved from https://www.lib.umn.edu/apps/instruction/ebp/

Warren, J. I., McLaughlin, M., Bardsley, J., Eich, J., Esche, C. A., Kropkowski, L., & Risch, S. (2016). The strengths and challenges of implementing EBP in healthcare systems. *Worldviews on Evidence-Based Nursing, 13*(1), 15–24.

Wilson, M., Ice, S., Nakashima, C. Y., Cox, L. A., Morse, E. C., Philip, G., & Vuong, E. (2015). Striving for evidence-based practice innovations through a hybrid model journal club: A pilot study. *Nurse Education Today, 35,* 657–662.

Wurmser, T. (2009). The financial case for EBP. *Nursing Management, 40*(2),12–14.

At the end of this chapter, you will be able to:

< List four characteristics of an innovator
< Provide examples of innovative behaviors in clinical practice
< Establish two goals to develop oneself in a new job
< Explain how to implement at least one characteristic for a team leader as applied to one's job

< Outline a plan to develop your professionalism as a nurse
< List three behaviors important to maintaining professional integrity over the course of your career

awareness
behavioral inventory for professionalism
career development
change agent
communication
critical thinking
developing oneself
flexibility to change

information overload
innovator
interprofessional collaboration
ladder program
leader
lifelong learning
mentor
personal development file

preceptors
professionalism
role model
self-awareness
sense of inquiry
socialization
team leadership skills
wheel of professionalism in nursing

CHAPTER 17

Developing Oneself as an Innovator

Diane McNally Forsyth

17.1 Who Is an Innovator?

At the end of this section, you will be able to:

‹ List four characteristics of an innovator
‹ Provide examples of innovative behaviors in clinical practice

An *innovator* is one who is willing to try new things in practice, using evidence, to enhance the quality of patient care and to foster nursing knowledge. According to Rogers (2003), "innovativeness is the degree to which an individual . . . is relatively earlier in adopting new ideas than other members of a social system" (p. 18). It is vital that a nurse be an innovator because one's practice is ever evolving in the fast-paced world of health care. Retaining and using new information is enhanced when one becomes an active participant in change (Scalon & Woolforde, 2016). Will you be the first to learn about something new on your unit? Will you wait to see how those who took a class earlier evaluate it before you register? Evolving into an evidence-based practice (EBP) *leader* on one's unit or practice area is a process that occurs with effort and time.

Innovator Characteristics

There are several characteristics of an innovator. These include (1) a *sense of inquiry* (Titler, 2001), (2) *flexibility to change* (Shaver, 2001), (3) *awareness* of self and of the unit (MacIntosh, 2003), and (4) good *communication* skills (Rogers, 2003).

Sense of Inquiry

First, an innovator needs a sense of inquiry or curiosity. Maintaining currency in practice is critical. How many nursing articles will a nurse read to stay abreast of changes in practice? When in nursing school, reading is automatic. However, as a graduate nurse, it is not uncommon to dislike reading nursing journals. New graduates tend to focus on technical nursing tasks, leaving less time to reflect on their practice. Bjorkstrom, Athlin, and Johansson (2008) explored new graduates' perceptions of their professionalism after graduation and found that they rated themselves low in "knowledge mastery" and "desire to contribute through research" (p. 1386). However, reading the latest information in one's field is vital for maintaining a fresh practice in the constantly changing nursing world.

Thinking critically about a nursing dilemma is a part of this characteristic. How might a practice problem be solved? What is new evidence to improve a practice? Following one's sense of inquiry can lead to improved patient care. One example is when a nurse noted that a policy about staff accompaniment for patients going off the unit for tests and procedures was flawed. This nurse discussed it with supervisors, gathered input for needed changes, and then moved the policy revisions through the necessary practice committees in that institution to make a change. In this example, both staff and patients benefited from the enhancement.

The decision to be an innovator begins with knowledge. According to Rogers (2003), information seeking and information processing are foundational and a means to gain an understanding about a proposed change or problem. Data to support EBP planning, implementation, and evaluation must be "credible and persuasive" (Bradley et al., 2004, p. 6), so practicing one's sense of inquiry should be a daily behavior. A sense of inquiry to continually seek knowledge and critique the evidence is key (Titler, 2001).

Having a sense of inquiry or curiosity is analogous to being a critical thinker. Inherent in obtaining knowledge for an innovator are *critical thinking* strategies. Richard Paul's (1990) theory of critical thinking includes a set of interdependent or micro skills. These skills include (1) identifying the problem for practice; (2) deciphering the purpose by reading critically to understand the why behind the problem; (3) uncovering assumptions that may include personal or institutional biases; (4) recognizing and using different paradigms, such as looking at the evidence in different ways; (5) demonstrating different methods of reasoning by examining values and rationale behind decisions for change; (6) examining data, which entails an understanding of statistical or other methods for critiquing; (7) creating alternate solutions using creativity to invent new options to the problem; and (8) evaluating one's thinking to improve it (Chubinski, 1996). Experienced nurses often use these skills automatically. Because research skills to review and evaluate the evidence and strength of evidence are foundational to EBP, such critical thinking skills will serve the innovator well.

Flexibility

The second innovator characteristic is flexibility to change. In any practice setting, change is constant, so being open to and maintaining a positive attitude about change makes it easier for oneself and one's peers. A successful change in the practice setting occurs when a skilled *change agent*, an innovator, manages the many feelings associated with change, such as feelings of achievement, loss, pride, and stress (Marquis & Huston, 2006). On one hand, flexibility is being willing to try a new product or implement a new policy; your peers and patients will benefit from trying this change. You will also benefit personally by updating your practice. On the other hand, if nurses do not try the new product or implement the new policy, their practices will stagnate. Flexibility to change also requires openness to failure because sometimes new ideas do not work as planned. One example occurred when a new graduate nurse read a research article about a new procedure and tried to implement it in her unit. Unfortunately, this change was rejected by most staff members on the unit. Reasons for this might have been that implementation of the new procedure worked fine in the research setting but did not carry through to the practice setting, this particular unit was different from the one in the research setting, or the nurse was a novice change agent and therefore unable to understand the process of making policy changes on her unit. Whatever the reason for failure, it is important to keep trying to implement new changes for the benefit of patients. Strive to evaluate why a proposed change did not work and use unit resources to try the new procedure in a different way. Rogers (2003) noted that the innovation–decision process may lead to rejection for a variety of reasons. Think of the many experiments that failed at first, such as Thomas Edison's search for electricity.

Awareness

Awareness is a third characteristic of an innovator. This awareness is about oneself and one's clinical practice area (MacIntosh, 2003). *Self-awareness* is about knowing yourself; how you think, act, use your senses to make decisions, and why you do these things. It entails your ethical, cultural, and spiritual values. Think about the reasons you became a nurse or why you opted to work

FYI

An innovator is one who is willing to try new things in practice, using evidence, to enhance the quality of patient care and to foster nursing knowledge. Evolving into an EBP leader on one's unit or practice area is a process that occurs with effort and time.

in a specific practice area. A better understanding of how one thinks leads to knowledge of why one acts in ways that ultimately affect practice decisions.

An example was when a nurse disagreed with an institutional policy change relating to withdrawal of food and fluids for terminally ill patients in specific circumstances because he had different beliefs about life and death. He spoke with his nurse manager and the chaplain assigned to that unit in an effort to alleviate his discomfort. By understanding the ethical rationale behind this institutional policy and devising strategies he could use when faced with such a situation, he was able to continue working on this unit. Because of his self-awareness, he was able to seek resources to understand the meaning of the new policy and promote his continued job satisfaction.

Awareness of one's unit is also an important component of self-awareness. This is also known as situational awareness, whereby nurses perceive, comprehend, and anticipate possible outcomes based on what is happening in their environments (Gluyas & Harris, 2016). On one level, knowing the names and some characteristics about coworkers is basic. On a higher level, understanding what motivates certain people or knowing how different people react to changes can assist the innovator when change education is needed. The unit, or social system, is where the staff shares a common culture. It is important to know this culture, because diffusion of innovation occurs within the social system (Rogers, 2003). MacIntosh (2003) noted the importance of realizing one's practice as a part of finding one's professional identity when beginning work as a new graduate. In this stage, she noted that "nurses begin to develop an awareness of their work contexts that enables them to recognize discrepancies, compare competence, experience dissonance, and attempt to balance differences" (p. 732). Having an awareness of one's unit and colleagues increases self-awareness that will enhance one's practice.

Socialization to the unit helps to assimilate the new nurse. Things that help with unit awareness include uncovering who the formal and informal leaders are, how education occurs, levels of communication for implementing practice changes, and possible motivators that are positive rewards for staff (often this is food). Awareness of both oneself and the unit assists the innovator to create positive changes that can improve patient care and allow the new nurse to be an effective team member.

Communication Skills

Another characteristic of an innovator is use of good communication skills. Although these are vital skills as a nurse and leader, they are also important as an innovator. Rogers (2003) defined communication as "a process in which participants create and share information with one another in order to reach a mutual understanding" (p. 335). Communication behavior of innovators includes increased social participation and being connected through interpersonal networks (Rogers, 2003). Two parts of communication are related to being an innovator for EBP. During day-to-day practice, one must communicate clearly to one's peers and patients; this is a natural part of one's professional practice and is learned in your nursing program. Communicating with those of varying backgrounds is vital to foster relationships and a positive work environment (Nelson-Brantley & Ford, 2017). The second part of communication as an innovator means communicating to a wider audience. For example, communicating practice changes to others is an important aspect of disseminating EBP. As you lead your peers in unit changes, communicating effectively to others will involve both parts of communication. When planning an EBP change, it is important to discuss proposed changes with peers to gather broader input. Later, communication might mean one-on-one sharing of information or teaching a large group, such as a class about the new topic. This could also entail diffusion of research from your institution at a conference, sharing current research related to a specialty practice, and/or publishing.

Communicating about EBP with peers can occur in many ways. Creating one's professional network not only assists the development of leadership skills but also contributes to positive growth as a professional. This might mean belonging to a specialty organization or getting involved in institutional committees. Frequently, these groups provide EBP discussions. Another way to discuss new practice ideas is through a journal club, either face to face or online. Journal clubs foster increased knowledge about practice change, as well as a better understanding of research designs (Baker, 2013). All of these characteristics of an innovator blend to enhance EBP. These are also characteristics of a leader. When one is an innovator, one is also a leader. This does not necessarily mean becoming a nurse manager; rather, it means leading your unit or specialty area or hospital in creating positive changes for nursing practice. When innovators manifest these characteristics in a confident manner, they become role models for other nurses, too. Nursing is a team practice. When going solo, you are less likely to be successful in creating change. The hospital may have educators or other advanced practice nurses who can assist you in creating changes for EBP. Use of a professional network and institutional resources can be helpful when solving a clinical issue.

CRITICAL THINKING EXERCISE 17-1

Think of a nurse you consider to be an innovator. What characteristics does this person have? How might you model these characteristics?

TEST YOUR KNOWLEDGE 17-1

1. Which of the following are characteristics of an innovator? (Select all that apply.)
    a. Sense of curiosity
    b. Cynical nature
    c. Inflexible
    d. Self-aware

True/False

2. Innovators are critical thinkers.
3. Change keeps nursing practice up to date.
4. All change is positive.
5. The culture of the social system can inhibit change.

How did you do? 1. a, d; 2. T; 3. T; 4. F; 5. T

17.2 Developing Oneself

At the end of this section, you will be able to:

‹ Establish two goals to develop oneself in a new job
‹ Explain how to implement at least one characteristic for a team leader as applied to one's job

Self-development benefits you as well as your employer and your patients. Each time you gain new knowledge, whether from reading or a formal class, your patients will benefit by receiving the latest information. Because this increases the quality of care, your institution benefits, too. Therefore, it is imperative that nursing professionals commit to long-term growth and development (Watson, 2005).

Lifelong Learning

Lifelong learning simply means to continue adding skills and knowledge about the profession as it continues to evolve. Students learn how to do basic nursing in their undergraduate program, but it is imperative to continue to evolve as a professional nurse. Florence Nightingale recognized this when she stated her reason for writing *Notes on Nursing* (1859/1969): "I do not pretend to teach her [*sic*] how, I ask her to teach herself, and for this purpose I venture to give her some hints" (p. 4). Continued learning is up to each person.

KEY TERM

lifelong learning: Adding skills and knowledge about the profession as it continues to evolve

The innovator characteristics described previously are developed through lifelong learning. Generally, one learns how to learn in school. The clinical and theory skills gained in college should be applied upon entering the nursing practice world. Just as you are learning to apply theory to patient situations throughout your nursing education, nurses must continue to do the same throughout their nursing careers. MacIntosh (2003) found in her research that as new graduates developed a "reputation for professional expertise" (p. 735), an important stage was pursuing learning and growth.

There are formal and informal ways of gaining knowledge and growing professionally throughout one's career. Explore whether your facility offers partial payment for this learning. Many facilities provide partial tuition reimbursement for graduate classes or continuing education credits. Many state boards of nursing require continuing education credits for registered nurse (RN) license maintenance; hourly classes, online modules, or daylong conferences provide this continuing education.

Formal means of learning are accomplished by enrolling in a higher degree program, such as a master's or doctoral program of study. There are four Advanced Practice Registered Nurse (APRN) certifications: certified registered nurse anesthetist, certified nurse–midwife, clinical nurse specialist, and certified nurse practitioner (APRN Joint Dialogue Group Report, 2008). APRNs then focus on at least one of six populations: family/individual across the life span, adult-gerontology, pediatrics, neonatal, women's health/gender-related, or psychiatric-mental health (APRN Joint Dialogue Group Report, 2008). Education for APRNs is available in master's, doctorate, and postgraduate certificate programs of study. Options for a master's degree include a focus in areas beyond clinical practice, such as education, leadership, or informatics, or the Clinical Nurse Leader (CNL) role. The CNL is "a leader in the healthcare delivery system in all settings in which healthcare is delivered. CNL practice will vary across settings" (American Association of Colleges of Nursing [AACN], 2013, p. 4). In general, nursing doctoral programs are of two types: Doctor of Philosophy (PhD) and Doctor of Nursing Practice (DNP). PhD programs focus on generating theory and research to build the body of nursing knowledge. DNP programs focus on creating expert clinicians who are able to apply research to clinical practice. In the future, the DNP degree may be necessary to become certified as an APRN. In the past, admission to doctoral programs required some practice experience in a specific clinical specialty; however, because of the need for educators and researchers in nursing, more doctoral programs admit new baccalaureate graduates directly into their programs (AACN, 2005). Explore possible graduate programs that fit your learning style (i.e., online programs or in-person classes), your future goals, and the potential job market in your area. Ultimately, choose the program that fits you best.

KEY TERMS

developing oneself: Engaging in activities that promote long-term professional growth and development

mentor: One who assists with professional growth

Attending structured learning programs is another formal way of *developing oneself* as a professional. Conferences are excellent opportunities for learning new practices. These have the added advantage of renewing one's spirit and enthusiasm for nursing. They also provide opportunities for networking that improve self-growth. Participating in practice updates or classes offered by your institution is vital. Often these are mandatory.

Informal methods for growth include reading journals or new nursing books, reviewing current literature (i.e., the Cochrane Database or Joanna Briggs Institute), participating in nursing journal clubs, or talking with peers and advanced practice nurses about innovations in practice. Professional organizations offer another excellent method to promote lifelong learning. Many times, speakers provide reports about current research at meetings. Specialty organizations include a variety of members, many with vast experiences in that specialty. Asking questions of these experts provides the novice nurse with increased learning. It is also possible to find in such organizations a *mentor* who will assist with your professional growth. A preceptor is an experienced nurse who is familiar with unit practices and who acts as a guide throughout the orientation process.

The timing of lifelong learning is a factor that enters into one's personal and professional lives. One must look for opportunities as they happen, even though the timing is not always right. For example, if you have an opportunity to attend a national conference in your specialty area but you think you cannot afford the time or money to go, think about the professional benefits if you attended. Look for resources to foster attendance, such as institutional funds, community agency scholarships, or grants. Discuss it with your supervisor and your mentor. Many times options open up to enable conference attendance.

It is important not to get into a rut with your work because this can stifle your lifelong learning. "In seeking and responding to stimulation, nurses actively look for and engage in activities to prod their development" (MacIntosh, 2003, p. 735). Discovering ways for professional stimulation, such as connecting with others in a similar practice at a national or regional conference, tends to bolster current practice.

CRITICAL THINKING EXERCISE 17-2

Consider a specialty organization that you might consider joining. Find the organization's home page on the Web and explore opportunities for networking.

Developing on the Job

It is a good idea to uncover the ways to move up the ranks in any new job. Maybe it is becoming a charge nurse or volunteering for a unit or institutional committee. Perhaps the institution has a process for promotion in a rank, such as a career *ladder program*. Try to uncover institutional promotional methods before starting a new job. Ask the human resources representative or your supervisor to go over these steps so that you know what they are before taking the job. For example, if your institution has a ladder-type promotion, ask what criteria are needed to move up the ladder. Often peer reviews factor into annual performance reviews, so cultivate peer relationships and get feedback as a routine part of your practice.

Orientation

Take full advantage of the orientation program in any new job and learn from all the classes offered. During orientation, seek out possible mentors. Frequently, these knowledgeable nurses do presentations during orientation sessions or act as *preceptors* during clinical orientation. A mentor is a seasoned nurse who acts as a competent *role model* and acts to support, guide, teach, and encourage (Mijares & Bond, 2013) the novice nurse. During this time of newness on your unit, be sure to observe other nurses and ask them questions about how they do certain procedures or use various resources.

Frequently, resource time is offered to new employees as a part of the orientation process. Use this time to look up resources at your new hospital, such as manuals, toolkits, the committee structure (i.e., unit, specialty divisions, or hospitalwide), opportunities to volunteer for committees, or other unit activities. Inquire about the research process and how evidence-based changes are implemented on the unit. Ask whether there are journal clubs or similar venues where practice updates are discussed. Many times facilities have interest groups whose purpose is to discuss specific practices.

Schedule a time during orientation to meet with nurses in advanced roles (such as clinical nurse specialists, nurse practitioners, or nurse researchers) who may be resources for your unit. Get to know these nurses because they can provide excellent resources and updates for your unit. Inquire whether nursing and/or interdisciplinary rounds or other learning opportunities are provided. If you have a professional development staff educator assigned to your unit, determine his or her role in EBP updates. Talk with your nurse manager or supervisor about how he or she sees EBP and how you will receive updates for your practice. Try to understand the level of support from senior leadership because operational support is important for maintaining an innovative environment (Nelson-Brantley & Ford, 2017).

Locate sources for maintaining practice updates. During your orientation, build in time to visit the hospital library or website for the latest practice updates. Frequently, practice or education committees discuss a current research article that is germane to that specialty. Ask your preceptor about such committees or councils and arrange to sit in on one of their meetings to observe how they field questions about practice changes. Try to learn about the process of how changes occur in your facility, such as the route that practice changes take for approval. One example of understanding EBP change is attending a specialty practice committee as a new employee and being impressed by the excellent debate about updating a practice policy. When the process for change is better understood, it is easier to prepare for new updates because you know where change information stems from.

Learning from role models is a good way to learn, provided it is positive role modeling. Role modeling can be informally observed by any nurses on the unit, or it may be formalized by having a preceptor or by asking someone to act as a mentor. Any or all of these role models are helpful to enhance *professionalism* for novice nurses. Ask positive role models how they use current evidence in their practice. However, be forewarned that the expert nurse might not be able to provide specifics because that person weaves change so inherently into practice that it is difficult for this nurse to share what the novice needs to know (Benner, 1984).

On the down side, new graduates may observe practices that are not desirable or even safe. A word of caution here: As the new person on the unit, you need to be careful about questioning those practices or your self-development could be stunted. You need to alert someone, especially if what you observe is unsafe, because there may be people who remain quite behind in their adoption of new practices. An example of this was when a new employee learned how to use correct body mechanics when moving patients. When she was first on the unit and assisted staff members with moving a patient from a bed to a cart, she commented that the others were not using correct body mechanics, as she had learned. An experienced nurse negated her comments, noting that this was the fastest way to move patients and the way it was always done. The new employee was puzzled by this comment because she understood the statistics behind back injuries, so she discussed this with her nurse educator. As a result, all staff members on the unit needed to relearn proper body mechanics to prevent injuries, thereby enhancing clinical practice for all, not just the new graduate. Talking to a preceptor or another trusted peer can offer insight into these observations. Be careful not to be overly critical of unit practice because there may be reasons behind the actions that are not readily apparent. As a new person on the unit, you need to gain some trust among your peers, and this takes time. Becoming aware of discrepancies between expectations and what actually occurs on the unit is a stage of becoming a professional and feeling comfortable with one's own practice (MacIntosh, 2003). Eventually, new nurses can work to change outdated practices through the proper channels.

After a short time in the orientation process, new employees begin to realize the vast amount that they do not know about their specific practice area. This is the time to read literature in this specialty practice area. Sometimes reviewing nursing texts and past notes is sufficient. Now that specific practices are seen on a daily basis in a new job, theory means more because it is applied. Explore current research about new practices. Glean all that you can as soon as you can to foster self-development in your new specialty area. Having a rationale for making a practice change is helpful both to convince yourself that the change can be effective and to convince others.

As their formal orientation is completed, new employees frequently experience a time of uncertainty. New nurses might question whether this is the right unit or specialty area. They long for their days of classes when they had more guidance as a student, and they struggle with learning the vast amount of information about quality patient care. Moving from a novice to a competent nurse can be frustrating, such as learning how to organize one's shift with the many tasks, delegating to unlicensed personnel, and managing patient crises. It is so easy to leave work and want to forget about it. Yet this is the time when a true innovator will set goals and strive toward enhanced professionalism. Learn all that you can about your new practice and facility. Take advantage of all learning opportunities. Push your comfort zone so that as you feel more confident about one type of patient care diagnosis, you can seek out new opportunities for learning about other nursing interventions. Perhaps this is the time to volunteer for a unit committee so that you can learn more about the inner workings of creating and changing policy or to offer to present a topic for a staff development class. Remind yourself that this is part of developing as a professional.

Performance Appraisals and Reviews

In any job, there is some type of appraisal and review. Usually it is tied to salary or other promotional mechanisms, so it is important to pay attention to the details applicable for your agency. This process is designed to provide an opportunity to reflect on your strengths, areas for improvement, what you have done since the last review, and what you plan to accomplish within the next time period. Normally, setting goals is a part of this review process. However, acting in a goal-centered manner provides a framework for practice as well. Goals might be individual, such as seeking a promotion, or getting more active in workgroups. Other goals might include activities to enhance professionalism,

KEY TERMS

personal development file: A compilation of career accomplishments

career development: Experience and education that contribute to one's professional growth

interprofessional collaboration: Engaging with other professionals to provide evidence-based care

such as active work in a nursing organization. Whether you set goals only once per year during your annual performance review with your supervisor or you have daily goals, they serve to offer reflection for your practice and foster increased awareness. All of nursing should be goal oriented, such as how goals are always present in any nurse–patient interaction. Goals should incorporate EBP, such as monthly exploring the use of a new EBP guideline or technique for your practice.

Frequently, input from peers or other supervisors is requested as a part of a performance review. This is the time to ask peers who have provided helpful feedback for your development, such as preceptors or mentors. It is also helpful to organize your input, enabling your supervisor to get a full picture of your accomplishments. Watson (2005) suggested a *personal development file* or folder as a means to compile what you accomplish in your career because those "little things . . . [merge] into a substantial amount of additional *career development* activity" (p. 992; emphasis added). Make notes or include documents to remind you to include those items as a part of your review process. If you expended a special effort to teach a nursing student on your unit, make a note about it at the time to include in this self-appraisal. If you assisted with data collection for a research project, try to obtain a study summary to include for your records. Keep an accurate file of your continuing education documents. Organized personal record keeping is important and provides objective data for the performance review.

Developing Team Leadership Skills

The impact of team effectiveness for one's unit is significant (Timmermans, Van Linge, Van Petegem, Van Rompaey, & Denekens, 2012). *Interprofessional collaboration* is engaging with other professionals to provide evidence-based care. It is essential for quality patient care (Institute of Medicine, 2010) and requires a relationship between team learning and innovations in nursing (Timmermans et al., 2012). To implement EBP on a unit, all members need to be involved and work together to create the change. A small number of unit leaders can positively influence other unit staff members to enhance patient care with new evidence for practice change. Although nurses are likely involved in making decisions, the unit staff is directed to implement the changes. This is where awareness about one's unit is important. Use informal and formal leaders. Strategically organize common groups within the unit, such as those who work similar schedules. An example of this is "communication groups" within the unit where a small number of staff members are assigned to each group, a leader is assigned who acts as the communicator to the other members in that group, and the leader provides information, communicates about changes, and/or clarifies questions.

Another strategy is a change champion (Nelson-Brantley & Ford, 2017). At the unit level, change champions are staff members who continually promote new ideas for change and act as role models. Characteristics of successful change champions are the following: (1) expert clinician, (2) informal leader who is respected among peers, (3) positive working relationship with other interdisciplinary team members, (4) passionate about the topic of practice, and (5) commitment to improving the quality of patient care (Titler, 2006). These characteristics are important for any innovator as well. Innovators might be known as change champions or by any other title used by the institution to implement practice changes.

Developing *team leadership skills* occurs over time. This is also where innovator characteristics, a sense of inquiry, flexibility to change, awareness of self and of the unit, and good communication skills are needed. As you develop, your team leadership skills will emerge.

> **KEY TERMS**
>
> **team leadership skills:** Behaviors that collaboratively engage others while working toward a goal
>
> **behavioral inventory for professionalism:** A measure of education and training, skill, ethics, professional organization, and service

17.3 Professionalism

At the end of this section, you will be able to:

‹ Outline a plan to develop your professionalism as a nurse

Models of Professionalism

Professionalism is how one deports oneself within the nursing profession. Miller, Adams, and Beck (1993) developed a *behavioral inventory for professionalism* in nursing to measure the following: (1) education and training, including continuing education; (2) skill based on theoretical knowledge; (3) a code of ethics; (4) a professional organization; and (5) service. For example, their inventory

FYI

Perhaps the most important aspect of being a professional is to use what was learned in one's basic nursing program, especially the application of theory to clinical situations. Continuing to apply learning contributes to ongoing EBP as one uses newer research and theory as a part of one's practice.

measures continuing education attendance, the number of journals read, nursing books recently purchased, professional organization memberships, whether nursing theories are applied in one's practice, and participation in organization and community service. These authors surveyed more than 500 nurses and found that 92.3% reported reading from 1 to 10 nursing articles per month; however, only 15.9% belonged to a professional organization.

The *wheel of professionalism in nursing* (**Figure 17-1**) depicts components to enhance professionalism (Miller, 1984). The behaviors included in the wheel indicate degrees of professionalism; these behaviors might also be used as measures in working up a clinical ladder in one's facility. One example is that active participation in a specialty organization could assist with promotions in some institutions where such professional behaviors are a part of that institution's philosophy. Other examples include routinely reading articles related to one's practice to enhance theory application for practice, pursuing continuing education regularly for competence, and making practice changes for one's own practice to enhance professional autonomy.

Perhaps the most important aspect of being a professional is to use what was learned in one's basic nursing program, especially the application of theory to clinical situations. One can innovate; however, one is still obligated to use a theory base for safe patient care. Continuing to apply learning contributes to ongoing EBP as one uses newer research and theory as a part of one's practice.

A difficult component of professionalism for those new to the practice world involves *information overload*. Rogers (2003) defined this as "the state of an individual or system in which excessive communication inputs cannot be processed and utilized, leading to breakdown" (pp. 368–369). With added technology, healthcare professionals must manage an array of communication media and evidence for updated practice arriving at breakneck speed. Although it is complex enough for the new nurse to become proficient with patient care and learn to manage multiple patients, the additional expectations for keeping up with multiple modes of communication add increased stress. Learning how to manage technology is vital. Using all of the innovator characteristics can assist a new nurse to become an effective member of the team and provide quality patient care. Incorporating EBP will become a routine part of professional practice.

KEY TERMS

wheel of professionalism in nursing: A model depicting behaviors of the professional nurse

information overload: State of an individual in which excessive communication cannot be processed or used

A Final Word About Developing Oneself as an Innovator

Recognizing a possible gap between experiences in education programs and the actual workplace means that new graduates must seek resources to bridge

| FIGURE 17-1 | Wheel of Professionalism in Nursing |

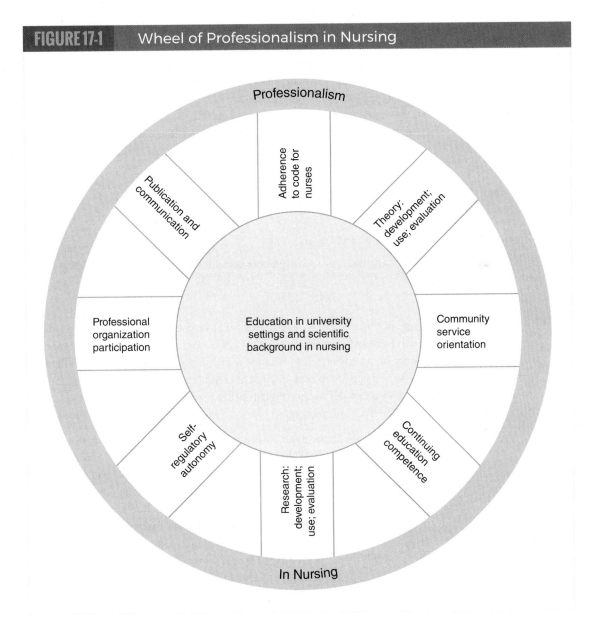

this gap. Welding (2011) noted that nurse residency programs are a formal means to bridge this gap, aiming to promote success and productivity for new graduates. Even without a residency program, being proactive eases this transition into practice for new graduates and puts them on the road to becoming innovators and leaders in practice. When nurses develop a strong sense of inquiry, are flexible toward change, become aware of self and of the unit, and implement good communication skills, they can be innovators, thus enhancing quality patient care for the facility. It is imperative that innovators continue to learn and assimilate ongoing changes about new evidence into their practice. Normally, practice is incorporated into education programs and initiatives by "what practitioners *do* (and choose not to do) but also what they *are* and the knowledge and thought that underpin their actions" (Coles, 2002, p. 8). In today's ever-changing world, knowledge is not always adequate; one must incorporate knowledge gained into one's practice.

17.4 Keeping It Ethical

At the end of this section, you will be able to:

‹ List three behaviors important to maintaining professional integrity over the course of your career

It may not be evident to you at this point in your career, but nursing professionals have an obligation to develop self-awareness. In your nursing program, you are being socialized to become a lifelong learner. Developing yourself is necessary if you are to remain current about practice issues and new technologies. A sense of self-awareness can bring a level of maturity that is necessary for ethical decision making.

Professional nurses need to promote themselves and the profession by making others aware of their accomplishments. There are many ways to achieve this. For example, when you earn a certification, be certain that your accomplishment is recognized by your organization. Make yourself available to promote nursing as a career through interactions with youth. Writing an editorial on a health topic that interests you or that you are passionate about is another way to make nursing more visible. The *Code of Ethics for Nurses with Interpretive Statements* (American Nurses Association

FYI

Nurses have a duty to give back to the profession. All nurses have a responsibility to assist novice nurses. EBP is more likely to thrive in environments where nurses feel supported and are provided with resources necessary to develop both personally and professionally.

CRITICAL THINKING EXERCISE 17-3

What is your professional ethical duty, according to the *Code of Ethics for Nurses* (ANA, 2001), when you see any unsafe practice or see another nurse "fudging" patient assessment data?

[ANA], 2015) holds nurses accountable for the development of the profession. For instance, if a student cheated on his or her work during nursing school, such "unprofessional behaviors developed in school . . . adversely . . . [affect] the nurse's ability to properly care for patients" once employed as an RN (Rhodes, Schutt, Langham, & Bilotta, 2003, p. 28).

At this point in your development, you have begun to build a personal development file. This will be especially important to you as you seek your first position as an RN and apply to graduate school. It is desirable to include a representative picture of your abilities. However, it would be unethical for you to overstate your capabilities. Records should never be falsified and must accurately reflect your work history.

As a nurse, you must take advantage of both formal and informal opportunities for professional growth. For example, your employer might provide educational benefits. Investigate conferences that will help to establish you as an expert in your field. Willingly accept responsibility for reporting back to your colleagues what you have learned.

Nurses have a duty to give back to the profession. All nurses have a responsibility to assist novice nurses to establish their practices. Recall the characteristics of a preceptor who was particularly helpful to you. Emulate this behavior with students you encounter. As your career progresses, make it a personal goal to always be mentoring at least one person. EBP is more likely to thrive in environments where nurses feel supported and are provided with the resources necessary to develop both personally and professionally.

TEST YOUR KNOWLEDGE 17-3

1. Which of the following are ethical behaviors? (Select all that apply.)
   a. Reading journal articles for a club meeting
   b. Skipping the afternoon conference sessions to go shopping
   c. Providing an accurate and meticulous resume
   d. Sharing information at a staff meeting about a new innovation that you heard about at a conference
   e. Ignoring a student assigned to your unit who has a question about a procedure
   f. Reporting a nurse who recorded vital signs when in fact they were not measured

How did you do? 1. a, c, d, f

Apply What You Have Learned

Do you have what it takes to be an innovator? Complete these assessments to learn more about your leadership styles.

1. The Emotional Quotient Assessment at http://www.ihhp.com/free-eq-quiz/
2. The New Enneagram Test at http://9types.com/rheti/index.php

RAPID REVIEW

» The four characteristics of an innovator are a sense of inquiry, flexibility to change, awareness of self and the unit, and good communication skills.

» A sense of inquiry is one's curiosity and can lead to seeking knowledge that improves patient care. This characteristic is analogous to being a critical thinker.

» Flexibility is the willingness to try something new, and it requires an openness to failure.

» Self-awareness is knowing yourself, and it helps you understand how you make decisions about practice. Awareness about the unit facilitates change because of understanding the social system.

» Communication skills are vital to leading and being a change agent.

» Lifelong learning takes place in formal and informal ways, both of which can contribute to EBP. Formal ways of learning include enrolling in graduate programs, attending conferences, and participating in in-services. Informal learning can involve reading literature, attending journal clubs, networking at meetings, and mentoring.

» Orientation, ladder programs, and personal development files are ways to develop oneself on the job.

» Setting goals and peer review are components of performance appraisals and employment reviews.

» EBP practice changes are facilitated when a team approach is used.

» The wheel of professionalism in nursing is a model that lists professional behaviors.

» Nurses are obligated to develop themselves as lifelong learners to thrive both personally and professionally.

REFERENCES

American Association of Colleges of Nursing. (2013). *Competencies and curricular expectations of the clinical nurse leader*ᴿᴹ *education and practice.* Retrieved from http://www.aacn.nche.edu/cnl/CNL-Competencies-October-2013.pdf

American Association of Colleges of Nursing Task Force on Future Faculty. (2005). Faculty shortages in baccalaureate and graduate nursing programs: Scope of the problem and strategies for expanding the supply. Retrieved from http://www.aacn.nche.edu/publications/whitepapers/facultyshortages.htm

American Nurses Association. (2015). *The code of ethics for nurses with interpretative statements.* Silver Springs, MD: Author.

APRN Joint Dialogue Group Report. (2008). *Consensus model for APRN regulation: Licensure, accreditation, certification and education.* Retrieved from http://www.aacn.nche.edu/education-resources/APRNReport.pdf

Baker, J. D. (2013). Journal club as a resource for practice. *AORN Journal, 98*(2), 102–106. doi:http://dx.doi.org/10.1016/j.aorn.2013.06.001

Benner, P. (1984). *From novice to expert: Excellence and power in clinical nursing practice.* Menlo Park, CA: Addison-Wesley.

Bjorkstrom, M. E., Athlin, E. E., & Johansson, I. S. (2008). Nurses' development of professional self—from being a nursing student in a baccalaureate programme to an experienced nurse. *Journal of Clinical Nursing, 17,* 1380–1391. doi:10.1111/j.1365-2702.2007.02014.x

Bradley, E. H., Webster, T. R., Baker, D., Schlesinger, M., Inouye, S. K., Barth, M. C., . . . Koren, M. J. (2004, July). Translating research into practice: Speeding adoption of innovative health care programs. *Commonwealth Fund,* 1–12. Retrieved from http://www.cmwf.org/programs/elders/bradley_translating_research_724.pdf

Chubinski, S. (1996). Creative critical-thinking strategies. *Nurse Educator, 21*(6), 23–27.

Coles, A. (2002). Developing professional judgment. *Journal of Continuing Education in the Health Professions, 22,* 3–10.

Gluyas, H., & Harris, S. J. (2016). Understanding situation awareness and its importance in patient safety. *Nursing Standard, 30*(34), 50–58.

Institute of Medicine. (2010). *The future of nursing: Leading change, advancing health* (Report Brief). Retrieved from https://www.aana.com/advocacy/federalgovernmentaffairs/Documents/Future%20of%20Nursing%202010%20Report%20Brief.pdf

MacIntosh, J. (2003). Reworking professional nursing identity. *Western Journal of Nursing Research, 25,* 725–741.

Marquis, B. L., & Huston, C. J. (2006). *Leadership roles and management functions in nursing: Theory and application* (5th ed.). Philadelphia, PA: Lippincott Williams & Wilkins.

Mijares, L., & Bond, M. L. (2013). Mentoring: A concept analysis. *Journal of Theory Construction and Testing, 17*(1), 23–28.

Miller, B. K. (1984). *Professionalism in nursing in nurse educators in baccalaureate and associate degree programs in Texas* (Doctoral dissertation). *Dissertation Abstracts International, 46,* 1118B.

Miller, B. K., Adams, D., & Beck, L. (1993). A behavioral inventory for professionalism in nursing. *Journal of Professional Nursing, 9*, 290–295.

Nelson-Brantley, H. V., & Ford, D. J. (2017). Leading change: A concept analysis. *Journal of Advanced Nursing, 73*, 834–846.

Nightingale, F. (1969). *Notes on nursing: What it is, and what it is not.* New York, NY: Dover. (Original work published 1859).

Paul, R. (1990). *Critical thinking: What every person needs to survive in a rapidly changing world.* Rohnert Park, CA: Center for Critical Thinking and Moral Critique.

Rhodes, M. K., Schutt, M. S., Langham, G. W., & Bilotta, D. E. (2003). The journey to nursing professionalism: A learner-centered approach. *Nursing Education Perspectives, 33*(1), 27–29.

Rogers, E. M. (2003). *Diffusion of innovations* (5th ed.). New York, NY: Free Press.

Scanlon, K. A., & Woolforde, L. (2016). Igniting change through an empowered frontline: A unique improvement approach centered on staff engagement, empowerment, and professional development. *Nurse Leader, 14*(1), 38–46.

Shaver, J. L. F. (2001). Looking to the future of academic administrative leadership. In N. L. Chaska (Ed.), *The nursing profession: Tomorrow and beyond* (pp. 931–943). Thousand Oaks, CA: Sage.

Timmermans, O., Van Linge, R., Van Petegem, P., Van Rompaey, B., & Denekens, J. (2012). Team learning and innovation in nursing, a review of the literature. *Nurse Education Today, 32*, 65–70. doi:10.1016/j.nedt.2011.07.006

Titler, M. (2001). Research utilization and evidence based practice. In N. L. Chaska (Ed.), *The nursing profession: Tomorrow and beyond* (pp. 423–437). Thousand Oaks, CA: Sage.

Titler, M. (2006). Developing an evidence-based practice. In G. LoBiondo-Wood & J. Haber (Eds.), *Nursing research: Methods and critical appraisal for evidence-based practice* (pp. 439–481). St. Louis, MO: Mosby.

Watson, R. (2005). Self-development and self-appraisal. In L. Caputi & L. Engelmann (Eds.), *Teaching nursing: The art and science* (Vol. 2.) Glen Ellyn, IL: College of DuPage Press.

Welding, N. M. (2011). Creating a nursing residency: Decrease turnover and increase clinical competence. *MEDSURG Nursing, 20*(1), 37–40.

Confirmation

Evaluating outcomes and networking with others substantiate adoption or rejection of innovations.

CHAPTER OBJECTIVES

At the end of this chapter, you will be able to:

- Define outcome
- Discuss ways outcomes can be classified
- Discuss factors that should be considered when selecting outcomes
- Discuss how data are used to evaluate outcomes
- List three dilemmas that can arise when nurses are involved in testing protocols

KEY TERMS

benchmarking
care-related outcomes
continuous quality improvement
Forces of Magnetism
indicators
intermediate outcomes

long-term outcomes
mandated reporting
nursing outcomes
nursing-sensitive outcomes
organizational priorities
outcome

outcomes research
patient populations
patient-related outcomes
performance-related outcomes
short-term outcomes
team membership

CHAPTER 18

Evaluating Outcomes of Innovations

Kathleen A. Rich

18.1 What Is an Outcome?

At the end of this section, you will be able to:

< Define outcome
< Discuss ways outcomes can be classified

Implementing an innovation, policy, or procedure does not necessarily guarantee that it will become the standard of care. Ongoing evaluation of an innovation through outcome measurements is necessary to ensure successful incorporation into clinical practice. According to Webster's, an *outcome* is defined as a consequence or visible result. *Nursing outcomes* measure states, behaviors, or perceptions of individuals, families, or communities (Moorehead, Johnson, Maas, & Swanson, 2013). *Outcomes research* examines the end results of health services on individuals and is intended to provide scientific evidence relating to decisions made by all who participate in health care. It also takes into account the patient's preferences and values (Krumholz, 2009). In nursing research, the outcome is frequently known as the dependent variable (Polit & Beck, 2014).

Outcomes may be classified by several different methods. One way outcomes can be classified is by focusing on who is being measured. Nurses may measure outcomes for individuals, groups, or organizations.

KEY TERMS

outcome:
Consequence or
visible result

nursing outcomes:
Measures of
states, behaviors,
or perceptions of
individuals, families,
or communities
as they relate to
nursing and health

outcomes research:
Studies about the
effects of care and
treatments on
individuals and
populations

**care-related
outcomes:** A
category of
outcomes that
measures the
effect of nursing
interventions

**patient-related
outcomes:** A type of
outcome related to
patient behaviors or
actions

**performance-
related outcomes:**
A type of outcome
related to how
nurses perform
their job

**short-term
outcomes:** Results
achieved in a brief
period of time

**intermediate
outcomes:** Changes
that occur after
an innovation is
introduced

Another way that outcomes can be grouped is by type: *care-related*, *patient-related*, and *performance-related outcomes* (Kleinpell, 2009). An example of a care-related outcome is the rate of pressure ulcer formation in patients on bed rest for more than 24 hours. Patient knowledge related to fluid restriction is an example of a patient-related outcome. Nursing staff adherence to best practice guidelines when providing discharge education to a heart failure patient is an example of a performance-related outcome.

Time is another way of classifying outcomes. *Short-term outcomes* are results achieved in a relatively brief period of time that usually involve a change in condition, such as absence of postoperative pain, or an increase in knowledge or skills, such as a patient's ability to draw up insulin. Another category of outcome classified by time is *intermediate outcomes*. They exist when changes occur after an innovation is introduced. Lifestyle modifications, such as weight loss and smoking cessation after enrolling in a wellness program, can be examples of intermediate outcomes. *Long-term outcomes* are primary changes in patients' behaviors or status, such as compliance with statin therapy resulting in a lower cholesterol level (Mauskop & Borden, 2011).

Nursing administrators are responsible for reporting *nursing-sensitive outcomes* at their institutions to demonstrate effectiveness of nursing care. Outcomes of nursing care should be measurable. These measurements can assist in determining responsibility in patient care (Micik et al., 2013). One nursing-sensitive outcome considered a National Patient Safety Goal mandated by the Joint Commission is to reduce the risk of healthcare-associated infections with central line bloodstream infections (Joint Commission, 2017b). The Joint Commission requires healthcare organizations to have education and evidence-based policies/protocols relative to central lines. Hospitals are also required to provide their central line infection rate to key participants. Two desirable outcomes that result from these practices are an improved communication among all involved healthcare providers regarding central lines and an associated reduction in hospital-acquired central line bloodstream infections.

Outcome-based measurements are a means used to establish evidence-based practice (EBP) and to evaluate the care delivered. In healthcare organizations, many activities are outcome driven. The rising costs of health care, increasingly stringent accreditation standards, and public reporting are several reasons why outcomes are closely scrutinized and are integral to ensuring the successful implementation of an innovation. In health care, outcomes are typically quantitative, not qualitative. Legislated in 2010, the Patient Protection and Affordable Care Act has improvement in healthcare quality among its goals. Within this legislation is a mandate regarding the development of a shared-savings program promoting accountability to a patient population (Patient Protection and Affordable Care Act, 2010). Termed Accountable Care Organizations (ACOs),

CRITICAL THINKING EXERCISE 18-1

Consider your last clinical experience. Are you aware of any outcomes that are being monitored on the unit or in the facility? If so, what are they and how would you classify them?

TEST YOUR KNOWLEDGE 18-1

Match the type of outcome with the indicator. (Select all that apply.)

1. Performance-related outcome
2. Patient-related outcome
3. Care-related outcome
4. Long-term outcome
5. Short-term outcome

a. Patient will not hemorrhage after delivery
b. Patient will maintain weight loss over 2 years
c. Patient will be afebrile after surgery
d. The rate of hospital-acquired infections
e. Patient satisfaction will be 90% or greater

How did you do? 1. e; 2. a, b, c; 3. d; 4. b; 5. a, c

the intent is to develop partnerships between hospitals and physicians to provide efficient quality care. The Centers for Medicare and Medicaid Services (CMS) reimburses ACOs based on patient outcomes. There are currently 33 CMS quality outcome measures that ACOs are held accountable to that affect reimbursement (CMS, 2015).

Evaluating outcomes is not static, but rather an ongoing process. Outcomes must be well defined for the evaluation to be meaningful. The effectiveness of any innovation is measured by the outcomes that result. These results are compared to baseline data in order to draw conclusions about the effectiveness of the innovation. The process continues as the innovation becomes standard practice.

KEY TERMS

long-term outcomes: Primary changes in patient behaviors or status over time

nursing-sensitive outcomes: Results that demonstrate the effectiveness of nursing care

18.2 Choosing Outcomes

At the end of this section, you will be able to:

‹ Discuss factors that should be considered when selecting outcomes

Choosing outcomes that appropriately fit an innovation is vital. This allows for an accurate evaluation of practice changes. During the selection process, outcomes should be considered for their significance and scope. Considerations may include disease-specific outcomes, response to interventions, quality of life, and fiscal impact

FYI

Outcome-based measurements are a means used to establish EBP and to evaluate the care delivered. The effectiveness of any innovation is measured by the outcomes that result.

TABLE 18-1	Outcomes and Indicators
Outcome	**Indicator**
Dyspnea reduction	Dyspnea rating scale
Decrease in postoperative pain	Pain numeric rating scale
Absence of skin ulcers	Pressure sore staging
Reduction in patient falls	Falls risk assessment tool
Knowledge: blood pressure medication	Blood pressure

(Burns & Grove, 2015). Outcomes should be measured using specific quantitative criteria, sometimes referred to as *indicators*. For example, if postoperative pain control is of interest, then pain should be quantified through a recognized indicator such as the numeric rating scale. If an outcome such as quality of life is the focus, then using an established instrument, such as the SF-36, which is a validated multipurpose health survey tool, is preferred (Contopoulos-Loannidis, Karvouni, Kouri, & Ioannidis, 2009). Instruments that have been tested for reliability and validity improve credibility of the evaluation process. **Table 18-1** lists examples of outcomes and associated indicators.

When determining outcomes to be measured, there are four major factors to consider: *patient populations*, *team membership*, *organizational priorities*, and *mandated reporting*. It is best when the selected outcomes address multiple factors. Journals, books, and websites are available to assist. **Table 18-2** lists selected organizations with their associated websites that contain health outcome information.

Patient Population

It is necessary to select outcomes that reflect the patient population served by the healthcare facility. Use of a generic patient outcome is a good strategy to measure outcomes when populations are diverse. For example, measuring symptom control or increased knowledge may apply to many disease conditions (Burns & Grove, 2015). The Nursing Outcomes Classification (NOC), developed at the University of Iowa College of Nursing, is a standardized list of generic patient outcome classifications that can be used to evaluate the efficacy of nursing interventions (Moorehead et al., 2013). Currently, 490 outcomes in the NOC system are associated with the North American Nursing Diagnosis Association and the nursing interventions classification. Each outcome is coded

TABLE 18-2	Selected Health Outcome Information Websites

Organization	Website
AcademyHealth	http://www.academyhealth.org
Agency for Healthcare Research and Quality	http://www.ahrq.gov/clinic/outcomix.htm
Centers for Medicare and Medicaid Services	http://www.cms.gov/Medicare/Medicare-Fee-for-Service-Payment/sharedsavingsprogram/Quality_Measures_Standards.html
Harvard College Library Health Data Resources	http://guides.library.harvard.edu/content.php?pid=176649&sid=1487349
Institute for Healthcare Improvement	http://www.ihi.org
The Joint Commission	http://www.jointcommission.org
National Cancer Institute	https://healthcaredelivery.cancer.gov/about/orb/
National Committee for Quality Assurance	http://www.ncqa.org/
Patient-Centered Outcomes Research Institute	http://www.pcori.org/research-results/patient-centered-outcomes-research
University of Iowa College of Nursing	http://www.nursing.uiowa.edu/cncce/nursing-outcomes-classification-overview

and consists of several components: a definition, a list of numeric indicators from which the nurse selects to evaluate the patient's status, a target outcome rating, and a 5-point Likert-type scale for measuring the status. "Knowledge: Healthy Diet" is an example of an NOC patient outcome and is defined as the extent of understanding conveyed about the recommended diet. The outcome may be applied to a diverse group of patients in a wide spectrum of healthcare settings. Included in this outcome are indicators that the nurse may choose for evaluation purposes, such as description of diet and description of potential for food and medication interaction (Moorehead et al., 2013). The Likert-type scale yields data ranging from none (1) to extensive (5) for each indicator.

Team Membership

When selecting an outcome, consideration should be given to the composition of members who form the team responsible for monitoring the outcome (Minnick, 2009). This includes the personnel members and capabilities that would be involved in implementing the innovation and outcome measurements. Utilizing an interdisciplinary approach including nursing, education, ancillary support services, and quality improvement allows for incorporation of different viewpoints and knowledge. It may also result in recommendation of new outcomes that were not previously considered. The creation of interdisciplinary relationships in the formulation and approval of policies and protocols is required to achieve American Nurses Credentialing Center (ANCC) Magnet Recognition (ANCC, 2017).

Advanced practice nurses (APNs) are integral members of interdisciplinary teams. The APN has expert clinical knowledge about rapidly occurring changes in the healthcare environment. APNs are familiar with institutional data and are able to assist with comparison to national benchmarks. APNs can assist with selecting realistic outcomes. An outcome that is realistic has a base definition that is true to life (Minnick, 2009). For example, selecting an outcome such as "improved quality of life in heart failure patients" is vague and has a multitude of meanings dependent upon the individual and the severity of the associated disease condition. People with slight limitation of physical activities might have a different perception of quality of life than do individuals who are unable to carry out physical activities without discomfort or symptoms at rest. Therefore, the vaguely written outcome cannot be realistically evaluated. APNs can assist to narrow the focus, thus making an outcome more measurable.

Staff nurses may be involved at several different levels during outcome selection and subsequent measurements. Nurses are familiar with the *continuous quality improvement* (CQI) process through participation with internal quality improvement measures. Staff nurses are often members of the interdisciplinary team involved in protocol development. They frequently provide insightful suggestions about approaches that can be used in the clinical setting to obtain outcome measurements. Staff nurses can identify patients who meet criteria for inclusion in the protocol. They can also collect data such as reviewing charts for compliance in documentation.

Organizational Priorities

A second consideration is selecting outcomes that address organizational priorities (Burston, Chaboyer, & Gillespie, 2013). Sometimes outcomes can be linked to the mission of the healthcare organization. For example, a faith-based hospital may focus attention on ensuring that all patients receive a spiritual assessment. Organizations may also use outcomes to evaluate specific areas that need improvement. CQI activities are an evaluation of existing practices that

CRITICAL THINKING EXERCISE 18-2

Your nurse manager selects you to represent the unit on a team monitoring patient safety. What outcomes would you suggest the team monitor?

involve delivery of services to the people (Newhouse & Pettit, 2006). The goal of CQI is to improve service. CQI measures can be generic indicators or can be narrowed into disease-specific outcomes.

Mandated Reports

Multiple publicly reported nursing indicators can be used to measure outcomes of EBP protocols. Hospitals and other healthcare agencies are required to gather data about specific disease entities and to report their findings to public agencies. Outcome data, available on State Boards of Health and the CMS websites, are published to make comparisons among healthcare facilities. Organizations use these data to gain a picture of how they compare to similar facilities. This is known as *benchmarking*. Clinical practice guidelines or standards of care recommended by professional organizations can also drive outcome selection.

There is often overlap among the various organizations that mandate reporting. For example, consider health care related to the use of aspirin for patients with cardiac disease. The American College of Cardiology (ACC) and American Heart Association (AHA) have issued guidelines delineating the performance measures for patients experiencing an ST-elevation or non-ST-elevation acute myocardial infarction (AMI) (AHA, 2008). These performance measures require that healthcare providers instruct patients to continue on an aspirin regimen after discharge (AHA, 2008). The Joint Commission requires hospitals to report on eight core measure sets, one of which is AMI (Joint Commission, 2017a). One of the 33 CMS ACO outcomes includes use of aspirin or other antithrombotics in patients with ischemic vascular disease that includes those with a discharge diagnosis of MI (CMS, 2015). Achieving an acceptable score on this outcome requires a multidisciplinary effort by physicians, nurses, and pharmacists.

In addition to reporting mandatory CMS and Joint Commission data, many healthcare facilities are members of not-for-profit organizations to benchmark indicators. For example, hospitals can subscribe to databases maintained by the ACC and the Society of Thoracic Surgeons. The ACC (2014) has eight databases that include acute myocardial infarction treatment, outpatient cardiovascular care, and diabetes and cardiometabolic treatments among others. The Society

KEY TERM

benchmarking: Comparison of organizational outcome data to other organizations or national databases

of Thoracic Surgeons (2013) provides statistics about adult and congenital heart surgery and for thoracic surgery patients. Organizations such as these provide EBP guidelines for various disease entities, allowing subscribers to review the latest information for protocol development and implementation within the facility.

Another such organization is the Institute for Healthcare Improvement (IHI). The IHI is a not-for-profit organization that targets healthcare improvements on a global level (IHI, 2013). IHI promotes the concept known as "bundles" that are defined as a group of disease-specific interventions that together have a larger impact on prevention of a complication or disease (Resar, Griffin, Haraden, & Nolan, 2012). As an example, a reduction in the incidence of ventilator-associated pneumonia (VAP) was proposed through implementation of five interventions grouped together known as the "ventilator bundle." VAP is defined as a nosocomial pneumonia that develops 48 hours or longer after a patient has an artificial airway such as a tracheostomy or endotracheal tube inserted (Centers for Disease Control and Prevention, 2017). VAP is the most serious complication of a three-tier surveillance definition for ventilator-associated events developed by the Centers for Disease Control and Prevention (Magill et al., 2013). The mortality rate for patients diagnosed with VAP ranges from 25% to 40%, and the diagnosis adds an estimated cost of up to $40,000 to a hospital admission (Greene & Sposato, 2009). The ventilator bundle consists of these strategies: keeping the head of the bed elevated at least 30 degrees at all times unless clinically contraindicated, daily sedation vacations with assessments of weaning readiness, peptic ulcer prevention, and deep vein thrombosis prophylaxis (AHRQ, 2011). To evaluate VAP protocol, based on the ventilator bundle, an outcome could be to reduce the incidence of VAP by 75%.

In the Magnet Recognition Program (ANCC, 2013), healthcare organizations are required to provide examples of nurse-sensitive quality indicators as part of the application process or to maintain Magnet Recognition. There are 14 components, known as *Forces of Magnetism*, that exhibit nursing excellence. **Table 18-3** lists these forces. For example, for a healthcare organization to meet Force 7, Quality Improvement, evidence must show that nursing staff members participate in CQI activities and that CQI is perceived to improve care within the facility (ANCC, 2013). In addition, the organization must provide examples of a change in nursing practice that occurred as a result of data originating from fiscal, satisfaction, or clinical outcomes. The following scenario demonstrates how one outcome can be used to address mandates from the Joint Commission, IHI, and the Magnet Recognition Program.

KEY TERM

Forces of Magnetism: Qualities that exhibit nursing excellence

TABLE 18-3	Fourteen Forces of Magnetism
Force 1	Quality of Nursing Leadership
Force 2	Organizational Structure
Force 3	Management Style
Force 4	Personnel Policies and Programs
Force 5	Professional Models of Care
Force 6	Quality of Care
Force 7	Quality Improvement
Force 8	Consultation and Resources
Force 9	Autonomy
Force 10	Community and the Healthcare Organization
Force 11	Nurses as Teachers
Force 12	Image of Nursing
Force 13	Interdisciplinary Relationships
Force 14	Professional Development

Continuing with VAP as an example, suppose the infection prevention nurse in your facility reports that, despite implementing the ventilator bundle, the VAP rate has not decreased in the last two quarters. A multidisciplinary committee consisting of nursing, respiratory therapy, infection prevention, quality improvement, and staff education examines the evidence. The committee determines that regularly scheduled oral hygiene, including teeth brushing, while on the ventilator has been linked with a reduction of plaque and oropharyngeal colonization.

The committee decides to change oral care products currently used in your facility and recommends a change in protocol. The new ventilator oral care protocol is developed and presented to the staff along with a review of related infection control findings related to VAP. The staff are enthusiastic about the change in oral care products and the new protocol. Over the next few months, follow-up reporting will be provided to the nursing staff. The quarterly VAP rate will be compared to the rate prior to the implementation of the new protocol to determine the effectiveness of the practice change.

TEST YOUR KNOWLEDGE 18-2

1. Which of the following are considerations when selecting outcomes? (Select all that apply.)
   a. Organizational mission
   b. Publicly reported benchmarks
   c. Type of patients served at healthcare facility
   d. Expertise of team members
2. Which of the following statements is false?
   a. Journals, books, and websites are available to assist nurses in selecting outcomes.
   b. NOC outcomes could be used in evaluation plans.
   c. Benchmarking is a way to compare facility with national data.
   d. Clinical guidelines are only suggestions and are not evidence based.

How did you do? 1. a, b, c, d; 2. d

18.3 Evaluating the Outcomes

At the end of this section, you will be able to:

< Discuss how data are used to evaluate outcomes

After an outcome has been selected and measured, data are compiled and evaluated to draw conclusions. Demonstrating the effectiveness of an innovation is a challenge, and conclusions must not extend beyond the scope of the data. Evaluation is facilitated when appropriate outcomes and associated indicators are chosen. If the outcome is not clearly defined, then the measurements and subsequent evaluation will be flawed. For example, suppose that you are a member of an interdisciplinary team that has developed a nursing protocol that reduces the amount of time the patient remains on bed rest after a cardiac catheterization procedure from 6 hours to 4 hours. The outcome selected is absence of bleeding from the femoral arterial puncture site. No other indicators are measured. The results obtained after implementing the protocol revealed that there was an increase in bleeding at the femoral arterial site in the 4-hour bed rest patients compared to the 6-hour bed rest patients. Before concluding that a shorter bed rest time leads to an increase in femoral bleeding, a few additional questions need to be considered. First, was

FYI

After an outcome has been selected and measured, data are compiled and evaluated to draw conclusions. Evaluation is facilitated when appropriate outcomes and associated indicators are chosen—conversely, if the outcome is not clearly defined, then the measurements and subsequent evaluation will be flawed.

CRITICAL THINKING EXERCISE 18-3

You are asked to join an interdisciplinary committee formed to examine glucose management in intensive care unit (ICU) patients. You note that the current ICU practice is to administer a sliding scale subcutaneous insulin dose based on the bedside glucose obtained at 6-hour time intervals. A retrospective chart review of 50 ICU patients receiving the sliding scale insulin dosage for 24 hours reveals that glycemic control in ICU patients is not present. Consequently, the committee develops an evidence-based intravenous (IV) insulin protocol based on hourly glucose measurements. Glycemic control in ICU patients is the outcome selected, and you are going to use a blood sugar result of less than 180 mg/dL within 8 hours of instituting the IV protocol as a measurement indicator. Staff nurses collect data on 50 patients over a 3-month time period and compare those to the baseline data shown here:

	Mean Blood Glucose Level Before Change	Mean Blood Glucose Level After Change
On admission	250	248
8 hours after admit	235	194
12 hours after admit	230	180
24 hours after admit	212	181

Although these reductions were statistically significant ($p = .02$), the outcome was not met. What other variables could be accounting for the fact that the outcome was not met? Would you continue to use the IV insulin protocol?

absence of bleeding defined in a measurable way? Because bleeding might be interpreted in several different ways, a precise definition of bleeding should have been provided to ensure consistency in reporting. Second, when should patients be assessed for absence of bleeding? Is the absence of bleeding to be assessed when the patient first ambulates or at a later time? Input from the staff prior to changing the nursing protocol could have clarified these questions, resulting in more reliable results.

Another consideration in outcome evaluation is to obtain data relative to current practice for comparison purposes. To document the need for a practice change and to support a new protocol, baseline data might need to be collected to demonstrate limitations of the current standard of care. Consideration must be given to all extraneous variables that may be influencing the outcome, such as time, equipment, safety, and costs. It could be helpful to involve a statistician to perform complex analyses.

18.4 Keeping It Ethical

At the end of this section, you will be able to:

‹ List three dilemmas that can arise when nurses are involved in testing protocols

As a staff nurse, it is likely that you will be involved at some point in evaluating patient care outcomes. At the very least, your documentation will be a source of data. There are other ways for you to become involved in evaluation. When nurses are involved in testing protocols, ethical dilemmas can arise. Issues can concern the selection of the sample, data collection, and reporting.

When considering the recruitment of patients to participate in protocol testing, you must make certain that they fit the criteria and are not included simply to reach the sample size needed. You are obligated to collect data as directed by the protocol. Reflect back to the example of reducing the number of hours on bed rest following cardiac catheterization. Suppose you were to assess for bleeding in one of your patients but were unable to do that assessment because of an emergency on the unit. You might be tempted to guess or enter data collected at a later time. But for the integrity of the process, it would be preferable to indicate that the data are missing. Another issue that can arise is that sometimes nurses have a tendency to change behaviors when they are aware that data are being collected. For example, a hospital is implementing a smoking cessation program. Because the nursing staff know that their unit is being compared to other units in the facility, they are very careful to follow the program exactly as outlined. However, after data collection is concluded and the protocol is found to be effective, it would not be in the best interest of patients for nurses to return to using former protocols.

FYI

When nurses are involved in testing protocols, ethical dilemmas can arise. Issues can concern the selection of the sample, data collection, and reporting.

TEST YOUR KNOWLEDGE 18-4

1. Which of the following behaviors is unethical? (Select all that apply.)
    a. Ensuring patients enrolled in a protocol meet criteria
    b. Filling in all missing data at the conclusion of your shift
    c. Refusing to participate in outcome measurement
    d. Continuing to follow protocols after data collection ends

How did you do? 1. b, c

Apply What You Have Learned

It has been 6 months since the hand hygiene policy was implemented throughout your facility. Now it is time to evaluate whether the desired outcomes have been met. You invite the chair of the Quality Assurance Committee to attend the next meeting of the EBP committee. You ask the chair to report on the monthly hand hygiene compliance rates for the past 6 months and rates prior to when the policy was implemented. This will allow EBP committee members to compare compliance rates before and after implementation of the policy. Review the chair's report within this text's digital resources. What conclusions can you draw about the effectiveness of the policy?

Quality Assurance Committee Hand Hygiene (HH) Compliance Report

Units	Baseline Percentage of HH Compliance Rate	Percentage of Hand Hygiene Compliance Rates After Policy Change						
	Total	Jan	Feb	Mar	April	May	June	Total
Critical Care	50.75	84.25	86.5	84.75	83.75	84.75	84.5	84.75
CCU	50	88	86	80	78	85	83	83.33
ICU	44	80	85	83	80	79	80	81.17
ER	39	78	80	81	81	80	83	80.5

(continued)

Apply What You Have Learned *(continued)*

Units	Baseline Percentage of HH Compliance Rate	Percentage of Hand Hygiene Compliance Rates After Policy Change						
	Total	Jan	Feb	Mar	April	May	June	Total
OR	70	91	95	95	96	95	92	93.83
Med-Surg	43.2	87.6	88.4	85.6	78.6	77.4	71.2	81.47
Tele	43	90	90	88	86	85	83	87.0
Onc	50	83	87	87	80	78	75	81.67
Ortho	39	92	90	85	80	75	60	80.33
Gen med	44	88	90	85	75	74	70	80.33
Gen surg	40	85	85	83	72	75	68	78.0
Maternal Child	47.0	83.0	85.75	82.75	79.5	65.0	72.0	78.0
NICU	65	95	93	90	91	90	89	91.33
Peds	38	65	80	78	73	50	62	68.0
L & D	45	87	85	80	74	70	72	78.0
Mother-Baby	40	85	85	83	80	50	65	74.67
TOTAL	46.98	84.95	86.88	84.37	80.62	75.72	75.9	81.41

⚡ *RAPID REVIEW*

» An outcome is a consequence or a visible result. Nursing outcomes measure states, behaviors, or perceptions of individuals, families, or communities.

» Outcomes research examines the effect of care on individuals and populations.

» Outcomes can be classified by focusing on who is to be measured: individuals, groups, or organizations. They can also be grouped as care-related, patient-related, and performance-related. They also may be classified according to time: short term, intermediate, and long term.

» Outcomes that demonstrate the effectiveness of nursing care are known as nursing-sensitive outcomes.

» Indicators specify how the outcome should be measured. Usually, quantitative measures are used.

» Four major factors should be considered in regard to outcomes: patient populations, team selection, organizational priorities, and mandated reporting.

» Outcomes may be derived from a variety of sources such as NOC, clinical practice guidelines, standards of care, and Forces of Magnetism. CQI and benchmarking are processes that involve outcome evaluation.

» Conclusions are best drawn when outcomes are clearly defined, data are carefully collected, and findings are compared to baseline data. Considerations should be given to possible extraneous variables.

» Ethical issues can concern selection of the sample, data collection, and reporting.

REFERENCES

Agency for Healthcare Research and Quality. (2011). Ventilator bundle checklist. Retrieved from https://innovations.ahrq.gov/qualitytools/ventilator-bundle-checklist

American College of Cardiology. (2014). National cardiovascular data registry. Retrieved from https://www.ncdr.com/WebNCDR/docs/default-source/public-more-info -enrollment-landing-page-docs/ncdr-brochure.pdf?sfvrsn=2

American Heart Association. (2008). ACC/AHA performance measures for adults with ST-elevation and non-ST-elevation myocardial infarction. *Circulation, 118*, 2596–2648.

American Nurses Credentialing Center. (2017). Forces of Magnetism. Retrieved from http:// www.nursecredentialing.org/Magnet/ProgramOverview/HistoryoftheMagnetProgram /ForcesofMagnetism

Burns, N., & Grove, S. (2014). *Understanding nursing research: Building an evidence-based practice* (8th ed.). Maryland Heights, MO: Elsevier.

Burston, S., Chaboyer, W., & Gillespie, B. (2013). Nurse-sensitive indicators suitable to reflect nursing care quality: A review and discussion of ideas. *Journal of Clinical Nursing.* Advance online publication. doi:10.1111/jocn.12337

Centers for Disease Control and Prevention. (2017, January). *Ventilator-associated pneumonia (VAP) event.* July 1, 2013 CDC/NHSN Protocol Clarifications. Retrieved from http://www.cdc.gov/nhsn/pdfs/pscmanual/6pscvapcurrent.pdf

Centers for Medicare and Medicaid Services. (2015). Quality measures and performance standards. Retrieved from http://www.cms.gov/Medicare/Medicare-Fee-for-Service -Payment/sharedsavingsprogram/Quality_Measures_Standards.html

Contopoulos-Loannidis, D., Karvouni, A., Kouri, I., & Ioannidis, J. (2009). Reporting and interpretation of SF-36 outcomes in randomized trials: Systematic review. *British Medical Journal, 338*, a3006.

Greene, L. R., & Sposato, K. (2009). *Guide to the elimination of ventilator-associated pneumonia.* Washington, DC: Association for Professionals in Infection Prevention. Retrieved from http://www.apic.org/Resource_/EliminationGuideForm/18e326ad -b484-471c-9c35-6822a53ee4a2/File/VAP_09.pdf

Institute for Healthcare Improvement. (2013). About IHI. Retrieved from http://www .ihi.org/about/pages/default.aspx

Joint Commission. (2017a). Core measure sets: Acute myocardial infarction. Retrieved from https://www.jointcommission.org/core_measure_sets.aspx

Joint Commission. (2017b). National patient safety goals—Hospital Accreditation Program. Retrieved from http://www.jointcommission.org/assets/1/6/HAP_NPSG _Chapter_2014.pdf

Kleinpell, R. (2009). Measuring outcomes in advanced practice nursing. In R. Kleinpell (Ed.), *Outcome assessment in advanced practice nursing* (2nd ed., pp. 1–61). New York, NY: Springer.

Krumholz, H. (2009). Outcomes research: Myths and realities. *Circulation: Cardiovascular Quality and Outcomes, 2*, 1–3.

Magill, S., Klompas, M., Balk, R., Burns, S., Deutschman, C., Diekema, D., & Lipsett, P. (2013). Developing a new national approach to surveillance for ventilator-associated events. *Critical Care Medicine, 41*(11), 2467–2475.

Mauskop, A., & Borden, W. (2011). Predictors of statin adherence. *Current Cardiology Reports, 13*(6), 553–558.

Micik, S., Besic, N., Johnson, N., Han, M., Hamlyn, S., & Ball, H. (2013). Reducing risk for ventilator associated pneumonia through nursing sensitive interventions. *Intensive and Critical Care Nursing, 29*(5), 261–265.

Minnick, A. (2009). General design and implementation challenges in outcomes assessment. In R. Kleinpell (Ed.), *Outcome assessment in advanced practice nursing* (2nd ed., pp. 107–118). New York, NY: Springer.

Moorehead, S., Johnson, M., Maas, M., & Swanson, E. (Eds.). (2013). *Nursing outcomes classification (NOC): Measurement of health outcomes* (5th ed.). St. Louis, MO: Mosby.

Newhouse, R., & Pettit, J. (2006). The slippery slope: Differentiating between quality improvement from research. *Journal of Nursing Administration, 36*(4), 211–219.

Patient Protection and Affordable Care Act. (2010). H.R. 3590. Retrieved from http:// www.gpo.gov/fdsys/pkg/BILLS-111hr3590enr/pdf/BILLS-111hr3590enr.pdf

Polit, D., & Beck, C. (2014). *Essentials of nursing research* (8th ed.). Philadelphia, PA: Lippincott Williams & Wilkins.

Resar, R., Griffin, F. A., Haraden, C., & Nolan, T. W. (2012). *Using care bundles to improve health care quality*. IHI Innovation Series white paper. Cambridge, MA: Institute for Healthcare Improvement. Retrieved from http://www.ihi.org/resources/Pages /IHIWhitePapers/UsingCareBundles.aspx

Society of Thoracic Surgeons. (2013). Executive summaries. Retrieved from http://www .sts.org/sts-national-database/database-managers/executive-summaries

At the end of this chapter, you will be able to:

< Discuss the importance of dissemination of research findings to building evidence-based practice

< Recognize the importance of dissemination in the cycle of science

< Explain how poster presentations are useful to disseminate new knowledge

< List the essential components of a well-constructed poster

< Describe strategies that make oral presentations successful

< List elements that must be considered when preparing a manuscript

< Discuss the process for submitting a manuscript for publication

< Demonstrate professional behaviors when attending conferences

< List strategies to get the most out of conference attendance

< Discuss why nurses are obligated to participate in the process of dissemination

KEY TERMS

authorship
call for abstracts
dissemination

manuscript
networking
papers

posters
presentations

CHAPTER 19

Sharing the Insights with Others

Janet M. Brown and Nola A. Schmidt

19.1 Dissemination: What Is My Role?

At the end of this section, you will be able to:

‹ Discuss the importance of dissemination of research findings to building evidence-based practice

‹ Recognize the importance of dissemination in the cycle of science

Recently, national efforts have been aimed at realizing the goal of dissemination for the purpose of improving patient outcomes and reducing costs (Coleman, Rosenbek, & Roman, 2013). Evidence-based practice (EBP) cannot be successful if nurses fail to read or hear about new knowledge. Evidence must be made available in accessible and comprehensible ways so that innovations are adopted. *Dissemination* is the communication of clinical, research, and theoretical findings for the purpose of transitioning new knowledge to the point of care. EBP cannot evolve unless communication channels in the societal system are used effectively to bring about change. Dissemination of findings is most successful if multiple methods are used over time. These methods need to be systematic, coordinated, and efficient (Kerner, Rimer, & Emmons, 2005). In the profession of nursing, there are three major ways that new knowledge is disseminated: posters, presentations, and papers. These are often referred to as the 3 Ps of dissemination.

FYI

Dissemination is the communication of clinical, research, and theoretical findings for the purpose of transitioning new knowledge to the point of care. EBP cannot evolve unless communication channels in the societal system are used effectively to bring about change.

KEY TERM

dissemination: Communication of clinical research and theoretical findings to transition new knowledge to the point of care

Every healthcare discipline faces the challenge of conveying research findings to clinicians in a timely manner. Dissemination is facilitated when activities are carefully and appropriately considered. A dissemination plan, targeted at the needs of the nurses who will use the information, is critical to ensuring efficient adoption of an innovation. Researchers should craft messages in a way that is understandable to clinicians (Gagnon, 2011).

Warren et al. (2016) noted that although most nurses are familiar with EBP, they have little time to keep up with new knowledge or implement best practice changes in healthcare settings. This challenge to dissemination is not new. As far back as 1995, Cronenwett suggested that attention be given to: (1) what information should be disseminated, (2) whom the information should be targeted to, and (3) the most effective way for nurses to access the information. One can readily see how her three points are congruent with Rogers's (2003) theory of diffusion of innovation. For example, suppose an EBP guideline for the provision of mouth care to terminally ill patients is revised. For this practice to be effectively disseminated, details about what products to use, appropriate techniques, and patient outcomes should be communicated over time to members of the social system. Therefore, in this example, it would be most important to get this information to hospice, long-term care, and home care nurses. Disseminating the revised guideline in professional journals targeted to these types of nurses would be appropriate. Also, involving their professional organizations, such as the Hospice and Palliative Nurses Association, in the dissemination process, by posting the revised guideline on their websites, would be beneficial. Coleman et al. (2013) have emphasized the importance of organizational commitment to ensuring translation of research findings to practice. To ensure dissemination, they recommended several key strategies:

» Engaging organizational leadership, both clinical and administrative
» Identifying ways to support adoption of new practices
» Collecting, analyzing, and presenting outcome data to demonstrate change
» Explaining how social and political factors influence adoption

Recall the four phases of the cycle of scientific development: theory development, research, dissemination, and application to practice. All nurses must be accountable for professional activities that facilitate dissemination. Just as theorists and researchers have responsibilities to communicate findings, nurses have responsibilities to actively seek and apply new knowledge. Without dissemination, there is no reason to develop theories and conduct research because nurses would not read and hear about the latest findings.

1. New knowledge is effectively disseminated through: (Select all that apply.)

    a. Papers
    b. Posters
    c. Proclamations
    d. Presentations

2. Dissemination is important for which of the following reasons?

    a. Publishers need to make a profit.
    b. Most research grants require reporting.
    c. New knowledge is transmitted to patient care.
    d. Theorists and researchers need something to do.

3. Dissemination is an important phase in

    a. The cycle of scientific development
    b. The Krebs cycle
    c. The cycle of life
    d. The cycle of professional nursing

How did you do? 1. a, b, d; 2. c; 3. a

19.2 The 3 Ps of Dissemination

At the end of this section, you will be able to:

‹ Explain how poster presentations are useful to disseminate new knowledge
‹ List the essential components of a well-constructed poster
‹ Describe strategies that make oral presentations successful
‹ List elements that must be considered when preparing a manuscript
‹ Discuss the process for submitting a manuscript for publication

Posters

Posters are an important scholarly venue for disseminating evidence (Bindon & Davenport, 2013). A major advantage of poster presentations over other methods is that opportunities for *networking* exist. Poster sessions allow for interactions among professionals. Presenters receive immediate feedback from a variety of individuals who attend the poster session. Interactions allow for the exchange of ideas about areas of common interest (Bingham & O'Neal, 2013).

KEY TERM

posters: A scholarly venue for disseminating evidence

The versatility of the poster as a medium for dissemination makes it effective in a variety of situations. Posters are often used in the clinical arena to convey innovations or describe EBP. At professional conferences, research studies are often summarized in a poster display. Nurses may have opportunities to display posters at their places of employment. A poster could be displayed on a unit or in an area where staff members are likely to gather, such as the cafeteria or hallway.

Because dissemination from individuals in clinical practice is essential to building nursing knowledge, unit-based posters are an excellent opportunity for nurses to disseminate the unique knowledge they possess. Evidence-based projects, quality improvement, and interesting patient case studies lend themselves to poster presentations. For example, a nurse notes that a better way is needed for securing scalp needles used with infants. Over time, he devises a technique that is superior to other taping methods. A poster presentation would be an ideal way to share his innovation with other nurses.

Poster presentations are a mainstay of professional conferences. Most all major conferences include at least one poster session, and such sessions are growing in popularity to the point that it is not uncommon to have several sessions throughout a conference. Because poster submissions are usually competitive, it is an honor to have a poster selected for display.

How to Be a Poster Presenter

There is a typical process for selecting individuals to present at poster presentations. To be considered for presentation, individuals are required to submit an abstract summarizing the project. Abstracts are peer reviewed using stringent criteria. To increase the likelihood of having an abstract selected, attention to poster guidelines when writing an abstract for submission is critical. For example, it would be expected that the abstract contain the exact headings as specified in the guidelines. Another way to increase the chances of having an abstract accepted for presentation is to consider whether the poster would be appropriate for the audience expected at the conference. Notices, also known as a *call for abstracts*, publicize that submissions for abstracts are being sought. Calls for abstracts typically include information about submission and provide clues about the intended audience. Information in the call for abstracts can help one decide whether a topic is congruent with the conference objectives. A title that communicates the significance of content being disseminated is likely to capture the interest of the reviewer (Garner, Morey, Yang, & Faruque, 2012). For example, if childhood obesity is the focus of a conference, it is unlikely that a poster about obesity in older adults would be selected. Carefully matching one's scholarly work to the appropriate

BOX 19-1	Tips on How to Write a Good Abstract

Target appropriate audience and conference aim

Ensure abstract is submitted by the deadline

Carefully follow directions for formatting

Use appropriate font and font size (Arial and Times New Roman 10 and 12 allow maximum wordage in a limited space)

Adhere to the word limit specified

Provide biographical and contact information as requested

Keep title clear and concise using fewer than 10 words

Write in past tense

Provide key information in a succinct manner

Correct errors

Ask a colleague to provide feedback

Check for spelling mistakes

Take 5 minutes to conduct a final check

conference can reduce wasted effort and disappointment. See **Box 19-1** for tips on how to write a good abstract.

Individuals who submit abstracts for consideration at a conference are notified about the outcome of the review. With the acceptance of an abstract come several professional obligations. It is important to indicate acceptance of the invitation. If circumstances have changed and it is necessary to decline, doing so in a timely manner will allow the selection committee to fill the spot. When a commitment to present is made, it is essential to fulfill that commitment. Conference attendees become disgruntled if presenters are absent. If circumstances warrant an absence, having a colleague present is an acceptable alternative. Registration and payment of conference fees are required of most presenters, but sometimes a reduced fee is available.

When at the conference, presenters have a responsibility to fulfill the obligations of being a presenter. There are designated times for setting up and taking down posters. Presenters should adhere to these scheduled times. Presenters should make themselves available next to their posters during poster sessions to answer questions and convey excitement about the topic (Ellerbee, 2006). It is not unusual for attendees to seek out specific presenters who have similar interests. This type of networking is invaluable. Poster sessions provide an excellent forum for nurses from different settings to meet and exchange information

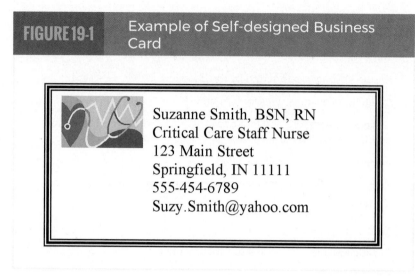

FIGURE 19-1 Example of Self-designed Business Card

(Ilic & Rowe, 2013). Having handouts containing information not included in the abstract promotes dissemination. It is often helpful to offer business cards to individuals who are interested in your work (Ellerbee, 2006). If your organization does not provide business cards, it is easy to make your own (**Figure 19-1**).

Speed posters offer a new variation to traditional poster sessions (Wagnes, 2016). This is modeled after speed dating. Posters are grouped in a room according to specialty groups. A rotation schedule is published to allow all attendees to hear about each poster in the specialty. Attendees gather before a poster while the author discusses, for about 5 minutes, main points made in the poster. This is followed by a 2-minute question and answer session. When a bell rings, attendees rotate to the next poster. The use of speed posters effectively engages attendees in discussion and improves networking.

A new approach to the traditional presentations of posters is presenting posters at an e-poster conference (Pierce, 2016). Posters are uploaded to a website and a discussion thread is created for each poster. This allows dissemination of information while providing opportunities for participants to dialog about the key points. Additionally, participants are asked to provide feedback about the design and organization of the posters, which presenters may find helpful.

Tips for Creating Effective Posters

Regardless of the environment or setting in which posters will be displayed, they should be created to communicate ideas effectively. Attention to both content and appearance is necessary because evidence shows that nurses are more likely to look at posters that have a title that is easy to read and a presentation that is aesthetically pleasing (Siedlecki, 2017). Creating posters requires more skill and effort than is usually anticipated, but although it is time consuming, most nurses find the process to be rewarding (Singh, 2013). Hand (2010) recommended starting work on a poster about 2 months before presentation.

Many strategies can be used to enhance delivery of the message. No matter how attractive a poster appears, if attention is not given to content, dissemination of information is diminished. Siedlecki (2017) found that interest in the content often determines which posters attendees will view. It is helpful to ask, "What is it that viewers should know after reading this poster?" Having this outcome in mind focuses the scope of the content to be presented. The message should be straightforward, and the text should be written in a common and meaningful language. Complete sentences are not needed, and content can be mixed with charts and graphs. Staggering bullets in an outline format is an effective way to present content and avoid redundancy. Jargon, abbreviations, and symbols should be avoided unless it is certain that the intended audience will recognize them. The goal is to be succinct yet to deliver a complete message (Bindon & Davenport, 2013). It should take viewers no longer than 5 minutes to read a poster (Hand, 2010).

Specific content to be included on a poster is often outlined in the call for abstracts. Every poster should have a title and indicate the authors and their affiliations. It is acceptable to include a logo of the affiliation. Abstracts are not included on posters unless it is required by the conference guidelines (Kohtz, Hymer, & Humbles-Pegues, 2017). Most posters also include a purpose statement. Other content is determined by the type of information that is being presented. See **Table 19-1** for a listing of content typically included in posters. Acknowledgment should be given to organizations that provided funding for the project. It is also acceptable to acknowledge individuals who provided assistance for the project.

No matter how well content is articulated in a poster, if the display is not visually appealing, individuals will not be enticed to read it. Consideration should be given to the layout, font, color, and graphics. Because effective use of white space draws attention to poster content, a balance of 20% text, 40% figures, and 40% white spaces is recommended (Kohtz et al., 2017). A good resource for making a poster can be found at http://downloads.graphicsland .com/how-to-make-a-scientific-poster.pdf.

Arranging poster elements in a logical sequence allows the viewer to move easily from one section to another through the material. Title, author, and affiliation are usually centered at the top of the poster. Layout of the poster should be balanced with content flowing from top to bottom of each section. Typically,

| TABLE 19-1 | Content Typically Included in Posters | | |

Research	EBP	Clinical Case Study	Quality Management Project
Title/Author/ Affiliation	Title/Author/ Affiliation	Title/Author/ Affiliation	Title/Author/ Affiliation
Research Aim, Question, Hypothesis	PICO Question	Clinical Problem	Clinical Issue
Review of Literature	Review of Literature	Background Information	Description of Team
Conceptual Model	Method	Assessment	Preparation
Research Design	Synthesis of Findings	Nursing Diagnosis	Planning
Sample	Decision About Practice	Plan	Assessment
Results	Implementation	Implementation	Implementation
Limitations	Evaluation	Evaluation	Diversification
Discussion of Findings	Discussion	Discussion	Discussion

displays are divided into three sections. For example, 6 by 4 feet is a common poster size. The center section should be 4 feet wide, leaving a 1-foot section on each side (see **Figure 19-2**). Important information should be placed at eye level at the center of the poster. Arrows can be used to direct viewers, and it is acceptable to vary the orientation of the pages (Bindon & Davenport, 2013; Ellerbee, 2006). Layouts should appear scholarly and professional. Presenters should avoid cluttering layouts with items such as ribbons, lace, and flowers because these items distract from the information being presented.

It is important to select fonts that make the content easy to read (Ellerbee, 2006). Titles and headings should be easily visible from 3 to 6 feet away. This means that letters should have a font size of 96 points or more (2–3 inches high). Other text should be visible from 2 to 4 feet away; therefore, font sizes of 24 to 36 points (about 1 inch high) are recommended. A simple way to test whether the font is large enough is to place the poster on the ground. If it can be read while standing over it, the font size is sufficiently large. Fonts should be limited to one or two different styles. A roman-style font with a serif type is recommended. It is easier to differentiate similar-looking letters and numbers because serif typefaces have tails or feet (Kohtz et al., 2017). Using bullets and

FIGURE 19-2   Logical Layout for EBP Posters

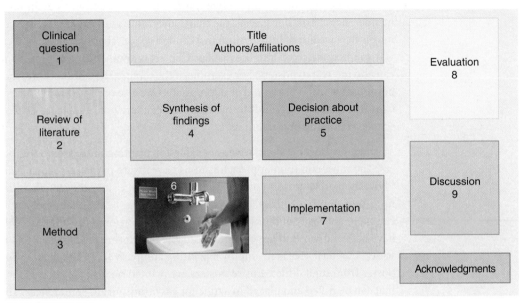

Image © Photos.com

avoiding full sentences makes best use of space. When each line is limited to no more than 30 characters and no more than six lines of text per heading, content can be kept organized and succinct. Consistency in the use of capitalization and punctuation should be maintained. Capital letters are usually used for titles and headings.

Although selecting colors for posters is fun, choices should make material more attractive and emphasize important content (Bindon & Davenport, 2013). Sometimes easels are provided for poster displays. If this is the case, background colors are not easily altered and will usually be brown, dark blue, or dark gray (Ellerbee, 2006). Selecting three to four colors that complement standard backgrounds is advised (Bindon & Davenport, 2013). Dark-colored fonts on lighter backgrounds are the easiest to read. Bright colors attract, and complementary colors provide the greatest contrast (Singh, 2013). Red and green are often used to highlight critical information; however, use of these two colors should be limited because some individuals have difficulty distinguishing them (Ellerbee, 2006). Sometimes presenters select colors because they represent a particular topic. For example, a poster on breast cancer may include pink as an accent color because this color is associated with breast cancer. Because color choices have both scientific and artistic implications, presenters can make color choices based on evidence from the literature.

Including graphics is an effective way to present content in a parsimonious manner. Bar charts, line graphs, pie charts, diagrams, and scatter plots can communicate a wealth of information in a limited space. They are also an effective way to integrate color into the display. Clip art is another kind of graphic that can add interest to posters. For example, if the topic is about infant care, then a border showing babies would be appropriate. Overuse of clip art is discouraged. Clip art of nurses' caps and the medical caduceus are not suitable to include in scholarly nursing presentations.

There are several alternatives available for printing and assembling posters. The most common approach is to use a software package, such as Adobe Photoshop or Microsoft PowerPoint (Singh, 2013). Using software also allows for experimenting with spacing, colors, and layouts. Additionally, corrections can be made easily and business logos can be incorporated. Some presenters have access at work to large printers capable of printing on paper up to 4 feet wide. An alternative is to employ a printing company that can quickly print a poster from digital files. Entire posters are printed on a single sheet of paper that can be rolled and placed in a tube for easy transport to conferences. There are some disadvantages to this approach. Because large printers are slow and require skill to use, printing ahead of time is advisable. If typographical errors are found and revisions are needed, the entire poster, rather than a single slide, could require reprinting. Another drawback to using large printers is that presenters have a tendency to include too much information, making it difficult to read the posters.

A cost-effective alternative to printing on one large poster is to print PowerPoint slides out individually. These can then be placed directly on the bulletin board. Printing the slides on higher grade paper conveys a sense of quality and professionalism. Some presenters laminate their slides to protect them; however, glare may result, making reading more difficult. Office supply companies can print and laminate PowerPoint slides, but it is wise to obtain price quotes before engaging in these services. Construction paper, color-coded art paper, or commercial paper with preprinted designs are inexpensive ways to add color. Picture mattes can be used to frame slides and offer another way to add color, dimension, and distinct boundaries for content sections. Preformed letters or stencils are sometimes used on picture mattes for the title, author, and affiliation. Although mattes can be more costly than construction paper, they can be reused over a number of years. Regardless of the method selected to print materials, it is never acceptable to handwrite posters for a professional presentation.

Presenters often use Velcro, push pins, or staples to attach their posters to display boards. Regardless of the method used, it is important to securely anchor the poster. Coming prepared with extra supplies is helpful because it is not uncommon to encounter problems when hanging posters. If traveling to conferences by air, it is wise to carry aboard posters to ensure that materials arrive with you.

KEY TERM

presentations:
Scholarly oral presentations to disseminate new knowledge

No matter how many times presenters proofread their posters, it is still possible for an error to be overlooked. Completing posters with sufficient time for obtaining feedback from colleagues is invaluable. For feedback to be constructive, colleagues must be comfortable offering criticism and suggestions. It is recommended that after assembling posters, presenters step back and critically appraise their work. Referring back to submission criteria while appraising can ensure that posters meet conference goals.

Oral Presentations

Like posters, oral *presentations* are an effective way to disseminate new knowledge. There is a growing expectation for nurses who practice at the bedside to engage in conference presentations (Happell, 2009). The submission process for an oral presentation is very similar to poster abstract submissions. In fact, nurses must often decide whether to deliver a poster or presentation when submitting an abstract to a conference. Authors elect to present orally when the topic is too complex to present in the space of a poster. Philosophical and theoretical work is best suited for oral presentations. Whereas posters work especially well for disseminating information about pilots and work in progress, completed work may be disseminated best through oral presentations.

There are professional responsibilities, similar to poster presentations, that must be fulfilled when accepting invitations to present papers. Many times presenters must submit their PowerPoint slides and handouts in advance of the conference. Objectives for presentations are often requested so that conference planners can apply for continuing education credits. Late fees might be assessed to presenters failing to meet deadlines. Should presenters find themselves unable to attend a conference, sending colleagues to substitute is preferable to canceling.

Successful oral presentations are a result of careful preparation and attention to detail. A multitude of sites offering suggestions for presenting can be found on the Web, such as http://www.wordstream.com/blog/ws/2014/11/19 /how-to-improve-presentation-skills and https://www.mindtools.com/pages /article/newCS_96.htm. Principles related to layout, font, color, and graphics of poster preparation are applicable to the preparation of slides that accompany oral presentations. Presentations begin by showing a title slide (Wax, Cartin, & Pinette, 2011), followed by a slide acknowledging funding sources and contributors. It is recommended to have one slide for every 30–60 seconds (Wax et al., 2011). Time should be allotted for questions at the end of the presentation. It is recommended that the last slide of the presentation be blank. This serves as a cue to the audience that the presentation is concluded. Novice presenters are advised to read papers from typed scripts rather than ad-libbing. Without experience, ad-libbing frequently results in a disorganized presentation that goes beyond the time limits (Happell, 2009). One can expect that one double-spaced typed page with 1-inch margins using an average sized font equals 2 minutes of speaking time. The best way to gauge the length of the presentation, however, is to rehearse the presentation aloud while using the visual aids. Typically, people speak faster when presenting than when rehearsing. Inserting visual cues into the script, such as "slow down" or "breathe," serves as a reminder for maintaining an appropriate speaking pace. Another helpful strategy to aid delivery is to enlarge the font so that the script is easier to read. Also, large font and familiarity with content can be invaluable if there is inadequate lighting at the podium (Happell, 2009; Wax et al., 2011). It is recommended to rehearse alone the first few times, followed by practicing in front of a small group of people. It may be helpful to use a laser pointer to draw attention to important points on your slides. For hints about how to use a pointer effectively, see **Box 19-2**.

As with posters, steps can be taken to avoid disaster. For example, having the presentation loaded on a flash drive can serve as a backup if needed. While traveling, never put presentation materials into checked baggage; always keep it on your person. Before presenting, it is wise to take advantage of the speaker ready room to ensure that presentation slides are functioning. To reduce anxiety, it may be helpful to observe other presentations that occur in the assigned presentation room. This allows for observing lighting, podium, microphone, and the slide management system (Wax et al., 2011).

BOX 19-2	Tips for Using Laser Pointers

Use device sparingly.

Do not wave the beam around the screen or room.

Brace the pointer against the podium to minimize tremor.

Once the point is made, turn the laser off.

Provide your own pointer.

Bring spare batteries.

It is smart to avoid the two most common mistakes made by presenters. First, when presenters read directly from slides, the audience can become disengaged from the presentation. Keeping PowerPoint slides bulleted with phrases discourages this practice. Presenters should strive to present more depth and detail about the topic through speaking rather than through visual aids. The second most common mistake occurs when presenters disregard time constraints. It is expected that presenters adhere to the time limitations for their presentations (Wax et al., 2011). It is inconsiderate to continue speaking after room moderators have indicated that the time has expired. Another way presenters disregard time constraints is by failing to be present during the entire paper session. Four to six papers are typically grouped together over 90 minutes. Presenters should arrive well before paper sessions begin and confirm their presence with room moderators and confirm that last-minute scheduling changes have not been made. Arriving early also allows an opportunity to test audiovisual aids. Presenters are expected to make themselves available at the conclusion of paper sessions because attendees might wish to network. Having business cards to share with colleagues during this time is advisable.

Papers

Scholarly *papers* are published in a variety of venues and are essential for disseminating knowledge. Nurses in clinical areas are in an excellent position to write and submit papers about case studies, EBP, and quality management projects. Researchers, theorists, and nurse educators also publish papers for the purpose of extending nursing's body of knowledge. Although there are many types of scholarly papers, the process of submission tends to be the same and is similar to the process of submitting a poster abstract. Several helpful strategies can assist novice writers to get started. One strategy is to submit a paper based on an already presented poster because the abstract and outline are already prepared. Gray (2005) recommended writing daily for 15–30 minutes and provided some tips for accomplishing this (see **Box 19-3**). Writing daily helps to form good habits about writing and leads to feelings of accomplishment. Another strategy is to recruit a colleague and have standing appointment times designated for writing. Collaborating with others creates accountability

KEY TERM

papers: Manuscripts published in professional journals

CRITICAL THINKING EXERCISE 19-1

You have been asked by a professor at your college to collaborate on a paper for publication in a peer-reviewed nursing journal. The professor expects you to do all of the research and writing and stated that you will be acknowledged for your assistance but that your name will not appear as an author on the article. What ethical issues need to be discussed in this situation? What action, if any, would you take?

> **BOX 19-3** Tips for Writing for 15–30 Minutes a Day
>
> Write in the same place every day.
>
> Write at the same time every day, preferably in the morning.
>
> Put your writing time in your calendar as an appointment.
>
> Start your writing session in the same way each day.
>
> Learn to stop internal and external interruptions.

KEY TERMS

authorship: List of authors in an order that reflects the amount of their contributions

manuscript: A scholarly paper prior to its publication

and can also be fun. It can be productive when novice writers collaborate with more seasoned writers.

When collaborating with others, it is important to determine *authorship* at the onset. Authors are listed in terms of their contribution to the paper. Usually the idea for the paper was generated by the first author. Other authors are listed in an order reflecting the amount of their contributions to writing. Others who participated in the project, but not in the writing, can receive an acknowledgment rather than authorship (Valente, 2013). When writing teams have good collegial relationships, authorship may be rotated among members of the team. Early in one's career, it is advisable to give consideration to the way one's name will appear in publications. For example, some authors include a middle name or initial. Consistently using the same format builds publication recognition and facilitates citation chasing.

After the decision to publish has been made, the next decision is to determine where the *manuscript* will be submitted (Valente, 2013). *Manuscript* is the term used for a scholarly paper prior to its publication. Just as with poster abstracts, consideration should be given to matching the topic and the intended audience with the purpose of the publication. Reading articles in journals to get a feel for their styles can help in determining whether the manuscript would be a good fit. With the expanse of the Web, open-access journals have proliferated. Although some open-access journals are reputable, there are others that are known as "predatory journals." It may be tempting to submit to predatory journals because a manuscript is more likely to be accepted due to questionable peer review processes. For example, authors may be misled because editorial boards may be fabricated or articles may be plagiarized from other publications (Haug, 2013). Be aware that exorbitant fees may be required after an article is accepted, so it is helpful to know if fees are required before submitting an article. A list of predatory journals can be found at http://beallslist.weebly.com/.

Once a journal for publication has been selected, query letters can be sent to journal editors to receive feedback about their interest in publishing the manuscript. It is accepted practice to send query letters to several editors simultaneously because the letter does not obligate the author to publish in a particular journal. Journal editors use query letters to decide whether to accept manuscripts for their journal. See **Box 19-4** for an example of a query letter.

When a decision is made about where the manuscript will be submitted, reviewing author guidelines is necessary. Adhering to the guidelines from the beginning saves time by eliminating the need to adjust a manuscript later. Journals specify the type of style to be used for preparation of manuscripts and expect that authors adhere strictly (Garner et al., 2012). For example,

---

BOX 19-4   Example of Query Letter

December 1, 2017

Ms. Brenda Tipton

Senior Editor, Nursing Division

Kraft and Frank Learning

53 Hall Street

Harrington, TN 32167

Dear Ms. Tipton,

I am in the process of preparing a manuscript entitled "How to Publish for Nursing: Tips for Getting It Done." This manuscript is important because the national trend is for nurses in clinical practice to publish in the specialty areas. The intended audience is staff nurses, and the manuscript will be about 15 pages in length. It is not under review by any other journal. It is my original work and there is no conflict of interest to declare. Would you be interested in reviewing this manuscript for *Hot Issues in Nursing*? Please contact me regarding your interest as indicated below.

Cordially,

Suzanne Smith, BSN, RN

Critical Care Staff Nurse

123 Main Street

Springfield, IN 11111

555-454-6789

Suzy.Smith@yahoo.com

CRITICAL THINKING EXERCISE 19-2

When you publish an article, how do you want your name to appear?

some journals require American Psychological Association style, while others may require Modern Language Association style. Guidelines also specify the number of words in an abstract, page limits, font, headings, and other criteria. It is essential that the guidelines be followed meticulously because manuscripts can be rejected when authors fail to follow the criteria. Familiarity with the language and tone used in the journal will also facilitate writing. For example, it is preferred in some journals to use the term *nurses*, whereas the term *clinicians* is used in other journals. Resources, such as Garner and colleagues (2012) and Holmes, Hodgson, Nishimura, and Simari (2009), provide suggestions for writing effective research reports or other types of articles.

Obtaining feedback from colleagues during the writing process can be invaluable. Gray (2005) suggested sharing early drafts with nonexperts and later drafts with experts. Nonexperts can include family members, students, or colleagues in other disciplines. Because these individuals are less likely to understand the content, problems with organization and clarity are more likely to be identified. Experts are individuals with advanced degrees in nursing. Such individuals can provide reviews about the content as well as organization and clarity. Another way to obtain feedback is to join a writing circle (Gray, 2005). In writing circles, writers convene weekly, giving feedback on only a few manuscript pages. The group is given 5 minutes to read the work of one member. Discussion follows during which members indicate for each paragraph the topic sentence, providing rationales for their choices. If the writing is clear and organized, there will be agreement about the topic sentences. For nurses affiliated with universities, writing centers offer another resource for obtaining feedback. Just as with submission of poster abstracts, it is essential to review manuscripts many times prior to actually submitting them for publication.

There are many similarities between the process of submitting an abstract for presentation at a conference and submitting a manuscript for publication. It is important to review the author guidelines for instructions about submission. Many journals only accept submissions online. Editors of peer-reviewed journals send blinded copies of manuscripts to several experts for review. Peer reviewers may be selected because of their expertise about the topic, research method, method of analysis, or theory. For journals not using a peer review process, manuscripts are reviewed by the editor. The length of time it takes for the review varies among journals, but one can expect to wait 3–6 months for a response. It may be tempting to submit manuscripts to multiple journals at the same time, but this is absolutely unacceptable practice. A manuscript cannot be submitted to a second journal unless it is rejected by the first or the author withdraws the manuscript submission. Eventually, authors receive notice about the status of manuscripts. Editorial decisions about manuscripts usually fall into one of four categories: accept, accept with minor revisions, accept with major

TEST YOUR KNOWLEDGE 19-2

1. When making a poster, which of the following should you do?
   a. Use full sentences and avoid using bullets.
   b. Use color to emphasize important points.
   c. Use fancy or script font because viewers find them attractive.
   d. Avoid including acknowledgment of funding sources because of space limitations.

2. Which of the following are strategies that are helpful when beginning to write a paper? (Select all that apply.)
   a. Writing 15–30 minutes a week
   b. Collaborating with others
   c. Selecting a journal for submission
   d. Adapting a poster presentation

3. When delivering oral presentations, presenters should do which of the following? (Select all that apply.)
   a. Respect time constraints.
   b. Remain to the end of the paper session to network.
   c. Read from the PowerPoint slides.
   d. Ad-lib to make the presentation more conversational.

How did you do? 1. b; 2. b, c, d; 3. a, b

revisions, and not accepted for publication. Feedback from peer reviewers is usually included with notification of the decision. It is rare for a manuscript to be accepted for publication outright. Most often, minor or major revisions are required. Using feedback from peer reviewers to make revisions is often an effective way to ensure acceptance of the manuscript on a second submission. Although it is natural for authors to be disappointed when manuscripts are rejected, they should immediately investigate other opportunities for submission. Feedback from peer reviewers can be used to make revisions, and another journal can be targeted.

19.3 Using Technology to Disseminate Knowledge

At the end of this section, you will be able to:

‹ Describe how technology can aid in dissemination
‹ Discuss three different technologies that can be used to disseminate new knowledge

In this digital age, information and news can be communicated throughout the world in a matter of minutes (sometimes even in seconds!). For the U.S. general public, the Internet has become the main source of information about science and technology (National Science Board, 2012). Americans rely equally on television and Internet for the answers. Thus, it raises the question, Why does it take so long to disseminate research findings into practice given the multitude of technologies available for use? Reliance on traditional methods, such as presentations, posters, and papers, by healthcare providers could be one barrier to dissemination. To address this barrier, the use of more sophisticated communication technologies to reach a larger audience is needed. For example, the Internet enables nurses to extend the focus of EBP to include public policy and public health, and it provides greater exploration, understanding, and management of EBP initiatives (Paxton, 2013). Although using technology for dissemination sounds easy, it requires much more than simply placing a resource on an Internet site. Successful dissemination requires special skills researchers and clinicians typically do not possess. Therefore, collaborating with professionals who have a strong understanding of advertising and the use of media and websites is essential.

Nurses must capitalize on current and emerging technologies and their uses. Whereas websites have become commonplace, many forms of media can be used to engage individuals. Participatory media involving blogs, wikis, video blogs, social networking sites, microblogging sites, podcasts, and mashups offer various ways to engage others (Haigh & Costa, 2012). For example, Craig and Wong (2013) found that students, using wiki technology for an assignment, reported that the global nature of this technology enhanced their ability to collaborate internationally. Another example is the use of online videos. One well-known collection of videos is posted on the TED (Technology, Entertainment, Design) website (Sugimoto & Thelwall, 2013). Social media networks, such as Facebook and Twitter, provide the potential to facilitate dissemination of evidence. For example, Harris (2013) found that social media networks promoted effective dissemination of effective public health practice among state health departments nationwide.

Electronic journals, as communication channels, are developing as new information platforms; however, promotional activities are essential to effective use (Vasishta, 2013). Although library websites are the best way to promote electronic journals, Vasishta found that most library websites fall short of providing an effective platform for electronic journals. Because clinicians find it difficult to access these resources, communication of new ideas is limited. Until the visibility of electronic journals is increased, they will fail to reach their potential audiences.

19.4 Making the Most of Conferences

At the end of this section, you will be able to:

< Demonstrate professional behaviors when attending conferences
< List strategies to get the most out of conference attendance

Not only are conferences excellent venues for dissemination of new knowledge, but they also provide opportunities for developing connections with colleagues who have similar interests, meeting experts in the field, and exploring career opportunities. Nurses are drawn to conferences with themes that are compatible with their interests so they can participate in meaningful exchanges of ideas (McIntyre, Millar, & Thomas, 2007). Sometimes, employers send nurses to conferences that fit with organizational goals (Brown & Schmidt, 2009). For example, a hospital administrator may send several nurses to a conference on how to apply for Magnet Recognition. Nurses may also be sent to conferences if education is needed to comply with governmental or accrediting regulations (Murray, 2008). If nurses are active in professional organizations, they may attend conferences as delegates. Conferences that assist nurses to meet professional goals merit consideration (Murray, 2008). For example, it may be wise for nurses to select conferences that offer continuing education units if that is required for license renewal. Conference participants should take full advantage of networking opportunities to make the most of their experiences (Brown & Schmidt, 2009).

Maintaining a professional demeanor at all times is advantageous because you never know who you might meet or what opportunities could arise (Brown & Schmidt, 2009). For example, it is possible to be offered the opportunity to interview for a position with a leading expert in your specialty. Invitations to collaborate on papers and research studies are not uncommon. For individuals considering

FYI

Not only are conferences excellent venues for dissemination of new knowledge, but they also provide opportunities for developing connections with colleagues who have similar interests, meeting experts in the field, and exploring career opportunities. Professional behaviors always make favorable impressions and should be practiced when attending conferences.

graduate study, networking with students and faculty from programs under consideration can be helpful. Questions about various programs can be answered when conversing with these individuals. It pays to be professional at all times. For example, individuals may find themselves sitting next to the dean of the graduate program under consideration. It would be quite uncomfortable to have an admission interview with this dean if the image portrayed is unfavorable.

Professional behaviors always make favorable impressions and should be practiced when attending conferences. Participants should dress professionally. Although attending a conference is a day away from work, it should not be considered a day off. Wearing sweatpants or jeans to be comfortable is not acceptable. It is customary for individuals to wear business suits or skirts or trousers that are paired with conservative blouses, sweaters, or jackets. Layering clothing is always wise because presentation rooms can vary in temperature. Arriving on time, introducing yourself to others, and offering a handshake make excellent first impressions. Inquiring where someone is from or why they chose to attend this conference is a good way to begin a conversation. If individuals find areas of common interest, having a business card to share facilitates networking. Allowing cell phones to ring during presentations shows disrespect for both presenters and members of the audience. Phones should be either turned off or silenced. It is also rude to converse with other attendees during presentations.

It is best to take full advantage of conferences because they can be costly to attend (Brown & Schmidt, 2009). Reviewing conference programs in their entirety allows participants to select sessions that pertain to their interests. Abstracts contain valuable information that helps identify presentations and posters of interest. Highlighting or writing out a schedule of preferred sessions ensures that time is maximized. It can be disappointing to overlook a scheduled session of interest. When planning a schedule, keep in mind that it is acceptable to change rooms between presentations during the same session time. If attending conferences with colleagues, it can be tempting to attend all sessions together. However, to maximize exposure to new ideas, it is wise to split up and share information later.

In addition to the sessions, conferences offer many other opportunities for networking. Attending interdisciplinary conferences may offer an opportunity to foster a collaborative approach to EBP (Newhouse & Spring, 2010). Some of the most important exchanges of information occur during conversations in hallways or at receptions. Viewing poster sessions, visiting vendor exhibits, and attending meals and breaks provide opportunities to meet new people or renew friendships. If there is a respected authority you would like to meet, introduce yourself. Most experts are eager to discuss their work. Networking, like dissemination, is vital to building the discipline of nursing.

TEST YOUR KNOWLEDGE 19-4

1. When attending a conference, which of the following behaviors are acceptable? (Select all that apply.)

    a. Wear business attire.
    b. Keep cell phones on silent or vibrate.
    c. Feel free to come in and out of sessions at will.
    d. Share business cards with other attendees.
2. Which of the following strategies help make the most of conferences? (Select all that apply.)

    a. Attending receptions
    b. Attending all sessions with your friends
    c. Planning a schedule in advance
    d. Talking with experts

How did you do? 1. a, b, d; 2. a, c, d

19.5 Keeping It Ethical

At the end of this section, you will be able to:

< Identify ethical concerns when presenting or publishing
< Discuss why nurses are obligated to participate in the process of dissemination

Ethical principles related to the dissemination of EBP are as critical as ethical principles are in research conduct (Garcia, 2004). One critical ethical practice is to acknowledge authorship on all scholarly works. There are numerous guidelines to distinguish individuals who are authors from those who contributed to the study or project (Welker & McCue, 2006). To be an author, one should have made significant contributions to the ideas in the paper, participated in data analysis, contributed to the process of writing, and given approval on the final version of the paper (Ohler, 2003).

Another ethical consideration involving the 3 Ps relates to conflict of interest. Conflict of interest is a concept that refers to a situation when an individual may personally benefit from his or her actions. For example, a nurse may be paid by a company to promote a new device or drug during a presentation. It is not uncommon for presenters and authors to have to sign a form disclosing a conflict of interest, and sometimes presenters may have to add a slide to their presentation stating whether or not a conflict of interest exists (Ohler, 2003).

Presenters and authors also have to disclose off-label use of drugs if given during a study. When a drug is used in a different way than described in the

FDA-approved drug label, it is called "off-label." Off-label could apply to using a drug for unapproved age groups, doses, forms, or purposes. Like conflict of interest, forms or slides that disclose the off-label use of drugs may be expected.

The overall purpose of research dissemination is to begin the process of getting new knowledge used for the good of society (Cronenwett, 1995, p. 430). There are increased demands for healthcare providers and systems to be efficient and effective in providing patient care. Nurses can no longer plead ignorance of new knowledge. They must be accountable for creating best practice by rapidly moving new information to the point of care (Cronenwett, 1995).

Having accountability means that nurses must use their resources wisely. Opportunities for dissemination are limited; space in journals and presentation times at conferences must be allocated fairly. Authors should never simply tweak a manuscript that has already been published to resubmit to another journal for publication as original work. Furthermore, it is a waste of time and money for nurses to attend conferences but not participate fully. Nurses are obligated to fulfill expectations placed on them by employers who sponsor attendance at conferences.

Nurses have a responsibility to actively participate in the process of dissemination. Reading articles, attending conferences, presenting posters and papers, and networking with other professionals are expected activities. Nurses can organize scholarly events in their facilities such as research days where posters about unit-based projects are presented. The power of sharing information about unit-based activities should not be underestimated. The discipline of nursing is lacking dissemination from individuals in clinical practice. Dissemination of knowledge within nursing also raises the visibility of nursing to the public. To support these types of activities, nurses must advocate for budget dollars and release time from employers.

FYI

Nurses have a responsibility to actively participate in the process of dissemination. Reading articles, attending conferences, presenting posters and papers, and networking with other professionals are expected activities.

At the conclusion of the journey through this text, it is hoped that an appreciation for nursing research and its importance to EBP has ensued. With the knowledge and skills acquired through the content and application exercises, you are equipped to be an innovator by engaging in the process of moving evidence over time through the communication channels of social systems to improve patient care.

TEST YOUR KNOWLEDGE 19-5

True/False

1. Because information is growing at a rapid pace, it is acceptable for nurses to plead ignorance about new knowledge.

2. All nurses are obligated to participate in the process of dissemination.

How did you do? 1. F; 2. T

Apply What You Have Learned

Because the process that the EBP committee used was effective in creating a policy that reduced medication errors, several members submitted an abstract to a professional conference. You have just received notification that the abstract was accepted as a poster presentation. Within this text's digital resources, you will find the acceptance letter and guidelines for presentation of posters at this conference. While being certain to follow these guidelines, use the ideas in this chapter to create a poster that effectively disseminates your information.

RAPID REVIEW

» Dissemination is the communication of clinical, research, and theoretical findings for the purpose of transitioning new knowledge to the point of care. It is an important step of the cycle of scientific development.

» The 3 Ps of dissemination are posters, papers, and presentations.

» Posters are an excellent medium for disseminating information in a succinct and visually interesting manner. A mainstay of professional conferences, they can also be used at places of employment to communicate unit-based projects.

» Oral presentations are an effective way to disseminate new knowledge when the topic is too complex to present in the space of a poster. Presenters have professional responsibilities, such as adhering to the time allotted and making themselves available for networking.

» A manuscript is a scholarly paper prior to its publication. Like posters, many papers undergo a rigorous peer review process before being accepted for publication.

» Technology offers an efficient and expedient way to disseminate information; however, collaboration may be needed to effectively communicate through the Internet.

» Maintaining a professional demeanor at conferences is advantageous. There are many strategies for making the most of conference attendance such as writing out a schedule and talking with experts.

» Nurses have a responsibility to actively participate in dissemination by reading articles, attending conferences, presenting posters and papers, and networking with other professionals.

REFERENCES

Bindon, S. L., & Davenport, J. M. (2013). Developing a professional poster: Four "Ps" for advanced practice nurses to consider. *American Association of Critical Care Nurses, 24*(2), 169–176.

Bingham, R., & O'Neal, D. (2013). Developing great abstracts and posters: How to use the tools of science communication. *Nursing for Women's Health, 17*(2), 131–138.

Brown, J. M., & Schmidt, N. A. (2009). Getting the most out of conferences. *American Journal of Nursing, 39*(4), 52–55.

Coad, J., & Devitt, P. (2005). Research dissemination: The art of writing an abstract for conferences. *Nurse Education in Practice, 6*, 112–116.

Coleman, E. A., Rosenbek, S. A., & Roman, S. P. (2013). Disseminating evidence-based care into practice. *Population Health Management, 16*(4), 227–234.

Craig, J. A., & Wong, R. A. (2013). Student perceptions of the use and value of wiki technology for the creation and dissemination of an orthopedic physical therapy assignment. *Journal of Physical Therapy Education, 27*(1), 70–76.

Cronenwett, L. R. (1995). Effective methods for disseminating research findings to nurses in practice. *Nursing Clinics of North America, 30*, 429–438.

Ellerbee, S. M. (2006). Posters with an artistic flair. *Nurse Educator, 31*(4), 166–169.

Gagnon, M. L. (2011). Moving knowledge to action through dissemination and exchange. *Journal of Clinical Epidemiology, 64*, 25–31.

Garcia, A. M. (2004). Sixth version of the "uniform requirements for manuscripts submitted to biomedical journals": Lots of ethics, some new recommendations for manuscript preparation. *Journal of Epidemiology and Public Health, 58*(9), 731–733.

Garner, A., Morey, A., Yang, G., & Faruque, F. (2012). Ten points to address when publishing a manuscript. *Internet Journal of Allied Health Sciences and Practice, 10*(1), 1–7.

Gray, T. (2005). *Publish and flourish: Become a prolific scholar.* Las Cruces, NM: Teaching Academy, New Mexico State University.

Haigh, C., & Costa, C. (2012). Reconsidering the role of participatory media in nursing research and knowledge dissemination. *Journal of Research in Nursing, 17*(6), 598–607.

Hand, H. (2010). Reflections on preparing a poster for a RNC conference. *Nurse Researcher, 17*(2), 52–59.

Happell, B. (2009). Presenting with precision: Preparing and delivering a polished conference presentation. *Nurse Researcher, 16*(3), 45–55.

Harris, J. K. (2013). The network of Web 2.0 connections among state health departments: New pathways for dissemination. *Journal of Public Health Management Practice, 19*(3), 20–24.

Haug, C. (2013). The downside of open-access publishing. *New England Journal of Medicine, 368*, 791–793.

Holmes, D. R., Hodgson, P. K., Nishimura, R. A., & Simari, R. D. (2009). Manuscript preparation and publication. *Circulation, 120*, 906–913.

Ilic, D., & Rowe, N. (2013). What is the evidence that poster presentations are effective in promoting knowledge transfer? A state of the art review. *Health Information and Libraries, 30*(1), 4–12.

Kerner, J., Rimer, B., & Emmons, K. (2005). Dissemination research and research dissemination: How can we close the gap? *Health Psychology, 24*(5), 443–446.

Kohtz, C., Hymer, C., & Humbles-Pegues, P. (2017). Poster creation: Guidelines and tips for success. *Nursing 2017, 47*(3), 43–46.

McIntyre, E., Millar, S., & Thomas, F. (2007). Convening a conference: Facilitating networking among delegates. *Australian Family Practice, 36,* 659–660.

Murray, K. (2008). Leadership Q & A: Patient satisfaction, conference attendance. *Nursing Management, 39*(1), 56.

National Science Board. (2010). Chapter 7. Science and technology: Public attitudes and understanding. *Science and Engineering Indicators: 2010.* Retrieved from https://www.nsf.gov/statistics/seind12/c7/c7h.htm

Newhouse, R. P., & Spring, B. (2010). Interdisciplinary evidence-based practice: Moving from silos to synergy. *Nursing Outlook, 58,* 309–317.

Ohler, L. (2003). Improving authorship accountability: Ethical considerations in manuscript preparation. *Nurse Author and Editor Newsletter, 13*(2), 7–9.

Paxton, S. J. (2013). Dissemination in the Internet age: Taming a wild thing. *International Journal of Eating Disorders, 46*(5), 525–528.

Pierce, L. L. (2016). The e-poster conference: An online nursing research course learning activity. *Journal of Nursing Education, 55,* 533–535.

Rogers, E. M. (2003). *Diffusion of innovations* (5th ed.). New York, NY: Free Press.

Siedlecki, S. L. (2017). How to create a poster that attracts an audience. *AJN, 117*(3), 48–54.

Singh, A. (2013). How to develop a scientific poster for presentation. *Technic: The Journal of Operating Department Practice, 4*(3), 7–9.

Small Business Encyclopedia. (n.d.). Total quality management (TQM). Retrieved from http://answers.com/topic/tqm

Sugimoto, C. R., & Thelwall, M. (2013). Scholars on soap boxes: Science communication and dissemination in TED videos. *Journal of the American Society for Information Science and Technology, 64*(4), 663–674.

Valente, S. (2013). Transforming a presentation or poster into a publishable manuscript. *Nurse Author and Editor Newsletter, 23*(1), 5.

Vasishta, S. (2013). Dissemination of electronic journals: A content analysis of the library websites of technical university libraries in North India. *Electronic Library, 31*(3), 278–289.

Wagnes, L. D. (2016). Speed posters: An alternative to traditional poster and podium sessions. *Journal of Continuing Education in Nursing, 47,* 344–346.

Warren, J. I., McLaughlin, M., Bardsley, J., Eich, J., Esche, C. A., Kropkowski, L., & Risch, S. (2016). The strengths and challenges of implementing EBP in healthcare systems. *Worldviews on Evidence-Based Nursing, 13*(1), 15–25.

Wax, J. R., Cartin, A., & Pinette, M. G. (2011). Preparing a research presentation: A guide for investigators. *American Journal of Obstetrics and Gynecology, 205*(28e), 1–5.

Welker, J. A., & McCue, J. D. (2006). Authorship versus "credit" for participation in research: A case study of potential ethical dilemmas created by technical tools used by researchers and claims for authorship by their creators. *Journal of the American Medical Informatics Association, 14*(1), 16–18.

GLOSSARY

abstract   The first section of a research article that provides an overview of the study

accessible population   The group of elements to which the researcher has reasonable access

active rejection   Purposefully deciding not to adopt an innovation

adoption   Applying an innovation to practice

aggregate data   Data collected from individuals that are grouped to represent a population

AGREE II   Appraisal of Guidelines Research and Evaluation; internationally developed instrument to evaluate clinical practice guidelines

alpha level   Probability of making a type I error; typically designated as .05 or .01 at the end of the tail in a distribution

alternate form   A test for instrument reliability in which two different versions of new instruments are given. Scores are correlated, and strong positive correlations indicate good reliability; also known as parallel form

amodal   A data set that does not have a mode

analysis of variance   An inferential statistical test used when the level of measurement is interval or ratio and more than two groups are being compared

analytic epidemiology   Investigation of the determinants of disease

anonymity   Keeping the names of subjects separate from data so that no one, not even the researcher, knows subjects' identities; concealing the identity of subjects, even from the researcher

applied research   Research to discover knowledge that will solve a clinical problem

assent   Permission given by children to participate in research

associative relationship   A type of relationship such that when one variable changes the other variable changes

attrition rate   Dropout rate; loss of subjects before the study is completed; threat of mortality

auditability   When another researcher can clearly follow decisions made by the investigator, arriving at the same or comparable conclusions

audit trail   The documentation of the research process and researcher's decision making in qualitative studies

authorship   List of authors in an order that reflects the amount of their contributions

autonomous   Having the ability to make decisions

awareness   Understanding about oneself and the world

axial coding   The analysis of categories and labels after completion of open coding

barriers Factors that limit or prevent change

basic research Research to gain knowledge for the sake of gaining knowledge; bench research

behavioral inventory for professionalism A measure of education and training, skill, ethics, professional organization, and service

Belmont Report A report outlining three major principles (respect for persons, beneficence, and justice) foundational for the conduct of ethical research with human subjects

benchmarking Comparison of organizational outcome data to other organizations or national databases

beneficence The principle of doing good

between-groups design Study design where two groups of subjects can be compared

bias When extraneous variables influence the relationship between the independent and dependent variables

bimodal A data set with two modes

bivariate analysis The use of statistics to describe the relationship between two variables

Boolean operators Words, such as *and*, *or*, or *not*, that specify the relationship between search terms

bracketing A strategy used by qualitative researchers to set aside personal interpretations to avoid bias

call for abstracts Notices publicizing the desire for posters or presentations at conferences

call number Unique identification number assigned to items in a library by subject and author name

career development Experience and education that contribute to one's professional growth

care-related outcomes A category of outcomes that measures the effect of nursing interventions

case-control studies A type of retrospective study in which researchers begin with a group of people who already have the disease; studies that compare two groups: those who have a specific condition and those who do not have the condition

case reports or series Epidemiologic reports used to describe rare diseases or outcomes

case studies A description of a single or novel event; a unique methodology used in qualitative research that may also be considered a design or strategy for data collection

categorical data The lowest level of measurement whereby data are categorized simply into groups; nominal data

causal relationship When one variable determines the presence or change in another variable

causality The relationship between a cause and its effect

change A process that creates an alteration in a person or environment

change agent Individual who leads or champions change

change phases model An eight-phase process to describe organizational change

Chi square A common statistic used to analyze nominal and ordinal data to find differences between groups

CINAHL *Cumulative Index to Nursing and Allied Health Literature*; database for nursing and health-related literature

citation chasing Using a reference list to identify sources of evidence

clinical practice guidelines Recommendations based on evidence that serve as useful tools to direct clinical practice

cluster sampling Random sampling method of selecting elements from larger to smaller subsets of an accessible population; multistaging sampling

coding Assignment of labels to each line of transcript in qualitative analysis

coefficient of variation A percentage used to compare standard deviations when the units of measure are different or when the means of the distributions being compared are far apart

coercion The threat of harm or the offer of an excessive reward with the intent to force an individual to participate in a research study

cohort comparison Nonexperimental cross-sectional design in which more than one group is studied at the same time so that conclusions about a variable over time can be drawn without spending as much time

cohort studies Quasi-experimental studies using two or more groups; epidemiologic designs in which subjects are selected based on their exposure to a determinant

communication Process of creating and sharing information with one another to reach mutual understanding

community-based participatory action research Active involvement of community members throughout the research process

comparative designs Descriptive design type that compares two or more groups or variables

complex hypothesis A hypothesis describing the relationships among three or more variables

Computer Assisted Qualitative Data Analysis Software (CAQDAS) Computer software that assists in the management, coding, grouping, and analysis of qualitative data

concept analyses Scholarly papers that explore the attributes and characteristics of a concept

concepts Words or phrases that convey a unique idea that is relevant to a theory

conceptual definitions Definitions of concepts contained in a theory that sound like dictionary definitions

concurrent validity A test for criterion-related validity when a new instrument is administered at the same time as an instrument known to be valid; scores of the two instruments are compared, and strong positive correlations indicate good validity

conduct and utilization of research in nursing (CURN) Early study conducted about how nurses transition research findings into practice

confessionist tales Qualitative researchers' personalized accounts that provide insight about data collection and scientific rigor

confidence intervals Ranges established around means that estimate the probability of being correct

confidentiality The protection of subjects' identities from everyone except the researcher

confirmability One of four criteria for a trustworthy qualitative study that relates to the rigorous attempts to be objective and the maintenance of audit trails to document the research process; findings can be substantiated by participants

confounding variables Factors that interfere with the relationship between the independent and dependent variables; extraneous variable; Z variable

construct A word or phrase used to communicate a specific key idea to others

construct validity A threat to external validity when the instrument does not accurately measure the theoretical concepts

content validity A kind of validity to ensure that the instrument measures the concept; a test in which experts on the topic are asked to judge each item on an instrument by assigning a rating to determine its fit with the concept being measured

continuous data Interval- or ratio-level data that use a continuum of numeric values with equal intervals

continuous quality improvement A participatory process involving indicators that measure quality

control Ability to manipulate, regulate, or statistically adjust for factors that can affect the dependent variable

controlled vocabularies Standardized hierarchical lists that represent major subjects within a database

convenience sampling Nonprobability sampling method in which elements are selected because they are easy to access *convergent testing*   A test for construct validity in which new instruments are administered at the same time as an instrument known to be valid; scores of the two instruments are compared, and strong, positive correlations indicate good validity

correlated t test   A variation of the *t* test used when there is only one group or when the groups are related; paired *t* test

correlation coefficient   An estimate, ranging from 0.00 to +1.00, that indicates the reliability of an instrument; a statistic used to describe the relationship between two variables

correlational designs   Nonexperimental designs used to study relationships among two or more variables

cost-benefit ratio   Comparison of benefits to potential costs that might result from change

count data   The raw number of health phenomena under investigation in epidemiology

covary   When change in one variable is associated with change in another variable

credibility   One of four criteria for establishing a trustworthy qualitative study; refers to the truth or believability of findings

criterion-related validity   Degree to which the observed score and the true score are related

critical thinking   Skill set that involves critical appraisal of information

Cronbach's alpha   A test for instrument reliability used with interval or ratio items; all items are simultaneously compared using a computer

crossover designs   Experimental designs that use two or more treatments; subjects receive treatments in a random order

cross-sectional   Nonexperimental design used to gather data from a group of subjects at only one point in time; study design to measure exposure and disease as each exists in a population or representative sample at one specific point of time

cycle of scientific development   A model of the scientific process

data reduction   The simplification of large amounts of data obtained from qualitative interviews or other sources

data saturation   In qualitative research, the time when no new information is being obtained and repetition of information is consistently heard

Declaration of Helsinki   An international standard providing physician guidelines for conducting biomedical research

deductive reasoning   Thinking that moves from the general to the particular

degrees of freedom   A statistical concept used to refer to the number of sample values that are free to vary; $n - 1$

dependability   One of four criteria for a trustworthy qualitative study that relates to consistency in the findings over time; auditability; findings are reflective of data

dependent variable   Outcome or variable that is influenced by the independent variable; Y variable

descriptive correlational designs   Correlational design type used to explain the relationship among the variables or groups using a nondirectional hypothesis

descriptive designs   Designs that provide a picture of a situation as it is naturally happening without manipulation of any of the variables

descriptive epidemiology   Examination of the distribution of disease in a population in terms of person, place, and time

descriptive research   A category of research that is concerned with providing accurate descriptions of phenomena

descriptive statistics   Collection and presentation of data that explain characteristics of variables found in a sample

descriptive studies   Nonexperimental studies used to provide information about a phenomenon

determinants   Factors that are capable of bringing a change in health

developing oneself Engaging in activities that promote long-term professional growth and development

dichotomous Nominal measurement when only two possible fixed responses exist such as yes or no

direct observation Observing phenomena using the five senses; capturing information by watching participants

direction The way two variables covary

directional hypothesis Statement describing the direction of a relationship among two or more variables

discussion section Portion of a research article where interpretation of the results and how the findings extend the body of knowledge are discussed

dissemination Communication of clinical research and theoretical findings to transition new knowledge to the point of care

distribution The pattern of disease occurrence in and among populations or subgroups

divergent testing A test for construct validity in which new instruments are administered at the same time as an instrument measuring the opposite of the concept; scores of the two instruments are compared, and strong negative correlations indicate good validity

double-blind experimental designs Studies in which subjects and researchers do not know whether subjects are receiving experimental interventions or standard of care

early adopters Individuals who are the first to embrace an innovation

ecologic fallacy When false assumptions are made about individuals based on aggregated data and associations from populations

ecologic studies Correlational studies that are population-based rather than individual-based

effect size An estimate of how large a difference will be observed between the groups

effects of selection Threats to external validity when the sample does not represent the population

electronic indexes Electronic listings of electronic or print resources

elements Basic unit of the population such as individuals, events, experiences, or behaviors

emic The insider's or participant's perspective

empirical evidence Evidence that is verifiable by experience through the five senses or experiment

empirical indicators Measures of the variables being studied

empirical testing Collection of objectively measurable data that are gathered through the five senses to confirm or refute a hypothesis; hypothesis testing

endemic The expected occurrence of a particular disease within a community or population

epidemic A widespread occurrence of a disease in a community or population that is in excess of what is expected

epidemiology The study of distribution and determinants of disease in human populations

equivalence An attribute of reliability in which there is agreement between alternate forms of an instrument or alternate raters

ethnography A type of qualitative research that describes a culture

ethnonursing Systematic study and classification of nursing care beliefs, values, and practices in a particular culture

ethnoscience A method used in anthropology to discover new knowledge

etic The outsider's perspective; the perspective of the researcher

etiology The cause of disease

evidence-based practice (EBP) Practice based on the best available evidence, patient preferences, and clinical judgment

evidence hierarchies Predetermined scales that guide decisions for ranking evidence; levels of evidence

exclusion criteria Characteristics of elements that will not be included in the sample *exempt* Certain studies may be low enough risk not to require consent from individuals

expedited review A type of review by an institutional review board that can occur quickly; an IRB may conduct an expedited review if there is minimal risk to human subjects

experimental designs Designs involving random assignment to groups and manipulation of the independent variable

explanatory research Research concerned with identifying relationships among phenomena

exploding Technique for searching subject headings that identifies all records indexed to that term

exploratory designs Nonexperimental design type used when little is known about a phenomenon

ex post facto Research design in which researchers look back in time to determine possible causative factors; retrospective research design

exposure The contact with a disease or disease-producing agent

external validity The degree to which the results of the study can be generalized to other subjects, settings, and times

extraneous variables Factors that interfere with the relationship between the independent and dependent variables; confounding variable; Z variable

face validity A test for content validity when colleagues or subjects examine an instrument and are asked whether it appears to measure the concept

factor analysis A test for construct validity that is a statistical approach to identify items that group together

factorial designs Experimental designs allowing researchers to manipulate more than one intervention

false negative When a screening gives a negative result despite the presence of the disease

false positive When a screening gives a positive result even though the disease is not present

fieldwork The time researchers spend interacting with participants through interviews, observations, and detailed records

flexibility to change Being open and positive about change

focus groups A strategy to obtain data from a small group of people using interview questions

follow-up A longitudinal design used to follow subjects, selected for a specific characteristic or condition, into the future

Forces of Magnetism Qualities that exhibit nursing excellence

full review A type of review by an institutional review board that requires all members of the board to participate; an IRB conducts a full review if there is potential risk to human subjects

gatekeeper Person who facilitates or hinders the entry of the researcher into a particular group or setting

generalize Applying findings from a sample to a wider population

GRADE Grades of recommendations, assessment, development, and evaluation; an international, universal system for evaluating evidence

grey literature Unpublished reports, conference papers, and grant proposals

grounded theory A type of qualitative research that examines the process of a phenomenon and culminates in the generation of a theory

Hawthorne effect Subjects' behaviors may be affected by personal values or desires to please the experimenter; reactivity

health services research Research involving phenomena, such as cost, political factors, and culture, related to the delivery of health care

heterogeneous The degree to which elements are diverse or not alike

historical A type of qualitative research used to examine events or people to explain and understand the past to guide the present and future

history   A threat to internal validity when the dependent variable is influenced by an event that occurred during the study

homogeneity   The degree to which elements are similar or homogenous

homogenous   Elements that share many common characteristics

human rights   Freedoms to which all humans are entitled

hypotheses   Formal statements regarding the expected or predicted relationship among two or more variables

hypothesis testing   Collection of objectively measurable data that are gathered through the five senses to confirm or refute a hypothesis; empirical testing; a test for construct validity

impressionist tales   Qualitative researchers' storytelling and personal descriptions about the experience of conducting the study

incidence   The number of new cases of a disease in a population during a specified period of time

inclusion criteria   Characteristics that each element must possess to be included in the sample

independent t test   A variation of the *t* test used when data values vary independently from one another

independent variable   Variable that influences the dependent variable or outcome; intervention or treatment that is manipulated by the researcher; *X* variable

indexes   A listing of electronic or print resources

indicators   Quantitative criteria used to measure outcomes

individual nurse level   Practice changes that can be implemented by an individual nurse

inductive reasoning   Thinking that moves from the particular to the general

inferential statistics   Analysis of data as the basis for prediction related to the phenomenon of interest

informants   Individuals in a qualitative study; participants

information overload   State of an individual in which excessive communication cannot be processed or used

informed consent   An ethical practice requiring researchers to obtain voluntary participation by subjects after subjects have been informed of possible risks and benefits

innovation   Something new or novel

innovator   One who is willing to try new things

institutional review boards   Committees that review research proposals to determine whether research is ethical

instrumentation   A threat to internal validity when there are inconsistencies in data collection

integrative review   A scholarly paper that synthesizes published studies to answer questions about phenomena of interest

interaction of treatment and history   A threat to external validity when historical events affect the intervention

interaction of treatment and setting   A threat to external validity when an intervention conducted in one setting cannot be generalized to a different setting

interaction of treatment with selection of subjects   A threat to external validity where the independent variable might not affect individuals the same way

interlibrary loan   A service whereby libraries provide items in their collections to each other upon request; lending of items through a network of libraries

intermediate outcomes   Changes that occur after an innovation is introduced

internal consistency   An attribute of reliability when all items on an instrument measure the same concept

internal validity   The degree to which one can conclude that the independent variable produced changes in the dependent variable

international level   Changes that result from collaboration among nurses from different countries

interprofessional collaboration   Engaging with other professionals to provide evidence-based care

interrater reliability   A test for instrument reliability when two observers measure the same event. Scores are correlated, and strong positive correlations indicate good reliability

interval   A continuum of numeric values with equal intervals that lacks an absolute zero

intervention study   In epidemiology, a study that has a treatment that can be manipulated by the researcher

interviews   A method for collecting data in person or over the telephone

introduction   Part of a research article that states the problem and purpose

Iowa model for EBP to promote quality care   A systematic method explaining how organizations change practice

item to total correlation   A test for instrument reliability in which each item is correlated to the total score; reliable items have strong correlations with the total score

Jewish Chronic Disease Hospital study   Unethical study involving injection of cancer cells into subjects without their consent

journal   A scholarly or professional resource

journal club   A strategy for disseminating research among nurses by discussing articles in a small group

justice   The principle of equity or fairness in the distribution of burdens and benefits

key informants   Individuals who have intimate knowledge of a subject and are willing to share it with the researcher

keyword   A word used to search electronic databases; a significant word from a title or document used as an index to content

known group testing   A test for construct validity in which new instruments are administered to individuals known to be high or low on the characteristic being measured

Kuder-Richardson coefficient   A test for instrument reliability for use with dichotomous items; all items are simultaneously compared using a computer

kurtosis   The peakedness or flatness of a distribution of data

ladder program   An organizational process for promotion and career advancement

laggards   Individuals who are slow or fail to adopt an innovation

leader   One who takes initiative for change and empowers others

levels of evidence   Predetermined scales that guide decisions for ranking evidence; evidence hierarchies

levels of measurement   A system of classifying measurements according to a hierarchy of measurement and the type of statistical tests that is appropriate; levels are nominal, ordinal, interval, and ratio

lifelong learning   Adding skills and knowledge about the profession as it continues to evolve

Likert scales   Ordinal-level scales containing seven points on an agree or disagree continuum

list of references   Publication information for each article cited in a research report

lived experience   The perspective of an individual who has experienced the phenomenon

longitudinal designs   Designs used to gather data about subjects at more than one point in time

long-term outcomes   Primary changes in patient behaviors or status over time

magazine   A resource targeted to the general reading audience

magnitude   The strength of the relationship existing between two variables

mandated reporting   Data that must be shared with supervising or governmental agencies according to a specified timeline

manipulation   The ability of researchers to control the independent variable

manuscript   A scholarly paper prior to its publication

maturation   A threat to internal validity when subjects change by growing or maturing

mean   The mathematical average calculated by adding all of the data values and then dividing by the total number of values

measurement error   The difference between the true score and the observed score

measures of central tendency   Measures, such as the mean, median, and mode, that provide information about the typical case found in the data

measures of variability   Measures providing information about differences among data within a set; measures of dispersion

median   The point at the center of a data set

mediators   Extraneous variables that come between the independent and dependent variables

member checks   A strategy used in qualitative studies when the researcher goes back to participants and shares the results with them to ensure the findings reflect what participants said

memoing   A technique used in qualitative research to record ideas that come to researchers as they live with the data

mentor   One who assists with professional growth

meta-analysis   A scholarly paper that combines results of studies, both published and unpublished, into a measurable format and statistically estimates the effects of proposed interventions

metaparadigm   Four broad concepts core to nursing: person, environment, health, and nursing

meta-synthesis   A systematic review that contains only qualitative studies; a scholarly paper that combines results from qualitative studies

methodological   Studies for the purpose of creating and testing new instruments

methods section   Major portion of a research article that describes the study design, sample, and data collection

minimal risk   The probability and magnitude of harm from participating in a research study are not greater than those encountered in daily life

modality   The number of modes found in a data distribution

mode   The most frequently occurring value in a data set

model   Pictorial representation of concepts and their interrelationships

model of diffusion of innovations   Model to assist in understanding how new ideas come to be accepted practice

model of EBP levels of collaboration   A model explaining how five levels are intertwined to contribute to EBP

model testing   Correlational design to test a hypothesized theoretical model; causal modeling or path analysis

moderators   Extraneous variables that affect the relationship among the independent and dependent variables

mortality   A threat to internal validity when there is a loss of subjects before the study is completed; attrition rate

multiple experimental groups designs   Experimental designs using two or more experimental groups with one control group

multiple regression   An inferential statistical test used to describe the relationship of three or more variables

multitrait-multimethod testing   Test for construct validity in which a new instrument, established instrument of the same concept, and established instrument of the opposite concept are given at the same time; strong positive and negative correlations indicate good validity

multivariate analysis   The use of statistics to describe the relationships among three or more variables at interval and ratio levels

narrative reviews   Reviews based on common or uncommon elements of works without concern for research methods, designs, or settings; traditional literature review

national level Collaboration among nurses throughout the country to effect practice changes

Nazi experiments An example of unethical research using human subjects during World War II

negative case analysis A qualitative strategy involving the analysis of cases that do not fit patterns or categories

negatively skewed A distribution when the mean is less than the median and the mode; the longer tail is pointing to the left

nesting A strategy best used when a search contains two or more Boolean operators

networking Interacting with colleagues to exchange information and build relationships

network sampling Recruitment of participants based on word of mouth or referrals from other participants; snowball sampling

nominal The lowest level of measurement whereby data are categorized simply into groups; categorical data

nondirectional hypothesis Statement of the relationship among two variables that does not predict the direction of the relationship

nonequivalent control group pretest-posttest design A quasi-experimental design where two groups are measured before and after an intervention

nonequivalent groups posttest-only design A preexperimental design involving two groups measured after an intervention with little control for extraneous variables

nonexperimental designs Research designs that lack manipulation of the independent variable and random assignment

nonparametric Inferential statistics involving nominal- or ordinal-level data to make inferences about the population

nonprobability sampling Sampling methods that do not require random selection of elements

nonpropositional knowledge The art of nursing or knowledge that is obtained through practice

nonsignificant When results of the study could have occurred by chance; findings that support the null hypothesis

normal distribution Data representation with a distinctive bell-shaped curve, symmetric about the mean

null hypothesis A hypothesis stating that there is no relationship between the variables; the statistical hypothesis

Nuremberg Code Ethical code of conduct for research that uses human subjects

nursing outcomes Measures of states, behaviors, or perceptions of individuals, families, or communities as they relate to nursing and health

Nursing Quality Indicator Outcomes of nursing care, identified by the American Nurses Association, that address patient safety and quality of care

nursing-sensitive outcomes Results that demonstrate the effectiveness of nursing care

obligations Requirements to act in particular ways

observation A technique to gather data

odds ratio The statistic reported when epidemiologists conduct a case-control study

one-group posttest-only design A preexperimental design involving one group and a posttest with little control over extraneous variables

one-group time series design A quasi-experimental design where one group is measured prior to administering the intervention and then multiple times after the intervention

open coding The grouping of qualitative data into categories that seem logical

operational definitions Definitions that explicitly state how the variable will be measured or operationalized; empirical definitions

ordinal A continuum of numeric values where the intervals are not meant to be equal

organizational level When nurses in an organization effect practice changes

organizational priorities Situations of high importance because of volume of patients or costs

outcome Consequence or visible result

outcomes research Studies about the effects of care and treatments on individuals and populations

pandemic Epidemic that has spread worldwide

panel design Longitudinal design where the same subjects, drawn from the general population, provide data at multiple points in time

papers Manuscripts published in professional journals

parallel form A test for instrument reliability in which two different versions of new instruments are given. Scores are correlated, and strong positive correlations indicate good reliability; also known as alternate form

parametric Inferential statistical tests involving interval- or ratio-level data to make inferences about the population

participant observation Role of the researcher in qualitative methods when the researcher is not only an observer but also a participant during data collection

participants Individuals in a qualitative study; informants

passive rejection Lack of consideration given to adopting an innovation; hence, old practices are continued

patient populations A group of patients with similar characteristics

patient-related outcomes A type of outcome related to patient behaviors or actions

Pearson's r An inferential statistic used when two variables are measured at the interval or ratio level; Pearson product–moment correlation

peer debriefing A technique used in qualitative research in which the researcher enlists the help of another person, who is a peer, to discuss the data and findings

peer review When experts and editors rigorously evaluate a manuscript submitted for publication

percentage distributions Descriptive statistics used to group data to make results more comprehensible; calculated by dividing the frequency of an event by the total number of events

percentile A measure of rank representing the percentage of cases that a given value exceeds

performance-related outcomes A type of outcome related to how nurses perform their job

period prevalence The number of existing cases of disease in a population during a specified period of time

periodical A resource that is published on a set schedule

persistent observation When the researcher has spent sufficient quality time with participants while attempting to describe and capture the essence of the phenomenon

personal development file A compilation of career accomplishments

personal narrative A way of conveying the meaning of experiences through storytelling

phenomenology A type of qualitative research that describes the lived experience to achieve understanding of an experience from the perspective of the participants

physiological measures Data obtained from the measurement of biological, chemical, and microbiological phenomena

PICOT model A model in EBP used to formulate EBP questions; the acronym stands for patient population, intervention of interest, comparison of interest, outcome of interest, and time frame used to formulate EBP

pilot A small study to test a new intervention with a small number of subjects before testing with larger samples; adopting an innovation on a trial basis

plagiarism The use of another's work without giving proper credit

point prevalence The number of existing cases of disease in a population at a particular point in time

popular literature Works written to inform or entertain the general public

population The entire group of elements that meet study inclusion criteria

population parameters Characteristics of a population that are inferred from characteristics of a sample

positional operators Terms that specify the number of words that can appear between search terms

position of the median Calculated by using the formula $(n + 1)/2$, where n is the number of data values in the set

positive predictive value The probability that a person who screens positive actually has the disease

positively skewed A distribution in which the mean is greater than the median and the mode; the longer tail is pointing to the right

posters A scholarly venue for disseminating evidence

power analysis A statistical method used to determine the acceptable sample size that will best detect the true effect of the independent variable

practice guidelines Systematically developed statements to assist healthcare providers with making appropriate decisions about health care for specific clinical circumstances

preceptors Knowledgeable nurses who provide clinical orientation for new employees

precision A search strategy that narrows the parameters of the search

predictive correlational design Correlational design when researchers hypothesize which variables are predictors or outcomes

predictive research Research that forecasts precise relationships between dimensions of phenomena or differences between groups

predictive validity A test for criterion-related validity where a new instrument is given at two different times and scores are correlated; strong positive correlations indicate good validity

preexperimental A posttest-only design that involves manipulation of the independent variable but lacks control for extraneous variables

presentations Scholarly oral presentations to disseminate new knowledge

prevalence The number of existing cases of disease present in the population

primary sources Original information presented by the person or people responsible for creating it

print index Printed listing of electronic or print resources

probability Likelihood or chance that an event will occur in a situation

probability sampling Sampling method in which elements in the accessible population have an equal chance of being selected for inclusion in the study

problem statement A formal statement describing the problem addressed in the study

professionalism A set of behaviors that exemplify the role of the professional nurse

proportion A type of ratio where the numerator is included in the denominator

proposition A statement about the relationship between two or more concepts

propositional knowledge The science of nursing or knowledge that is obtained from research and scholarship

prospective designs Studies over time with presumed causes that follow subjects to determine whether the hypothesized effects actually occur

psychometrics The development of instruments to measure psychological attributes

purpose statement A statement indicating the aim of the study

purposive sampling Nonprobability sampling method used in qualitative studies to select a distinct group of individuals who either have lived the experience or have expertise in the event or experience being studied; sampling method to recruit specific persons who could provide inside information

pyramid of 5 Ss   A model showing how evidence can be categorized from strong to weak

qualification   Limiting fields of search, commonly using limits such as author, title, or subject

qualitative data analysis   The production of knowledge that results from analysis of words

qualitative research   Research that uses words to describe human behaviors

quantitative research   Research that uses numbers to obtain precise measurements

quasi-experimental designs   Research designs involving the manipulation of the independent variable but lacking random assignment to experimental and control groups

questionnaires   Printed instruments used to gather numerical data

quota sampling   Nonprobability sampling method involving selection of elements from an accessible population that has been divided into groups or strata

random assignment   Assignment technique in which subjects have an equal chance of being in either the treatment or the control group

random error   Error that occurs by chance during measurement

random sampling   Technique for selecting elements whereby each has the same chance of being selected

randomization   The selection, assignment, or arrangement of elements by chance

randomized controlled trials   Experimental studies that typically involve large samples and are conducted in multiple sites

range   The difference between the maximum and minimum values in a data set

rate   A measure of disease frequency in a defined population over a specified period of time

ratio   The highest level of measurement that involves numeric values that begin with an absolute zero and have equal intervals; in epidemiology a mathematical relationship between two numbers

reactivity   The influence of participating in a study on the responses of subjects; Hawthorne effect

realist tales   A real-life account of the culture being studied presented in a third-person voice that clearly separates researchers from participants

recall   A strategy used to search for the number of records retrieved with a keyword; the broad "catch" of retrieved records

record   Basic building block in an electronic or print database

referential adequacy   A technique used in qualitative research in which multiple sources of data are compared and the findings hold true

reflexivity   Using a journal to record thoughts, ideas, and decisions during qualitative data gathering

regional level   When nurses from a large geographic location collaborate to change practice

rejection   Decision not to adopt an innovation

relative risk   The statistic reported by epidemiologists when they conduct a cohort study

reliability   Obtaining consistent measurements over time

replicated   When another researcher has findings similar to a previous study

replication   Repeated studies to obtain similar results

representativeness   The degree to which elements of the sample are like elements in the population

research   Systematic study that leads to new knowledge and/or solutions to problems or questions

research hypothesis   A hypothesis indicating that a relationship among two or more variables exists

research imperative   An ethical rule stating that nurses should advance the body of knowledge

research problem   Area of concern when there is a gap in knowledge that requires a solution *research question*   An interrogatory statement describing the variables and population of the research study

research topic   A clinical problem of interest

research utilization   Changing practice based on the results of a single research study

respect for persons   Principle that individuals should be treated as autonomous and that those with diminished autonomy are entitled to protection

results section   Component of a research article that reports the methods used to analyze data and characteristics of the sample

retrospective designs   Research designs in which researchers look back in time to determine possible causative factors; ex post facto

review of literature   An unbiased, comprehensive, synthesized description of relevant previously published studies

role model   One who demonstrates desired characteristics and skills

Rule of 68–95–99.7   Rule stating that for every sample 68% of the data will fall within one standard deviation of the mean; 95% will fall within two standard deviations of the mean; 99.7% of the data will fall within three standard deviations of the mean

sample   A select group of elements that is representative of all eligible elements

sample statistics   Numerical data describing characteristics of the sample

sampling bias   A threat to external validity when a sample includes elements that over- or underrepresent characteristics when compared to elements in the target population

sampling distribution   A theoretical distribution representing an infinite number of samples that can be drawn from a population

sampling error   Error resulting when elements in the sample do not adequately represent the population

sampling frame   A list of all possible elements in the accessible population

sampling interval   The interval (k) between each element selected when using systematic random sampling

sampling plan   Plan to determine how the sample will be selected and recruited

scales   Used to assign a numeric value or score on a continuum

scholarly literature   Works written and edited by professionals in the discipline for other colleagues

scientific literature publication cycle   A model describing how research becomes disseminated in publications

screening   Testing people without known disease to determine whether they have a disease; used to reduce morbidity and mortality in populations

search field   Where each piece of information contained in the record is entered

secondary sources   Commentaries, summaries, reviews, or interpretation of primary sources; often written by those not involved in the original work

selection bias   A threat to internal validity when the change in the dependent variable is a result of the characteristics of the subjects before they entered a study

self-awareness   Knowing yourself

semiquartile range   The range of the middle 50% of the data

sense of inquiry   Curiosity

sensitivity   The ability of the test to correctly identify people with the disease by positive test results

short-term outcomes   Results achieved in a brief period of time

significance level   The alpha level established before the beginning of a study

simple hypothesis   A hypothesis describing the relationship among two variables

simple random sampling   Randomly selecting elements from the accessible population

skewed   An asymmetrical distribution of data

snowball sampling Recruitment of participants based on word of mouth or referrals from other participants

socialization Awareness about formal and informal rules of behavior

Solomon four-group design An experimental design involving four groups—some receive the intervention, others serve as controls; some are measured before and after the intervention, others are measured only after the intervention

specificity The ability of the test to correctly identify people without the disease by negative results

split-half reliability A test for instrument reliability in which the items are divided to form two instruments. Both instruments are given and the halves are compared using the Spearman-Brown formula

stability An attribute of reliability when instruments render the same scores with repeated measures under the same circumstances

standard deviation A measure of variability used to determine the number of data values falling within a specific interval in a normal distribution

statistical conclusion validity The degree that the results of the statistical analysis reflect the true relationship among the independent and dependent variables

statistical hypothesis A hypothesis stating that there is no relationship among the variables; null hypothesis

statistically significant When critical values fall in the tails of normal distributions; when findings did not happen by chance alone

Statistics The branch of mathematics that collects, analyzes, interprets, and presents numerical data in terms of samples and populations

statistics The numerical outcomes and probabilities derived from calculations on raw data

Stetler model Step-by-step instructions for integrating research into practice

stopwords Words, such as *a*, *the*, and *in*, that are so commonly used that they can hinder accurate record retrieval

storytelling A method of data collection associated with qualitative methods when researchers and participants tell their stories about the phenomenon of interest

strategic sampling Sampling in historical research to locate a small group of people who were either witnesses of or participants in the phenomenon being studied

stratified random sampling Selecting elements from an accessible population that has been divided into groups or strata

studies A level in the pyramid of 5 Ss that contains quantitative and qualitative studies, case studies, and concept analyses

study validity Ability to accept results as logical, reasonable, and justifiable based on the evidence presented

subject headings A set of controlled vocabulary used to classify materials; organization of databases according to topic

subject searching Searching databases using controlled vocabulary

subjects Individuals who participate in studies, typically studies using a quantitative design

summaries A level in the pyramid of 5 Ss containing detailed descriptions of evidence

survey designs Descriptive design type involving data obtained through subjects' self-report

synopses A level in the pyramid of 5 Ss containing brief descriptions of evidence

syntheses A level in the pyramid of 5 Ss containing evidence to present a whole depiction of a phenomenon

systematic error Error that occurs in the same way with each measurement

systematic random sampling Sampling method in which every *k*th element is selected from a numbered list of all elements in the accessible population; the starting point on the list is randomly selected

systematic review A rigorous and systematic synthesis of research findings about a clinical problem

systems A level in the pyramid of 5 Ss involving electronic medical records integrated with practice guidelines

t statistic Inferential statistical test to determine whether a statistically significant difference between groups exists

tailedness The degree to which a tail in a distribution is pulled to the left or to the right

target population All elements that meet the study inclusion criteria

team leadership skills Behaviors that collaboratively engage others while working toward a goal

team membership The composition of a team with respect to expertise and leadership

temporal ambiguity The inability to control for confounding variables and the inability to determine whether the exposure truly occurred before the disease

testing A threat to internal validity when a pretest influences the way subjects respond on a posttest

test-retest reliability A test for instrument reliability when new instruments are given at two different times under the same conditions; scores are correlated, and strong positive correlations indicate good reliability

theoretical framework The structure of a study that links the theory concepts to the study variables; a section of a research article that describes the theory used

theoretical sampling Nonprobability sampling method used in grounded theory to collect data from an initial group of participants

theory A set of concepts linked through propositions to explain a phenomenon

therapeutic imperative An ethical rule stating that nurses should perform actions that benefit the patient

trade literature Works written for professionals in a discipline using a more casual tone than used in scholarly literature

traditional literature review Article based on common or uncommon elements of works with little concern for research methods, designs, or settings; narrative literature review

transferability One of four criteria for a trustworthy qualitative study that relates to whether findings from one study can be transferred to a similar context; application of findings to a different situation

translational research Research for the purpose of linking research findings to the point of care

translational research model A model that provides specific strategies organizations can use to improve adoption of an evidence-based innovation

trend A type of longitudinal design to gather data from different samples across time

triangulation Use of different research methods in qualitative research to gather and compare data

truncation A search strategy that uses a symbol at the end of a group of letters that form the root search term

trustworthiness The quality, authenticity, and truthfulness of findings from qualitative research

Tuskegee study An unethical study about syphilis in which subjects were denied treatment so that the effects of the disease could be studied

two-group posttest-only designs Experimental designs when subjects are randomly assigned to an experimental or control group and measured after the intervention

two-group pretest-posttest design Subjects are randomly assigned to the experimental or control group and measured before and after the intervention; classic or true experiment

type I error When the researcher rejects the null hypothesis when it should have been accepted

type II error When the researcher inaccurately concludes that there is no relationship among the independent and dependent variables when an actual relationship does exist; when the researcher accepts the null hypothesis when it should have been rejected

uncertainty   Degree to which alternatives are perceived relative to the occurrence of an event and the probability of these alternatives

unimodal   A data set with one mode, such as a normal distribution

univariate analysis   The use of statistical tests to provide information about one variable

unstructured observations   A method of data collection associated with qualitative research in which phenomena of interest are allowed to emerge over time as observations are made

validity   The degree that an instrument measures what it is supposed to measure

visual analog scale   Ratio-level scale of a 100-mm line anchored on each end with words or symbols

vulnerable population   A special group of people needing protection because of members' limited ability to provide informed consent or because of their risk for coercion

wheel of professionalism in nursing   A model depicting behaviors of the professional nurse

wildcards   Symbols substituted for one or more letters in a search term

Willowbrook studies   An unethical study involving coercion of parents to allow their children to participate in the study in exchange for admission to a long-term care facility

within-groups design   Comparisons are made about the same subjects at two or more points in time or on two or more measures

z scores   Standardized units used to compare data gathered using different measurement scales

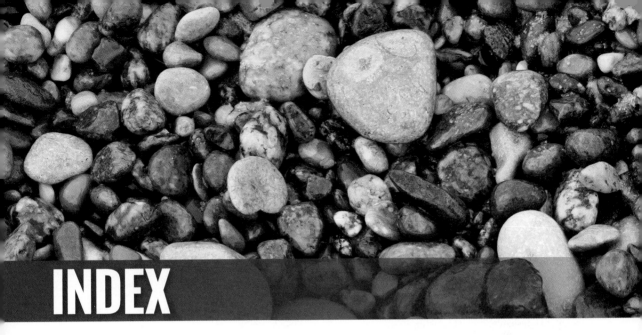

INDEX

Designs Organizational Chart

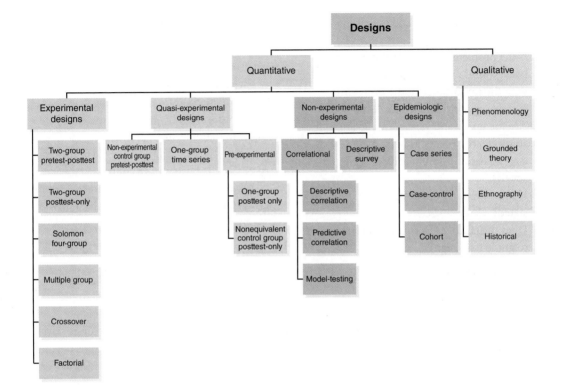

Questions to Consider When Appraising Nursing Studies

Introduction

1. Does the introduction demonstrate the need for the study?
2. Is the problem clearly and concisely identified?
3. Is the problem presented with enough background material to acquaint the reader with the importance of the problem?
4. Is the purpose of the study clearly stated?
5. Are the terms and variables relevant to the study clearly defined?
6. Are the assumptions clearly and simply stated?
7. If appropriate to the design, are hypotheses stated?
8. Does the study use a theoretical framework to guide its design?

Review of the Literature

1. Is the ROL relevant to the problem?
2. Is the review adequate in terms of the range and scope of ideas, opinions, and points of view relevant to the problem?
3. Is the review well organized and synthesized?
4. Does the review provide for critical appraisal of the contribution of each of the major references?
5. Does the review conclude with a summary of the literature with implications for the study?
6. Is the ROL adequately and correctly documented?

Methods

1. Is the research approach appropriate?
2. Was the protection of human subjects considered?
3. Are the details of data collection clearly and logically presented?
4. Are the instrument(s) appropriate for the study both in terms of the problem and the approach?
5. Are the instrument(s) described sufficiently in terms of content, structure, validity and reliability?
6. Is the population and the method for selecting the sample adequately described?
7. Is the method for selection of the sample appropriate?
8. Is the sample size sufficient?
9. Is attrition of sample reported and explained?
10. Does the design have controls at an acceptable level for the threats to internal validity?
11. What are the limits to generalizability in terms of external validity?

Results

1. Is the presentation of data clear?
2. Are the characteristics of the sample described?
3. Was the best method(s) of analysis selected?
4. Are the tables, charts, and graphs pertinent?

Discussion

1. Are the results based on the data presented?
2. Is the evidence sufficient to draw conclusions?
3. Are the results interpreted in the context of the problem/purpose, hypothesis, and theoretical framework/literature reviewed?
4. Are the conclusions and generalizations clearly stated?
5. Are the limitations of the findings clearly delineated?
6. Are the generalizations within the scope of the findings or beyond the findings?
7. Does the study contribute to nursing knowledge?